About IFPRI

The International Food Policy Research Institute (IFPRI), established in 1975, provides research-based policy solutions to sustainably reduce poverty and end hunger and malnutrition. The Institute conducts research, communicates results, optimizes partnerships, and builds capacity to ensure sustainable food production, promote healthy food systems, improve markets and trade, transform agriculture, build resilience, and strengthen institutions and governance. Gender is considered in all of the Institute's work. IFPRI collaborates with partners around the world, including development implementers, public institutions, the private sector, and farmers' organizations.

About IFPRI's Peer Review Process

IFPRI books are policy-relevant publications based on original and innovative research conducted at IFPRI. All manuscripts submitted for publication as IFPRI books undergo an extensive review procedure that is managed by IFPRI's Publications Review Committee (PRC). Upon submission to the PRC, the manuscript is reviewed by a PRC member. Once the manuscript is considered ready for external review, the PRC submits it to at least two external reviewers who are chosen for their familiarity with the subject matter and the country setting. Upon receipt of these blind external peer reviews, the PRC provides the author with an editorial decision and, when necessary, instructions for revision based on the external reviews. The PRC reassesses the revised manuscript and makes a recommendation regarding publication to the director general of IFPRI. With the director general's approval, the manuscript enters the editorial and production phase to become an IFPRI book.

nourishing MILLIONS

STORIES OF CHANGE IN NUTRITION

EDITED BY STUART GILLESPIE, JUDITH HODGE, SIVAN YOSEF, AND RAJUL PANDYA-LORCH

A Peer-Reviewed Publication

International Food Policy Research Institute
Washington, DC

International Food Policy Research Institute
2033 K Street, NW
Washington, DC 20006-1002 USA
Telephone: +1-202-862-5600
Fax: +1-202-467-4439
Email: ifpri@cgiar.org
www.ifpri.org

DOI: http://dx.doi.org/10.2499/9780896295889
ISBN: 978-0-89629-588-9

Cover design: Julia Vivalo
Book design and layout: David Popham
Suggested citation: Gillespie, S., J. Hodge, S. Yosef, and R. Pandya-Lorch, eds. 2016. *Nourishing Millions: Stories of Change in Nutrition*. Washington, DC: International Food Policy Research Institute.

Library of Congress Cataloging-in-Publication Data

Names: Gillespie, Stuart (Stuart R.), editor.
Title: Nourishing millions : stories of change in nutrition / edited by Stuart Gillespie, Judith Hodge, Sivan Yosef, and Rajul Pandya-Lorch.
Description: Washington, DC : International Food Policy Research Institute, [2016] | Includes bibliographical references.
Identifiers: LCCN 2016020023 | ISBN 9780896295889 (pbk. : alk. paper)
Subjects: LCSH: Malnutrition--Prevention. | Nutrition policy.
Classification: LCC RA645.N87 N68 2016 | DDC 363.8/7--dc23 LC record available at https://lccn.loc.gov/2016020023

Contents

Figures

Tables

Boxes

Foreword

The International Food Policy Research Institute (IFPRI) has spent four decades leading the way in high-quality evidence on food and nutrition security. Over the years, the institute has joined hands with local, national, and global partners in generating a rich body of knowledge that can help key decision makers—and implementers on the ground—improve the lives of poor and vulnerable people around the world.

As the international community enters the post-2015 development era, IFPRI's mission takes on a new sense of urgency. The costs of malnutrition are staggering, hindering macroeconomic growth on national and global scales and hampering the developmental, cognitive, and educational potential of children. We need to accelerate progress in ending hunger and malnutrition. Fortunately, the tools that will help us learn from past experiences, and allow us to apply these lessons to the future, are within our grasp. This is the unique contribution of *Nourishing Millions*: to add to the evidence base on nutrition by providing insight into what works, what does not, and the factors that contribute to success.

During the past five years, IFPRI has scaled up its commitment to achieving a world free of hunger and malnutrition by leading large initiatives such as the CGIAR Research Program on Agriculture for Nutrition and Health and the global research consortium Transform Nutrition, while undertaking cutting-edge impact evaluations of nutrition programs around the world through its Poverty, Health, and Nutrition Division. *Nourishing Millions* is a key element of the IFPRI-led Compact2025 initiative (www.compact2025.org), which brings stakeholders together to set priorities, innovate and learn, build on successes, and synthesize shareable lessons for the purpose of ending hunger and undernutrition by 2025. *Nourishing Millions* builds upon IFPRI's track record in sharing lessons—in 2009, IFPRI's *Millions Fed: Proven Successes in Agricultural Development* project examined 20 success stories of policies, programs, and investments in pro-poor agricultural development that helped to substantially reduce hunger across Africa, Asia, and Latin America.

The lessons contained in this book can help spark country-owned and country-led strategies and investments in nutrition, provide policy makers and practitioners with practical, evidence-based guidance on scaling up success stories, and inspire multiple actors to coordinate across sectors and disciplines.

Improvements in nutrition can secure the well-being of current and future generations, and also achieve gains in the many sectors that link to nutrition. With initiatives like *Nourishing Millions,* I have great hope that we can indeed end hunger and undernutrition by 2025.

Shenggen Fan
Director General, IFPRI

Preface

In recent years, the world has seen unprecedented levels of attention and political commitment to addressing malnutrition. Milestones such as the Scaling Up Nutrition (SUN) Movement, the *Lancet* Maternal and Child Nutrition Series, and the Second International Conference on Nutrition (ICN2) have underscored the rapid rise of nutrition on the global policy and research agenda.

Alongside these developments, it has become clear that the international community needs guidance on how to design, implement, and evaluate policies and interventions that promote nutrition for the world's poorest and most vulnerable people. In this context, stories on how to improve nutrition in real-world settings are needed—not only to inform action, but to inspire it too.

When we began *Nourishing Millions: Stories of Change in Nutrition,* we expected to assemble simple examples of effective nutrition programs and interventions. What has emerged is an extremely rich collection of narratives that highlight the successes—but also the challenges—associated with attempts to drive the nutrition agenda forward.

The stories in this book are diverse, spanning five decades and playing out in different arenas, from local to global. They take place in developing countries all over the world, and they involve many sectors and disciplines beyond nutrition itself, including health, agriculture, education, social protection, and water and sanitation. Most important, they paint a nuanced picture of success as a context-specific achievement that may, or may not, endure into the future.

One of our main take-aways from *Nourishing Millions* is that successes in nutrition depend on committed people to envision, implement, and evaluate interventions. We hope that this book inspires individuals—policy makers, practitioners, researchers, educators and students, and ordinary citizens—to replicate and scale up action against malnutrition and to generate further success for future generations.

Stuart Gillespie Judith Hodge Sivan Yosef Rajul Pandya-Lorch

Acknowledgments

The editors would like to thank the numerous individuals at the International Food Policy Research Institute (IFPRI) and beyond who contributed to the writing, review, and production of *Nourishing Millions*. We deeply appreciate their time and efforts.

Production of the book was led by IFPRI's Communications and Knowledge Management Division under the guidance of Katrin Park. Editing and coordination was led by Heidi Fritschel with additional editing support from Pamela Stedman-Edwards. Layout was completed by David Popham. Other communication-related activities were undertaken by Daniel Burnett, Michael Go, Milo Mitchell, Andrea Pedolsky, Peter Shelton, Julia Vivalo, and Sandra Yin. Djhoanna Cruz, Vickie Lee, Samantha Reddin (Transform Nutrition), Jessica White (independent consultant), and Laura Zseleczky provided additional support throughout the entire project.

The report underwent peer review by IFPRI's Publications Review Committee, chaired by Gershon Feder and supported by Corinne Garber. Many of the chapters were also initially reviewed by additional experts: Akhter Ahmed, Jean Baker, France Begin, Alan Dangour, Tim Frankenberger, Nemat Hajeebhoy, Kalle Hirvonen, Phuong Huynh, John Hoddinott, Karin Lapping, Emily Mates, Purnima Menon, Carlos Monteiro, Marie Ruel, Lisa Smith, Milo Stanojevich, and Boyd Swinburn.

The project's advisory committee members provided valuable guidance on the design of the project, including the selection of chapters and case studies: Alan Berg, Charlotte Dufour, Bonnie McClafferty, Purnima Menon, Robert Mwadime, Marie Ruel, Werner Schultink, Meera Shekar, and Patrick Webb. IFPRI researchers Harold Alderman, Derek Headey, and David Spielman provided critical feedback on the criteria for selecting case studies.

We are grateful to IFPRI's director general, Shenggen Fan, for his enthusiasm and support for the project.

The *Nourishing Millions* project was made possible through funding from the New Venture Fund. This work has also been supported by the Stories of Change project of the Transform Nutrition consortium, funded by the UK Department for International Development and by the Children's Investment Fund Foundation. The views expressed do not necessarily reflect those of the funders.

CHAPTER 1

How Nutrition Improves

Half a Century of Understanding and Responding to the Problem of Malnutrition

STUART GILLESPIE AND JODY HARRIS

MALNUTRITION IS A global challenge with huge social and economic costs. Undernutrition kills millions of young children annually, stunts growth, erodes child development, reduces the amount of schooling children attain, and increases the likelihood of their being poor as adults, if they survive. It also persists through the life cycle and beyond—underweight mothers are more likely to give birth to underweight children, perpetuating the transmission of malnutrition across generations. Undernutrition reduces global GDP by USD$1.4–2.1 trillion a year—the size of the total economy of Africa south of the Sahara.[1] And even though many countries are making progress in reducing child undernutrition, another form of malnutrition—overweight and obesity—is now changing the health landscape in every region of the world.

Over the past 50 years there have been many changes in how the problem of malnutrition has been conceptualized, analyzed, and addressed. Recent years have witnessed an unprecedented global rise in high-level political commitment and financing. Nutrition champions are making an increasingly effective case for investing in nutrition, and as we move into the new era of the Sustainable Development Goals (SDGs),[2] the wider development world is beginning to embrace nutrition as central to development programming and fundamental to achieving a whole range of development goals. Yet, although political momentum is essential for progress in nutrition, it is unquestionably not enough. In fact, it is in danger of fizzling out unless it leads to more and better action that yields results on the ground.

So, while much remains to be done to build and sustain national-level commitments to nutrition, policy makers and practitioners are increasingly grappling with the nuts-and-bolts challenges of turning the newfound global commitment into large-scale action at the country level. It is in this context that lessons on how to improve nutrition in the real world and in real time are needed. A recent multicountry review of scaling up impact on nutrition, undertaken by the international research consortium Transform Nutrition, summed up the challenge thus: "Although there is a strong

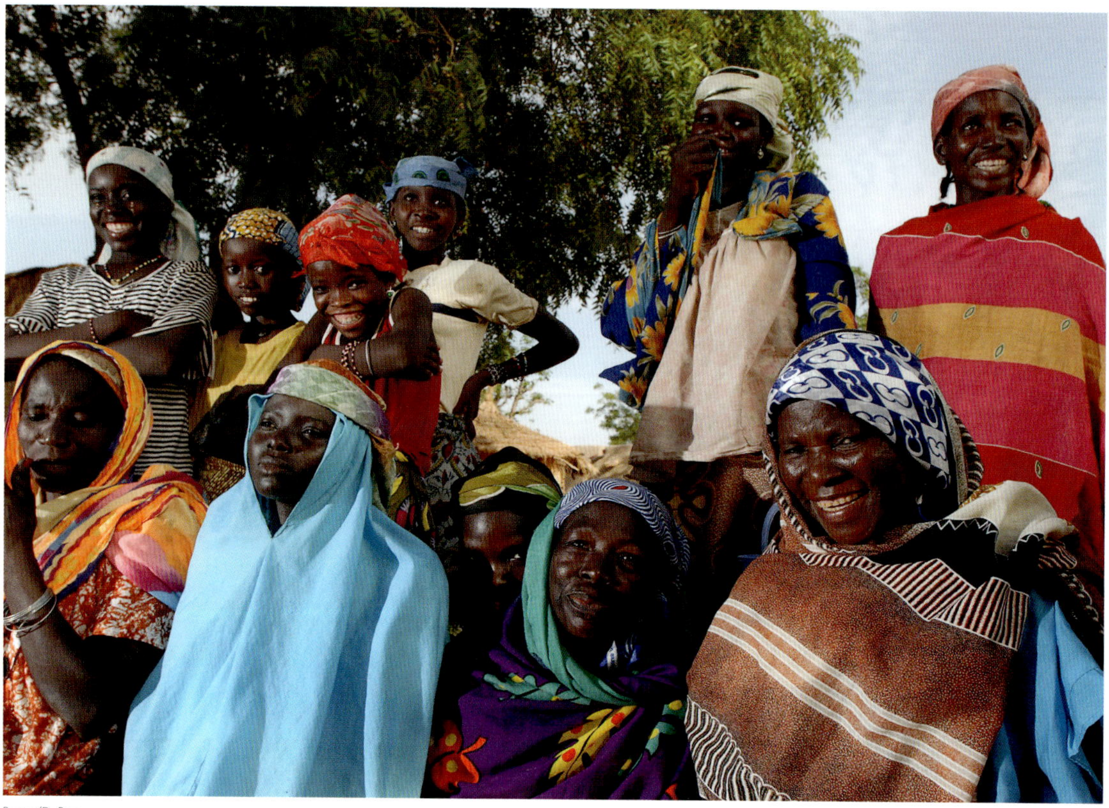

Panos/D. Rose

Community-driven nutrition programs aim to empower marginalized people.

consensus on what needs to be done, much less is known about how to operationalize the right mix of actions in different contexts, [and] how to do so at a scale that matches the size of the problem, in an equitable manner."[3]

The type of knowledge required to meet this challenge is as much about experience as it is about evidence. There is a growing demand for narratives of what has worked well (and what hasn't). Case studies of successful approaches to designing, implementing, scaling up, and sustaining an appropriate mix of nutrition-relevant actions are increasingly called for in global nutrition research and operations.

This book is an attempt to meet this demand by combining a review of various analyses and studies with a narrative approach to convey the drivers and pathways of success in nutrition in different contexts and at different times. It seeks to inspire as well as to inform. In recent years, there has been a growing focus on the potential of narrative and storytelling to inspire and promote change.[4] Stories can turn the key in ways that help the reader intuitively grasp why change is needed, what it involves, how it happens, and—crucially—how it can be made to happen. Stories enable listeners to extrapolate from case studies and to see analogies with their own backgrounds, their own contexts, and their own fields of expertise. Research has shown that stories catalyze change because they are natural and easy to tell, they show connections between things, and they cut through complexity. They are memorable, nonadversarial, and nonhierarchical. And because they engage feelings, they inspire, motivate, and energize people.[5]

There are many stories of change in this book—stories of how countries have accelerated progress in reducing malnutrition, of how successful interventions have been developed and implemented, and of how individual leaders and nutrition champions have emerged and changed the landscape. These stories fit within a larger context of the multiple narratives that have shaped global nutrition-relevant discourse and action during the past half-century since nutrition science emerged as a discipline. These narratives relate to the nature of the problem of malnutrition—its manifestations, causes, and consequences—as well as to the value of different approaches to addressing it. Representing, as they do, different perceptions and ways of framing malnutrition, they condition what is done and not done in different contexts and at different times. In this first chapter we seek to paint a picture, using a broad brush, of the evolution of approaches to understanding and responding to the challenge of malnutrition through the decades.[6]

Paradigms in International Nutrition: An Overview

Much has been written about the history of international nutrition from different subdisciplinary perspectives. Figure 1.1 summarizes a review of 11 nutrition history papers, grouped according to the broad perspective from which the authors chose to write.[7] Both differences and similarities between accounts are evident from this review, and

FIGURE 1.1 Historical evolution of approaches to understanding and responding to malnutrition

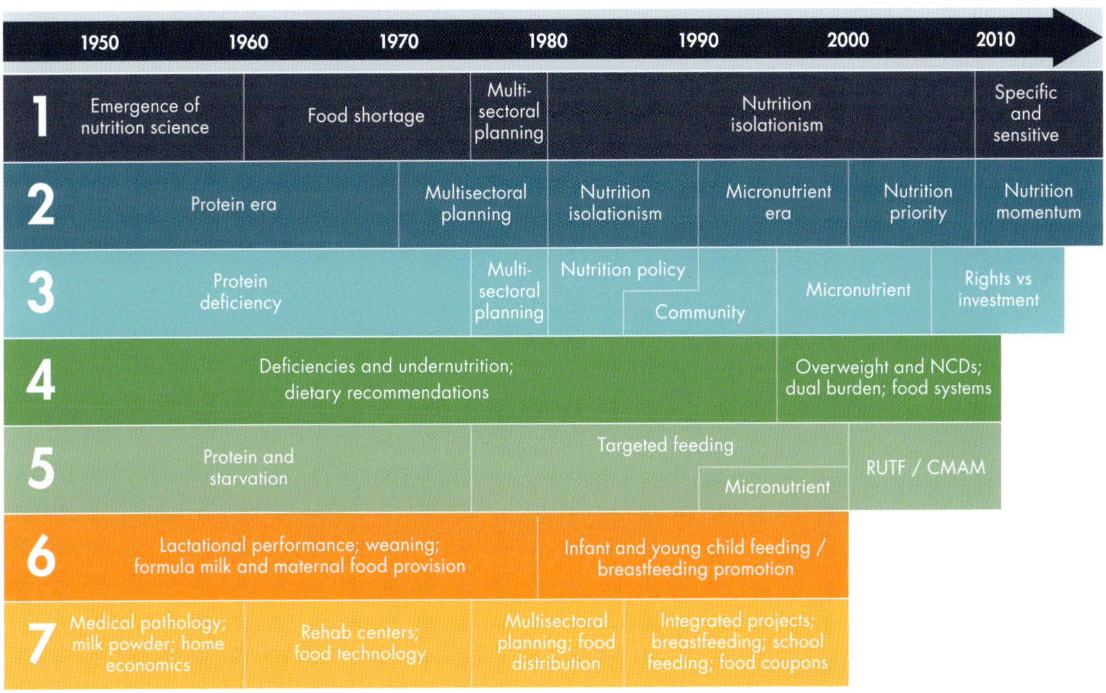

Source: Authors, based on sources listed in notes 8–18.

Note: RUTF = ready-to-use therapeutic food; CMAM = community-based management of acute malnutrition; NCDs = noncommunicable diseases.

it is useful to understand the origins and drivers of these differences and similarities before we begin to unfurl the history of international nutrition.

In terms of the differences, it is important to note at the outset that the nutrition community is not monolithic; indeed, it has been characterized by some as fragmented.[19] In recent decades, the international nutrition community has experienced a split between "emergency" nutritionists, who focus predominantly on treating malnutrition present in acute or recurring emergencies through various medical models, and "development" nutritionists, who focus on preventing malnutrition by addressing its more basic social, economic, and political drivers. This has also been characterized as a philosophical split between technocrats, with medical solutions to existing problems, and structuralists, who want to address why a problem emerges and is perpetuated—though the dichotomy between these two philosophies is rarely so clear-cut in practice. The discipline of nutrition stems from health and medicine, which in turn rest on classical theories from behavioral psychology, biomedical science, and public administration.[20] Nutrition training has therefore often struggled to bring in a broader social science perspective, which can help explain the complex interactions underlying malnutrition.[21]

In terms of the similarities, certain themes prevail across many of the histories. The practice of international nutrition is based in the discipline of nutrition science, which like any discipline has gone through distinct phases of understanding and action. The primary focus on starvation, protein, and medical models of intervention and treatment in the 1950s and 1960s gave way to multisectoral planning in the 1970s, before the focus shifted toward micronutrients (and subsequently what some termed the disciplinary isolationism of nutrition) in the 1990s and 2000s. In recent years the picture has become more complex as more actors, with a wider recognition of the multiple issues surrounding nutrition, have become involved. In what follows, we describe the key historical phases and try to explain how certain thematic or operational priorities emerged and evolved over time.

1950s–1960s: Famine, Hunger, and a Fixation on Protein

In the mid-20th century, the complexities of postwar reconstruction and an increasingly globalized world gave rise to the modern field of international development, concerned with improving the lives and economic prospects of "underdeveloped" countries. For many people working in development, hunger, and in particular the periodic famines that stalked these countries, was a particular preoccupation.

Alongside this focus on hunger, scientific research in nutrition targeted the biological role of particular nutrients in severe forms of undernutrition. The origins of a development focus on nutrition can be traced to an assumption that deficiencies of macronutrients—energy and protein—play a primary role in hunger and are the most visible manifestations of undernutrition in children. During the postwar years, the international community focused on the metabolic consequences and treatment of severe protein deficiency, which was the assumed mechanism for severe malnutrition. In 1955 the United Nations Protein Advisory Group was formed to advise the UN secretary-general on nutrition interventions. Right through to the 1970s, research continued to focus on the technological challenge of developing protein concentrates and isolates and on ways of increasing the protein content of conventional foods.

1970s: From Protein to Multisectoral Nutrition Planning

As the 1970s opened, some nutrition scientists were beginning to challenge the notion that protein deficiency was the main nutritional problem of the time. In groundbreaking work in India, Professor P. V. Sukhatme found that malnourished children improved not only when fed protein-rich foods, but also after consuming staple foods, including cereals.[22] In 1974, Donald McLaren published the article "The Great Protein Fiasco," which finally blew a hole in the notion that the main nutritional challenge was protein deficiency.

> The concept of the much-publicised world protein "gap," "crisis," or "problem" arose from the description of kwashiorkor in Africa in the 1930s and the assumption, which has turned out to be wrong, that malnutrition in children takes this form throughout the world. As a result, measures to detect protein deficiency and treat and prevent it by dietary means have been pursued until the present time. The price that has had to be paid for these mistakes is only beginning to be realised.[23]

Building on Sukhatme's findings, subsequent analyses showed that if people's diets were adequate in calories, then their protein intake too would be adequate. In a classic example of a collapsing paradigm, solutions to malnutrition began to be sought in the wider social and economic arena, well beyond technical nutrient fixes. The focus turned to alleviating hunger and poverty and assuring access to food.

McLaren's work also resonated with a wider movement underway to systematically diagnose and treat the underlying causes of malnutrition as part of a new field of nutrition policy and planning, which emerged from the first International Conference on Nutrition, National Development, and Planning in 1971.[24] This was a key moment when nutrition science began to connect with development policy and practice. In 1973, Alan Berg published *The Nutrition Factor,* advancing the idea that nutrition was an essential driver of economic growth, arguing that nutrition programs could be viewed as investments rather than simply consumption, and recommending specific actions that could be implemented relatively easily.

As the decade progressed, an increasing number of national governments and international agencies began to embrace nutrition objectives. Partly in response to food crises, nutritional surveillance initiatives emerged in which indicators of nutritional outcomes were tracked alongside those relating to their core determinants and sequelae, including food availability and health status.

In 1974 the World Food Conference focused on the global food crisis, and issues of distribution and access to food—rather than aggregate food supply—were increasingly perceived as drivers of hunger and malnutrition.[25] Two years later, the World Bank published an influential study showing that reliance on economic growth alone to assure dietary adequacy among the poor would take too long.[26] Amartya Sen's work on entitlements, which later won him a Nobel Prize, reinforced this shift away from a supply-side focus on food by emphasizing the distributional links between inequality, hunger, and famine.[27] In 1977 the UN Protein Advisory Group evolved into the UN Administrative Coordination Committee's Subcommittee on Nutrition (ACC/SCN or just SCN), with its attention now focused on improving breastfeeding, maternal and child nutrition, and complementary feeding.

The August 1973 publication of "The Baby Food Tragedy" in the *New Internationalist* was a pivotal event in nutrition that reverberates to this day.[28] The editorial in that issue started, "On the cover of this issue is a photograph of grave no. 19232. It is the grave of a Zambian baby. On it, the mother has placed a feeding bottle and an empty tin of milk-powder. They are symbols of infant death and of the mother's attempt to do her best for her child during its short life. What the

BOX 1.1 **Conceptualizing nutrition**

For more than a quarter century, the UNICEF conceptual framework of nutrition has been the gold standard for understanding the drivers of undernutrition.[29] The framework illustrates how these drivers operate at multiple levels, from immediate, individual-level causes, to underlying household- and community-level determinants related to food, health, and care, to basic or structural-level causes related to policy, politics, power, and capacity. Widely adopted and adapted,[30] the framework was the basis for the 2013 *Lancet* Maternal and Child Nutrition Series that shaped this book's structure.

The 1990 UNICEF nutrition framework

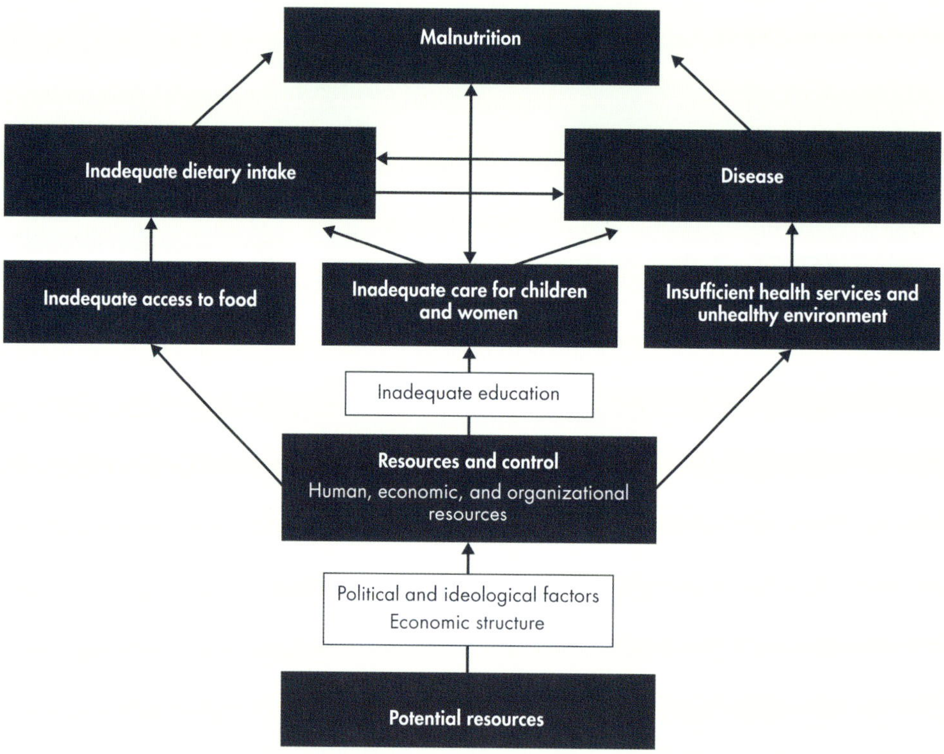

Source: Adapted from UNICEF, *Strategy for Improved Nutrition of Children and Women in Developing Countries* (New York, 1990).

mother does not know is that the way in which she used that same milk-powder and feeding bottle was also the main cause of her baby's death." Multinational companies (and Nestlé in particular) were accused of contributing to infant mortality in developing countries through the practices they adopted to market infant formula foods (see Chapter 3). This led to the World Health Assembly's passage of the International Code on the Marketing of Breast-milk Substitutes in 1981.[31] Ever since, these events have acted as lightning rod in the ongoing debate over the role of the private sector in nutrition.

As people's understanding of nutrition's etiological landscape continued to evolve, many raised the question of the most appropriate type of institutional arrangement for nutrition. Emerging notions of the multisectorality of nutrition and its causes, consequences, and solutions led, as Alan Berg succinctly put it, to nutrition being perceived as "everybody's business but nobody's main responsibility."[32] A growing understanding of this blind spot led to the concept of multisectoral nutrition planning, marking a reaction to largely food supply–oriented interventions that did not address the wider, nonfood drivers of malnutrition and had little impact. Program planning came to the fore. Nutrition institutes in many countries (such as Chile, Guatemala, India, Indonesia, Mexico, the Philippines, Tanzania, and Zambia) were now viewed as anachronistic because they treated malnutrition as a largely medical problem. To advocates of multisectoral planning, the challenge was not launching more and better *nutrition* interventions, but rather influencing policies and programs in a broad range of development sectors. This thinking led to the establishment of "nutrition cells," often in the office of a president or prime minister. A total of 26 nutrition planning entities were established in the 1970s, supported primarily by the U.S. Agency for International Development (USAID) and the Food and Agriculture Organization of the United Nations (FAO).[33]

1980s: From Multisectorality to Nutrition Isolationism

The decade of the 1980s dawned against a background of competing narratives on the provision of health care and on development more widely. The promotion of structural adjustment (focusing on removing state controls in national economies) did not sit easily with the World Health Organization's push for access to primary healthcare following the 1981 Alma Ata declaration. Against this backdrop, the notion of active community participation in nutrition program development began to take root (see Chapter 2). This aligned with wider participatory trends in development, as evidence emerged that programs with community-driven decision making had sustainable impacts. The Iringa program in Tanzania, launched in 1985, was a leading example that would have a major impact on nutrition thinking and action in years to come, stimulating the development of the pioneering UNICEF conceptual framework and nutrition strategy in 1990, as shown in Box 1.1.

By the 1980s most nutrition planning cells had ceased to function or been abandoned. The notion of multiple sectors somehow being coordinated in complex master plans by a nutrition cell that rarely had any political clout or funding was deeply flawed. In an important policy retrospective, John Osgood Field attributed this failure principally to unwarranted assumptions about political priorities, a focus on planning rather than action, and a lack of capacity and data for the systems analysis demanded by multisectoral planning.[34] The hard-learned lesson here was that a multifaceted challenge like malnutrition requires action from many sectors, but it does not necessarily require such actions to be elaborately choreographed by any one entity.[35] Analysis of such programs revealed a frequent lack of consideration of political determinants and resource availability.[36] The failure of multisectoral planning gave rise to the era of "nutritional isolationism" in which the pendulum swung back to nutritionists who increasingly focused on two sets of interventions that needed little involvement from other sectors: micronutrient supplementation and breastfeeding.[37]

The nutrition community itself, however, was not entirely harmonious at this time. Disagreements about responsibilities across sectors and agencies and an "either/or" mentality bedded in as debates on whether nutrition was primarily a health or a food issue became increasingly fractious. A commonly raised question was whether nutrition was better served by being incorporated into larger programs, divisions, or departments for health, agriculture, or social welfare or by maintaining its own identity in nutrition departments. Strangely, the notion that both options could be pursued was less common. There were debates too between practitioners, who argued that the field was too dominated by the science of nutrition, and academics, who questioned the rigor of conceptual constructs, data collection, and analysis used in practice.

During the 1980s, it became increasingly clear that certain micronutrients—that is, vitamins and minerals—were crucial for physical and cognitive growth and for preventing birth defects, morbidity, and mortality (see Chapter 4). In 1985 the UN SCN developed a 10-year plan for controlling vitamin A deficiency. The following year the International Coordinating Committee on Iodine Deficiency Disorders (ICCIDD) was formed and quickly became effective at bringing iodine deficiency disorders (IDDs) to international attention, developing support for wide-scale salt iodization, and promoting laws to enforce the participation of salt manufacturers.

1990s: The Birth of the UNICEF Framework and the Micronutrient Era

Conceptually, the start of the 1990s saw a giant step forward in the form of UNICEF's development of a coherent nutrition framework that provided a common language and indicated roles for different actors. The two pillars of UNICEF's new nutrition strategy—both deriving from experiences in the UNICEF-led Iringa program in Tanzania (described in Chapter 2)—comprised the conceptual framework describing the determinants and drivers of undernutrition at different levels (see Box 1.1) and a process for assessing, analyzing, and acting to address nutrition problems: the "triple A process." Both were to prove highly influential in the years to follow and remain so today (see, for example, Figure 1.2, showing the *Lancet* framework, which derives from the UNICEF framework). In 1990, UNICEF organized the UN World Summit for Children—a milestone in setting ambitious malnutrition reduction goals and building strong momentum around the human rights–based rationale for action, which UNICEF executive director James Grant called an "ethical imperative."[38]

The 1990s was also the decade of micronutrients, especially the "big three": vitamin A, iodine, and iron (see Chapter 4). The 1990 World Summit for Children set a goal of reducing anemia by one-third by the end of the decade (practitioners later concluded it could not be achieved because of the widespread difficulty of delivering supplements as well as recipients' poor adherence to supplementation due to side effects). It also established a goal of virtually eliminating IDDs by 2000, and many agencies, donors, and the salt industry took to this challenge. In 1991 the conference "Ending Hidden Hunger" helped strengthen micronutrient programming, and in 1993 the Micronutrient Initiative was formed. Overall, micronutrient control programs achieved considerable success during the 1990s: by the end of the decade, 60 percent of developing-country households were using iodized salt and 30 percent of children were receiving vitamin A capsules twice a year.[39]

In 1992 FAO and WHO co-convened the International Conference on Nutrition (ICN) in Rome. The conference endorsed the UNICEF conceptual framework and the World Summit for Children nutrition goals while laying further emphasis on household food security, nutrition surveillance, and micronutrient deficiency control. Countries were encouraged to prepare national plans of action for nutrition. Many were produced, but few were implemented.[40]

Up to this point, the literature on nutrition policy had been sparse since the first flush of publications on nutrition planning in the 1970s. Starting in the early 1990s, though, work on the political economy of nutrition began in earnest. In 1993 Per Pinstrup-Andersen edited a volume bringing together key thinkers in nutrition policy.[41] In one chapter, John Osgood Field summarized the factors behind nutrition's low political capital at the time (many of which still hold true today). These included the poor framing of issues; the relatively meager power of nutrition actors, who were unable to persuade political leaders to prioritize nutrition; entrenched structural or organizational issues, including nutrition's institutional homelessness; and the difficulty of defining or measuring political commitment.[42] Pinstrup-Andersen's summary posited that actors' goals, roles, and relative power are key to understanding and responding to nutrition policy challenges and concluded with a plea for more contextual political economy analyses to yield more useful and realistic results in the field.

Also in the early 1990s, the UN SCN convened several interagency workshops and undertook a series of eight country case studies that culminated in the synthesis entitled *How Nutrition Improves.*[43] The final chapter, which covered political economy, institutional capacity, and nutrition policy, pointed to the need for a mix of state- and community-led nutrition-relevant action, institutional support from both research and implementing partners and strong links between them, the use of a "functional classification" of data on nutrition and its drivers to catalyze and incentivize wider sectoral action, and a free press to shine a spotlight on emerging food and nutrition crises. The process of formulating the policy was increasingly viewed as at least as important as the final policy itself. Along these lines, the SCN frequently stressed the need to see policy as not just what it *says,* but what it *does* (following Clay and Schaffer's 1984 book[44]) in which the implementation mechanisms and processes developed by stakeholders needed to be clearly articulated. By the end of the 1990s, though, the field of the political economy of nutrition sank back into relative silence.

2000–2010: Emerging from the Development Shadows

From the mid-1990s to the mid-2000s, nutrition went through a lean policy period. Other major development challenges such as HIV/AIDS held the limelight, drawing donor dollars and generating media interest, as nutrition languished in the shadows. The spotlight shifted somewhat following a joint World Bank-UNICEF global assessment of nutrition-relevant policy and practice. The ensuing book argued that despite a growing consensus *within* the nutrition community on the key interventions that could be applied to tackle nutrition directly, *beyond* the nutrition community, knowledge about undernutrition, its consequences, and its relevance to poverty and other human development goals was fragmented and was being inconsistently applied.[45] It remained therefore for nutrition researchers, practitioners, and donors to demonstrate impact through rigorous evaluations and to communicate better outside their disciplinary comfort zone. In the same period, Richard Heaver of the World Bank wrote about management and capacity issues surrounding successful implementation of nutrition programs, focusing in particular on the role of higher-level nutrition "champions" and midlevel policy "entrepreneurs" in policy change.[46] Drawing from these various inputs, the World Bank published its highly influential nutrition strategy, *Repositioning Nutrition as Central to Development.*[47]

During this period, work was also underway at the International Food Policy Research Institute (IFPRI) on exploring the potential for "raising the floor" of a population's micronutrient status by developing and promoting biofortified crops, bred to be rich in vitamins and minerals. This work ultimately led to the launch of the HarvestPlus program in 2004.

Momentum picked up later in the decade with the publication of the first *Lancet* Maternal and Child Nutrition Series in 2008, which significantly raised the profile of nutrition. The series achieved several outcomes: it provided a structured, up-to-date evidence base on the trends, causes, and consequences of different forms of undernutrition and on the critical importance of the 6- to 24-month age group (which later led to the "1,000 days" concept). It focused on a package of direct, nutrition-specific interventions for which there was compelling evidence of efficacy, including micronutrient supplementation, fortification, infant and young child feeding, and prevention and treatment of severe acute malnutrition. Finally, it identified 36 countries in which 90 percent of the global burden of child stunting was located. The challenge, according to the *Lancet,* was to operationalize and scale up this package of interventions in these high-burden countries.

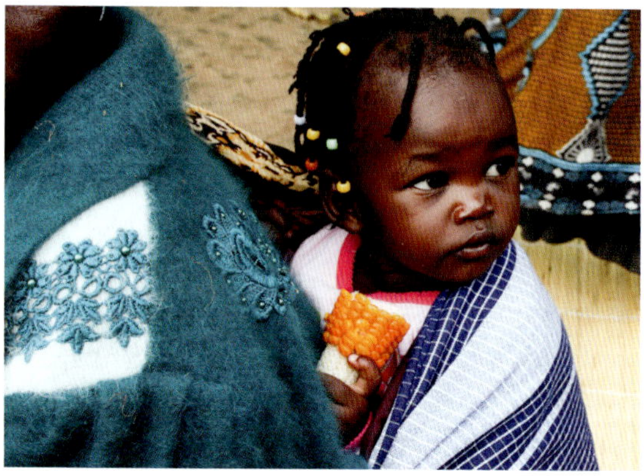

HarvestPlus/E. Simpungwe

Consuming biofortified orange maize can help children meet their daily vitamin A needs.

2010–2015: Ramping Up Political Commitment and Financing

In recent years high-level political commitment to address undernutrition has ramped up significantly among international UN, donor, and NGO organizations as well as many donor governments. Nutrition is no longer in the wings of the international development stage. Policies and strategy documents on nutrition proliferated among development agencies in this period, and overseas development assistance rose markedly.

This ascendancy has been brought about by a number of factors. Some of the impetus undoubtedly stemmed from the original 2008 *Lancet* Series and the ensuing discourse and media attention. The food price spikes of 2007–2008 also sparked renewed media and policy interest in undernutrition, and the 2008 Copenhagen Consensus (building on initial work in 2004 and later updated in 2012) concluded that nutrition interventions were among the most cost-effective in development.

One of the most important drivers, as well as beneficiaries, of the global momentum has been the Scaling Up Nutrition (SUN) Movement, launched in 2010, which now has membership from 57 countries worldwide. Founded on the principle that all people have a right to food and good nutrition, the SUN Movement seeks to "unite people—from governments, civil society, the United Nations, donors, businesses, and researchers—in a collective effort to improve nutrition."[48] Although the SUN Movement includes businesses as partners, the role of private-sector engagement—four decades after "the baby food tragedy" article in the *New Internationalist*—is still being vigorously debated.

In 2013 a second *Lancet* Maternal and Child Nutrition Series widened the scope of the 2008 series to review evidence and experience with "nutrition-sensitive" interventions from a range of sectors, including agriculture, social protection, education, and early childhood development.[49] It did so in light of evidence that direct interventions alone—if scaled up to 90 percent population coverage—would address only about one-fifth of the burden of child stunting in the highest-burden countries. This second series included an article on the politics of addressing malnutrition that raised the issue of enabling environments and reviewed experience.[50] The arena for nutrition-relevant action was broadening.

In the same year—2013—a major international Nutrition for Growth (N4G) summit led to unprecedented pledges of US$23 billion to address malnutrition. This was followed in 2014 by the Second International Conference on Nutrition (ICN2) and the launching of an annual series of *Global Nutrition Reports*. The *Global Nutrition Report* has positioned itself as not just a report, but a global accountability intervention. It highlights progress toward meeting nutrition goals and describes innovative approaches to addressing malnutrition and country experiences, but it also goes further to track the follow-up to the many pledges made at the 2013 N4G summit.

Such events, outputs, and policy windows have been underpinned and catalyzed by an international nutrition community of academics and practitioners that had been working in the background throughout nutrition's lean period and were thus poised to make links and grasp opportunities to advance an important part of the development agenda. The nutrition community has become more effective and more politically "streetwise" in making the case for investing in nutrition. It has done so by using a range of rationales including human rights, economic, and human development arguments. Other development sectors and actors are also now increasingly embracing nutrition—especially the agriculture community, which sought to put agriculture to work for better nutrition. In its reform process, the CGIAR network has placed a greater emphasis on nutrition than ever before, spearheaded by the Agriculture for Nutrition Health (A4NH) program, launched in 2010.

These international events and opportunities have also played out in national contexts. The emergence of a focus on how to implement, rather than simply what to implement, has led to a greater emphasis on the importance of political commitment from national governments, to efforts to build and measure commitment in various forms, and to implementation and scaling up of nutrition-relevant actions. The notion of "scaling up"—which only really surfaced in the nutrition world in the late 1990s (see Tom Marchione's 1999 book *Scaling Up, Scaling Down*[51])—is the SUN Movement's raison d'être. The focus is now shifting toward scaling up *impact* on nutrition—that is, not simply increasing coverage of a nutrition program, but rather focusing on what drives impact and then determining what mix of interventions must be applied to attain that impact.[52] This in turn emphasizes the need for a multisectoral, multilevel, and multistakeholder approach to generate a significant impact on malnutrition and to sustain it over time.

While high-level speeches in support of nutrition have been forthcoming, more concrete forms of financial and institutional commitment have in most cases been slower to materialize. Most high-burden countries still face significant gaps in their technical and strategic capacity to conceive, run, and scale up effective nutrition policies and programs—and as yet, there are few tangible, long-term plans or programs to strengthen capacity to improve nutrition.

But progress has been made and is being made. This book is intended to serve as a repository of experiences—to show what was done and how—in different contexts and at different times to address malnutrition and improve the lives of millions.

Structure of This Book

This overview's historical walk through 50 years of thinking and action on nutrition provides context for the stories that follow. The structure of the book, its themes, and the choice of chapters have been strongly influenced by, among other things, the *Lancet* 2013 Maternal and Child Nutrition Series' framework for actions (see Figure 1.2, adapted from the UNICEF framework in Box 1.1) and inputs from the *Nourishing Millions* advisory committee.

The stories in this book are divided into three sections, which correspond to the levels of response to malnutrition as shown in the *Lancet* framework. The first section—"Transforming Nutrition Interventions"—focuses on nutrition-specific interventions and programs that directly address malnutrition and target its immediate causes (light blue boxes in Figure 1.2). The chapters in this section focus on community-led programming (Chapter 2), interventions to ensure optimal infant and young child feeding practices (Chapter 3), micronutrient supplementation and fortification (Chapter 4), and community-based management of acute malnutrition (Chapter 5).

Section 2, "Transforming Sectoral Actions," covers nutrition-sensitive programs and approaches, which address the underlying determinants of malnutrition (green boxes). Nutrition sensitivity is not a new concept, but investment in developing, implementing, and evaluating nutrition-sensitive programs has intensified in the past few years. This section includes chapters focusing on agriculture (Chapter 6), social protection (Chapter 7), and water, sanitation, and hygiene (Chapter 8), all of which offer huge potential contributions to addressing malnutrition at scale. The final chapter in this section is on obesity prevention and control (Chapter 9), reflecting this growing global problem.

The third section—"Transforming National Policy and Programming"—focuses on how stories of change in nutrition play out at the country level. This permits us to highlight the role of the enabling environment (at the base of Figure 1.2 framework) and to show how the different levels of policy and practice come together, in different contexts and at different times, to drive change. Case studies have been developed for Thailand, Brazil, Bangladesh, Nepal, Peru, Vietnam, Ethiopia and the state of Odisha in India (Chapters 10–17). These all represent contexts in which a significant political commitment emerged, and actions were taken, to address a high burden of undernutrition. The chapters in this section attempt to unravel what happened and how change came about.

The choice of case studies highlighted within each chapter was determined by a set of criteria described in the Appendix.

Finally, before concluding, we devote a chapter (Chapter 18) to understanding the pivotal and transformational issue of leadership, highlighting stories of individuals who have successfully championed the cause of nutrition in different countries.

FIGURE 1.2 *Lancet* Nutrition Series framework for actions to achieve optimum fetal and child nutrition and development

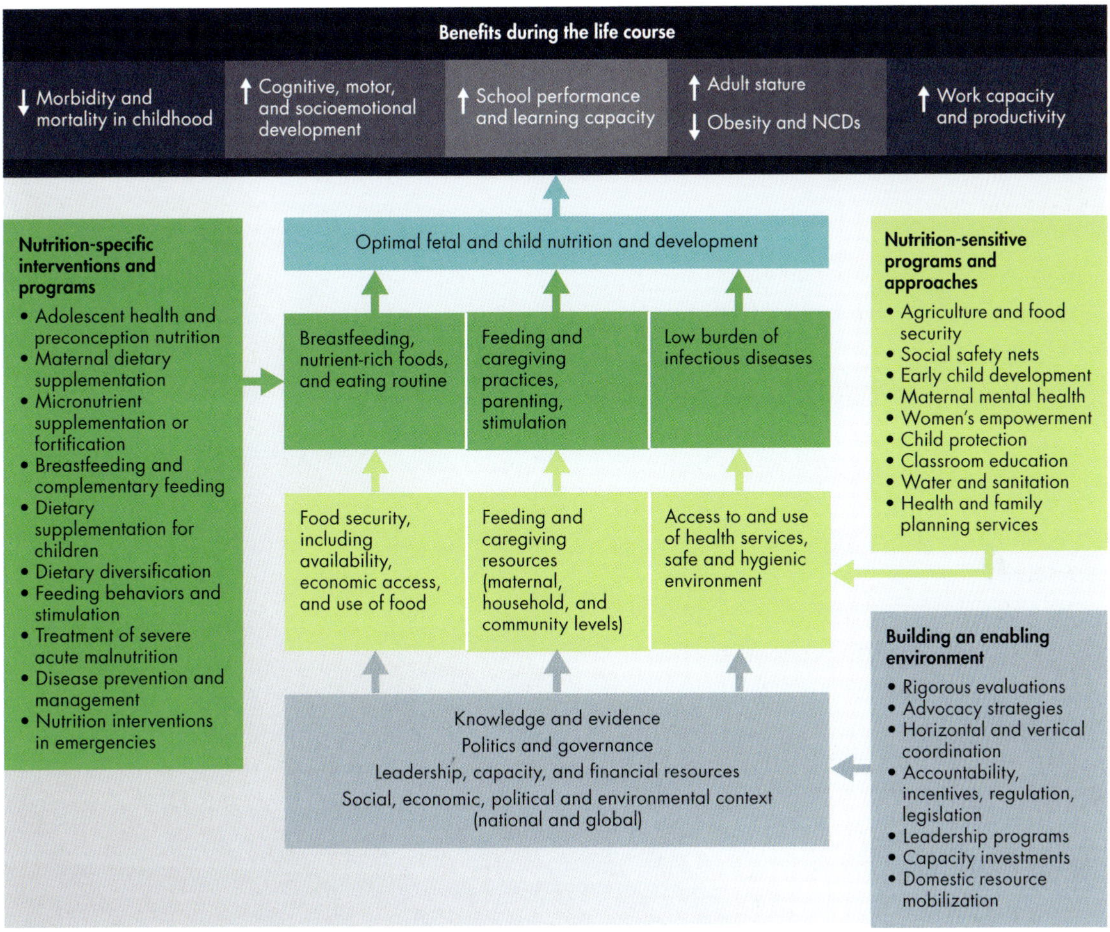

Source: R. E. Black, C. Victora, S. P. Walker, Z. A. Bhutta, P. Christian, M. de Onis, et al., "Maternal and Child Undernutrition and Overweight in Low-Income and Middle-Income Countries," *Lancet* 382, no. 9890 (2013): 427–451. Reproduced with permission.

Part I: Transforming Nutrition Interventions

CHAPTER 2

On the Front Line

Community Nutrition Programming

STUART GILLESPIE AND JUDITH HODGE

WHATEVER ADVANCES HAVE been made in terms of technologies, interventions, and their delivery platforms in recent decades, it is households and communities that remain on the front lines in combating malnutrition. During the past half century, several significant attempts have been made to initiate and implement community-based nutrition programs. This chapter assesses the evolution and performance of such approaches, highlighting several case studies.

In what follows, we differentiate between *community based* (which refers to the location of the intervention) and *community driven* (implying an active involvement of community members in designing and/or implementing the intervention). Several different communities may reside in any one village or urban slum—geography is only one of several factors that bring people together, or divide them. We also remind the reader that several of the interventions described in the first two sections of this book can be combined and delivered within community nutrition programs. In this sense, this chapter focuses more on the *how* of local nutrition-relevant action than on any one type of intervention (the *what*).

The literature on community nutrition programming includes various studies, evaluations, and reviews, with a particular concentration of scholarly studies in the 1990s. These include the following:

- three comprehensive reviews carried out by the United Nations Standing Committee on Nutrition, which attempted to unravel the dynamics underpinning success in nutrition, either at the national level or with regard to a specific program[1];
- a review of community-based programs that led to the formulation of the highly influential UNICEF nutrition strategy[2];
- a World Bank review of another four African programs[3];
- a questionnaire survey of 66 programs in Africa, also by the World Bank[4];
- a UNICEF-led appraisal of 22 community-based nutrition programs in South Asia[5];

- a review of 8 effective programs in Africa[6];
- a review of successful programs in Asia, undertaken by the International Food Policy Research Institute (IFPRI) for the Asian Development Bank[7];
- a USAID review of 10 community-based nutrition programs carried out in Kenya, Tanzania, and Uganda[8]; and
- further analyses undertaken as part of a joint World Bank–UNICEF assessment of nutrition policy and practice that culminated in the 2003 book *Combating Malnutrition: Time to Act.*[9]

The genesis of this 1990s attention to community nutrition in fact lay in experiments and experiences from the 1980s. Three of these were particularly influential: the Iringa program in Tanzania (see Box 2.1), the Tamil Nadu Integrated Nutrition Project (TINP) in southern India (see Box 2.2), and the Thai experience (described in Chapter 10).

In general, the assessments and evaluations listed above concurred in emphasizing the importance of four factors: the context, the process leading to the development of the program, the choice of activities, and the process adopted to manage and implement the program. Before highlighting

BOX 2.1 **Iringa: Africa's shining star**

Tanzania's Joint Nutrition Support Program in the country's Iringa region was a landmark success story in community-based nutrition programming during the 1980s. A collaboration between the Swedish International Development Authority (SIDA), the Tanzanian Food and Nutrition Centre, and UNICEF/WHO, the Iringa Nutrition Program was scaled up to cover more than 50 districts between 1983 and 1989.[10] The program emphasized social mobilization, local problem assessment and action planning, and tailor-made combinations of nutrition and food security interventions at the community level. Community workers monitored child growth to identify and assess families in which a child was malnourished and then worked with families to analyze possible causes and draw up an action plan in conjunction with local government organizations. Depending on the cause, interventions varied from counseling, to referral to the health service, to participation in a livelihood-creation, microcredit, or social protection program.[11]

Such active community involvement at each stage of the nutrition improvement process was pioneering (reflected in the use of the "triple A approach"—assessment, analysis, and action) and addressed the human rights of individuals and vulnerable groups.[12] In five years, the program almost eliminated severe child malnutrition (from 6.3 percent to 1.8 percent) and reduced moderate malnutrition by half.[13] Its dramatic success led to its national replication in the early 1990s as the Child Survival and Development Program, as well as to a number of lessons learned in terms of programming concepts and practice and to participatory development in general.[14] The program also became a leading community-based model, adopted in and adapted for many countries in Africa and Asia.

Aligning nutrition with community development, however, had a price. The Iringa experience was not sustained in Tanzania, and after a change in government in the late 1990s, it effectively fell through the institutional cracks.[15] In the new era of reform and cost-cutting, the community mobilization processes required for lasting change were considered too slow moving. Nutrition, increasingly equated with vertical micronutrient programs, was not considered an essential part of health reform.[16] Yet Iringa has had a lasting legacy by leading to the development of the hugely influential UNICEF conceptual framework of the causality of nutrition still in use today (see Chapter 1).

BOX 2.2 Community nutrition programming in India

In Indian nutrition programs, the practice of active community involvement has often lagged behind rhetoric—the programs may be community based, but few are community driven.[17] India's national Integrated Child Development Service (ICDS) scheme—the world's largest nutrition program—was launched in 1975 to address the health and nutrition needs of children under the age of six years. The program, which incorporates health, nutrition, and education interventions, operates through a network of *anganwadi* centers (AWCs) to provide services for adolescent girls, pregnant and lactating women, and children aged six months to six years. Individual or group counseling is delivered by community health workers or *anganwadi* workers. There is one AWC per village or for a population of 1,000 (700 in tribal areas).[18]

Although the ICDS has the potential to reach even the most vulnerable communities, evaluations suggest that gaps in program implementation result from factors such as poor targeting, poor coverage, and poor quality of service delivery.[19] Echoing findings across many evaluations of ICDS, a 2001 ethnographic study[20] found the ICDS to be concerned primarily with proper regulation, enumeration, and upward accountability rather than outcomes for children, and to be focused on delivering and documenting a narrow set of supplementary food outputs rather than the wider integrated services intended by the state.[21]

In sharp contrast, the Tamil Nadu Integrated Nutrition Project (TINP), launched in 1980 and developed alongside ICDS, achieved a significantly greater impact on child undernutrition than the national program. Between 1980 and 1989, the prevalence of children who were underweight dropped by approximately 1.5 percent a year in participating districts—twice the rate of nonparticipating ones.[22] The success of TINP was based on several factors, including selective feeding (the careful focus on supplementing the dietary intake of young children when their growth falters and until their growth resumes), favorable worker-to-supervisor ratios (see previous discussion of intensity), clear job descriptions, and a highly focused monitoring system.

The second evolution of TINP (TINP-2, launched in 1991 in 318 of Tamil Nadu's 385 rural blocks) sought to move beyond reducing severe malnutrition and to make a significant dent in the high prevalence of children suffering from moderate malnutrition by shifting toward a more preventive focus. Building on lessons learned from TINP-1, TINP-2 focused on strengthening local capacity, mobilizing the community, and targeting interpersonal communications, all aimed at improving home-based care and feeding of children younger than age 2 in order to prevent their becoming malnourished. This task was more difficult; some progress was made, but it was not as spectacular as that of TINP-1.[23] Later on, the TINP model became subsumed within the national ICDS program as the central government pursued universalization. As with Iringa, this high-intensity, time-intensive community program—however effective—did not sit easily with those pushing for scaling up a centralized program nationally. In the process, the political incentive to scale up coverage—in other words, a focus on quantity—trumped quality.

Although the ICDS, a national program that has been active for more than 40 years, has had limited success at the national level, there are signs of what can be done with higher-level commitment and stronger incentives for implementation and achieving results on the ground. The states of Odisha (described in Chapter 17) and Maharashtra are recent examples. In Maharashtra, key drivers associated with the rapid improvement in child nutrition included a doubling of spending on nutrition and a focus on filling vacancies among frontline workers in the ICDS scheme. Stunting in children under age five declined from 36.5 percent to 24.0 percent between 2005–2006 and 2012, and access to the ICDS was one of the determinants that improved the most between surveys.[24] Odisha, Maharashtra, and the earlier example of TINP show what can be achieved if community-based systems—supported by higher-level structures and incentives—are made to work effectively for communities.

several case studies and experiences, we dig deeper into these factors, listing key lessons and recommendations that emerged from these reviews.

Context

The degree to which program implementers can influence context is limited, at least in the short term. Several reviews have called for a two-pronged approach that involves catalyzing the development of programs where the context is favorable while promoting enabling environments through advocacy and social mobilization at all levels. Many reviews converged on the following contextual factors as being important:

- Political commitment at all levels of society and a conducive policy environment with supportive structures and policies. For programs to succeed in the long run, a context or environment that is enabling must be in place or created. Some of these contextual factors (for example, high literacy rate, women's empowerment, community organizational capacity and structures, appropriate legislation) may be particularly influenced by policy, others less so;
- The presence of complementary ongoing nutrition-sensitive programs from other sectors and/or local government;
- A culture of participation, particularly with regard to women;
- Community awareness, either existing or created, of the magnitude and consequences of malnutrition and a degree of commitment and knowledge to address them;
- Community organizations (such as women's groups, people's nongovernmental organizations [NGOs], credit associations, youth clubs, farmers' associations) along with adequate infrastructure for delivering basic services, including committed and capable staff; and
- Charismatic community leaders who can mobilize and motivate people to do more for themselves in a genuinely self-reliant way.

Process in Developing the Program

Community-driven programs are rarely initiated to improve nutrition alone (communities have broader priorities), so means must usually be found to foster multifaceted programs in which nutrition and health activities can be embedded (see the discussion of Bangladesh's SHOUHARDO program later in this chapter).

As mentioned, most reviews of community nutrition action cited have emphasized the processes involved—that is, the *how* questions of program development, implementation, and expansion. But what is a good process? Most reviews concurred that it is one in which participation, local ownership, and empowerment are driving forces. A focus on process tends to align with the human rights rationale for action, wherein beneficiaries are considered subjects of their own growth and development rather than passive recipients of transfers or handouts. In the past, top-down, outcome-focused service delivery or nutrition interventions (for example, the Integrated Child Development Service [ICDS] in the 1990s, discussed below) tended to dominate the field of nutrition. With limited community ownership and little attention, if any, to the strengthening of local nutrition-improving processes, their long-term effectiveness was low. In contrast, process-focused development projects emphasize working from the bottom up on participation and empowerment, are often supported by NGOs (as in the case of SHOUHARDO), and are often—at least initially—small scale.

The reviews highlighted the following factors as important to program development:

- Promoting and supporting a process whereby individuals and communities participate in *assessing* the nutrition problem, *analyzing* its causes and their available resources, and *acting* in response. This three-step iterative cycle—the "triple A" approach of assessment, analysis, and action—emerged from the Iringa experience in Tanzania described below and became the cornerstone of the UNICEF nutrition strategy[25];
- Finding an appropriate entry point that is relevant and responsive to the community's wishes and needs;
- Clearly identifying and defining time-bound goals and targets (young children, pregnant and lactating women, and adolescent girls are normally the focus);
- Identifying and supporting appropriate numbers and ratios of facilitators and community mobilizers, thereby providing a sense of joint ownership of the program or project by the community and the government (see the discussion of intensity under "Program Management and Implementation" below);
- Allocating adequate funding and time by donors and program managers to program development.

Program Design and Content

Community-based programs include a range of activities and interventions (see Chapters 3–5 in particular). For children, such programs could include any combination of the following: growth monitoring; infant and young child feeding; disease management, including feeding during and after diarrheal and oral rehydration therapy; micronutrient supplementation, such as promoting consumption of iodized salt; deworming; and possibly targeted food supplementation. For women, activities included in ante- and postnatal care strategies can encompass tetanus toxoid immunization, micronutrient supplementation (including iron and folic acid tablets for pregnant women and possibly a postpartum vitamin A megadose in cases where vitamin A deficiency is known to be a problem), iodized salt consumption, food supplementation during pregnancy, malaria chemoprophylaxis in endemic areas, and reproductive health education.

Along with program content, two key design considerations relate to program coverage and targeting. Coverage relates to the percentage of the at-risk population participating in the program, while targeting concerns the degree to which this

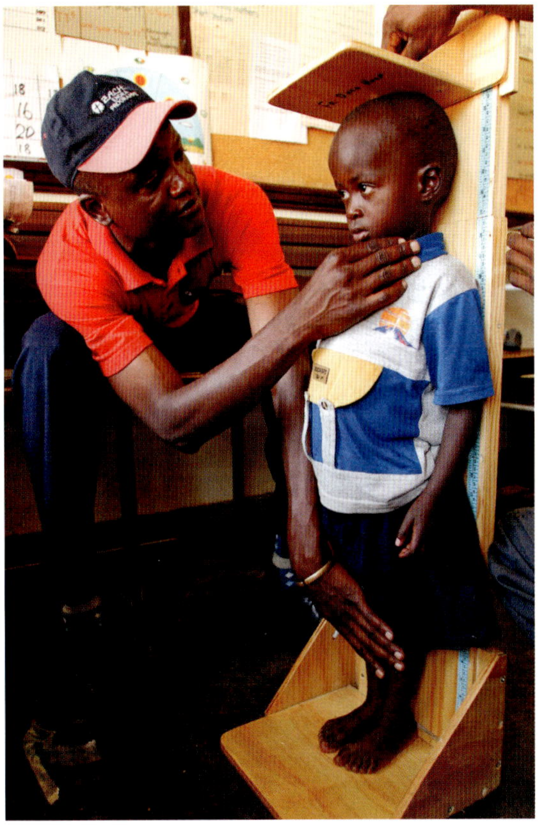

Panos/G. Pirozzi

A child is measured at a health clinic in Zimbabwe.

coverage is oriented toward the neediest among potential responders. Well-conceived programs may be ineffective simply because their coverage is too narrow to have a broad impact on the problem, they do not reach those most in need, or both. Coverage and targeting often work in opposite directions: that is, large-scale programs might have wide coverage but be poorly targeted, whereas small-scale programs (often run by NGOs) may be well targeted but have limited impact owing to their limited coverage.

Other key findings of reviews of community nutrition action are as follows:

- The promotion part of growth monitoring and promotion programs is key. Growth monitoring and promotion works better when it is group based, when proper feedback and counseling are provided, and when information is used efficiently at all levels;
- Nutrition education should be related to tangible resources, conveyed as behavior change communication (as in participatory educational theater) and as positive deviance;
- Credit and income-generating activities should be provided for women;
- Care for women and children should be improved by reducing women's workloads using appropriate technology, such as milling machines, solar dryers, and water wells; and
- A multisectoral approach should be adopted to maximize convergence with other relevant programs, such as those that deal with underlying food, health, and care-related causes of malnutrition.

Program Management and Implementation

The issue of intensity is key in program design and implementation. Intensity relates to resource use per participant, expressed either as dollars per participant per year or in population and worker ratios (for example, the number of children per community-level worker or mobilizer, or the number of facilitators or supervisors per mobilizer). Past experience suggests that effective programs require approximately $US5–15 per participant (at 1991 rates) per year excluding additional food, which roughly doubles the cost.[26]

With regard to personnel ratios, the successful example of Thailand (see Chapter 10) adopted a benchmark ratio of 1:20—that is, one community mobilizer per 20 households with young children, and one facilitator/supervisor per 20 mobilizers. In contrast, in India's ICDS in the 1990s, ratios approached 1:200—that is, one community-based *anganwadi* worker managed activities designed to cover approximately 200 households. Not surprisingly, the ICDS program was center-based and oriented to handing out food to individuals who attended (see Box 2.2). The critically important human dimension of counseling to improve home-based care and nutrition, tailored to the specific needs of individual children, was relatively neglected. In Tamil Nadu, on the other hand, TINP adopted a two-worker model (as opposed to just one worker) to increase intensity, with the second worker focusing primarily on home visits for the youngest growth-faltering children. Other key management and implementation factors underpinning successful programs included:

- Community involvement in program planning and implementation using participatory processes such as the triple-A approach, participatory rural appraisal, and community representation and voice within program hierarchies;
- Capacity development and training for programming staff and community members that is task oriented and part of the staff's professional development;

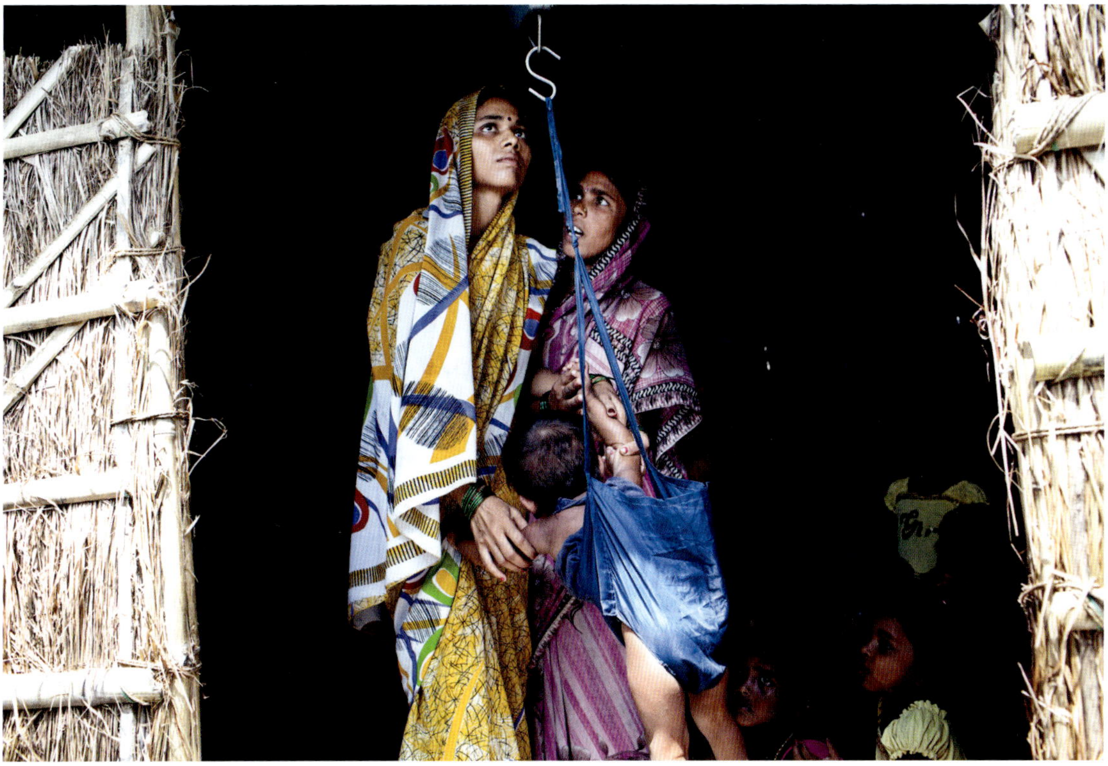

Panos/S. Das

Workers at an anganwadi center, which provides basic nutrition and health services, weigh an infant in Bihar, India.

- Strong leadership, training, and supervision of facilitators and mobilizers; an appropriate balance between top-down and bottom-up management; and links to effective community-based monitoring; and
- The involvement of local NGOs, which often provided excellent facilitators as well as culturally relevant training. They were usually accountable to the community, which facilitated sustainability.

SHOUHARDO in Bangladesh

Bangladesh's sustained success in reducing the prevalence of underweight and stunting among children during the past two decades (see Chapter 12) has not been linked to any particular nutrition intervention but rather to multidimensional drivers. Key likely contributors to this decline include improvements in household assets, parental education (both maternal and paternal), sanitation coverage, gender empowerment, and healthcare use.[27] Such a multipronged approach has been integral to the success of the SHOUHARDO (Strengthening Household Ability to Respond to Development Opportunities) community-based program.

SHOUHARDO I was a large-scale, five-year program (2004–2009) that aimed to reduce malnutrition and chronic food insecurity in vulnerable households in 18 of the poorest and hardest-to-reach districts of Bangladesh, serving a population of 2 million people.[28] The program provided both direct nutrition interventions, such as food aid and maternal and child health activities, and services for improving water, sanitation, and hygiene (WASH) and homestead food production. But what differentiated SHOUHARDO from other large-scale, community-based interventions was its use of a rights-based livelihoods approach for both addressing the conditions of poverty and promoting a "culture of equal citizenship rights."[29]

SHOUHARDO (which means friendship in Bengali) targeted the poorest and most vulnerable households living in the most poverty-stricken and remote chars and *haors* (unstable islands and wetlands formed of silt deposits) as well as coastal and urban slums. Household targeting within each village began with a participatory "well-being analysis." This involved grouping community members into economic categories based on criteria such as land ownership, income level, and food insecurity. The final participants chosen included 400,000 households, representing about three-quarters of all households in project villages.[30]

The program implemented a wide range of activities, recruiting community members to be facilitators and trainers in agriculture, fisheries, livestock, and other income-generating activities often focused on economic activities around the homestead.[31] A team of approximately 45 partner NGOs were responsible for implementing the program, with CARE Bangladesh playing the supervisory role.

Empowering Marginalized People

The program aimed to empower some of the most marginalized populations (women and adolescent girls in particular) to realize their basic rights, directing them to existing social protection schemes and mediating their interaction with duty-bearers (usually government officials).[32] This focus on rights was combined with a livelihoods approach, which takes a holistic view of people's lives to inform program design. The livelihoods perspective breaks down the traditional sectoral view that people's lives are composed of unconnected pieces; instead, it looks for synergistic impacts from cross-sector combinations of interventions based on an understanding of the strategies that households use to survive.[33] Within this model, SHOUHARDO also focused on factors that have a well-documented relationship with improved nutritional status and children's survival. These factors included education of women and girls and women's empowerment and control of resources.[34]

SHOUHARDO addressed not only the availability, access, and utilization issues that led to food insecurity but also the underlying structural issues that contributed to vulnerabilities specific to the population in its operational area.[35] Structural causes of food insecurity included not only poverty, poor sanitation, and frequent natural disasters but also power inequalities between women and men and between economic classes—politically sensitive areas that development agencies often steer clear of but that are crucial for tackling malnutrition in a sustainable manner. And such a radical departure from business as usual paid off. The program's results showed exceptionally large reductions in stunting between 2004 and 2009: a decline from 56 percent to 40 percent among children aged 6 to 24 months in the program's operational area. Furthermore, stunting reductions were far greater for the extreme-poor project households than for the poor (21.3 percent versus 12.7 percent). During the same period, levels of stunting remained unchanged in the country as a whole, and increases even occurred at some point owing to a food price crisis and extreme weather conditions.[36] So how did this community-based intervention achieve such success?

Understanding Success

Analysis (using a mixed-method approach) of SHOUHARDO's success highlighted the impact of various interventions. Improved nutritional status of children was associated with a combination of nutrition-specific (direct) and nutrition-sensitive (indirect) approaches. Direct interventions included food assistance (for children aged 6–24 months and lactating mothers) and health, hygiene, and nutrition support to mothers. SHOUHARDO's courtyard sessions on health, hygiene, and nutrition appeared to have made a significant impact on mothers' caring practices for their children and on their own antenatal care. More indirect interventions were those that improved households' economic conditions (for instance, participation in core occupational groups) and provided WASH support (that is, assistance with tubewells, a type of well in which a tube or pipe is bored into an underground aquifer to obtain safe water, and access to safe latrines).[37]

Many of the improvements in women's empowerment that occurred over the program's duration could be attributed to SHOUHARDO initiatives. The degree to which women participated in Empowerment, Knowledge, and Transformative Action (EKATA) and other program groups was linked to significant improvements in their influence on household decisions, freedom of movement, and reportedly, in patriarchal attitudes. In general, the more that household members had been involved in multiple SHOUHARDO interventions, the better off they became in terms of food security status, equality of power between female and male household members, and the nutritional status of young children.[38]

Building on Success: SHOUHARDO II

The program's second phase (SHOUHARDO II, 2010–2015) maintained a strong emphasis on improving livelihood security, food security, nutrition, and women's empowerment at the community level. However, this phase incorporated lessons learned from Phase I, with additional components aimed at strengthening local governance and improving adaptation to climate change. The program reached a further 370,000 households in 1,573 villages in 11 districts, targeting poor and extreme-poor households.[39] SHOUHARDO II prioritized community-based interventions, such as the capacity of village development committees to not only assess local factors constraining food security but to oversee program efforts to address them.[40] A final impact evaluation report suggests that SHOUHARDO II was associated with reducing stunting prevalence among children under age five from 61.7 percent at the time of the project's inception to 48.8 percent only four years later—a total reduction of 12.9 percentage points. Success was attributed to the program's nutrition-specific maternal and child health and nutrition interventions, as well as interventions designed to empower women, promote livelihoods, and improve health environments at the household level.[41]

Where Are We Now?

Compared with the 1990s, the importance of community-driven approaches in nutrition seems to have fallen behind in the wider literature on participation. While the *Lancet* Nutrition Series of 2013 discussed platforms at the community level for delivery, for example, it did not address community-*driven* approaches as they relate to active involvement of community members in program design and implementation. SHOUHARDO may be an exception (albeit one that was initiated more from a food security than a nutrition perspective). It stands in contrast to the frequent application of participatory approaches to livelihoods, agricultural development, women's empowerment, sanitation, and other sectors that only indirectly impact nutritional status.

In the 2000s, increasing attention was paid to the concept of community-driven development (CDD), with the World Bank supporting and evaluating a range of CDD approaches in different countries.[42] Reviews of these programs tended to focus on the crucial need to adapt interventions to the local context (including community-level perceptions of development) and on the importance of responsive state involvement in delivering public services and fostering downward accountability.[43]

While the issue of accountability in the delivery of public services has gained significant traction in recent years,[44] it had been relatively neglected in nutrition until recently. In identifying this gap, Nisbett et al.[45] pointed to the findings of a trial in Uganda that involved community meetings to reflect on scorecards of community healthcare provision in that country; the trial was associated with significant accelerations in decline in child mortality and wasting rates.[46]

Things are changing, however, and accountability in nutrition is moving to center stage. This trend was highlighted in a recent consultation among Scaling Up Nutrition (SUN) member countries[47] and through the way in which the annual *Global Nutrition Report*—in shining a light on the translation of stated commitments into action on the ground—positions itself as an accountability intervention, not just a simple report. Is community accountability for nutrition (building on past lessons described here and in Chapter 10 on Thailand) the new window of opportunity to ensure that the voice of local people will help them achieve their own nutrition security?

CHAPTER 3

Off to the Best Start

The Importance of Infant and Young Child Feeding

JUDITH HODGE

IN RECENT YEARS, nutrition interventions have focused on the critical first 1,000 days of life (from pregnancy up to the child's second birthday), a period which has been identified as a window of opportunity for preventing child morbidity and mortality and ensuring adequate growth. During this time, children have higher nutritional needs to support rapid growth and development; if these are not met (and supported by adequate care and access to health services), loss in linear growth is largely irreversible and the potential for intervention to promote catch-up growth later on is minimal.[1] Optimum nutrition in the first 1,000 days is also important for preventing overweight. Evidence suggests that infants with growth faltering in early life, followed by rapid weight gain in later childhood, might be at increased risk of adult obesity and noncommunicable diseases (NCDs), such as cardiovascular disease and hypertension.[2] Strategies to improve infant and young child feeding (IYCF) are therefore a cornerstone for the child survival and development programs of many countries.

Evidence for recommended feeding practices and about barriers to appropriate feeding has grown steadily, as has knowledge about interventions that have effectively promoted improved IYCF. Best practices for IYCF focus on *breastfeeding* (initiating breastfeeding within one hour of birth, exclusive breastfeeding (EBF)—only giving an infant breast-milk and no other food or water—for the first six months of life, and continued breastfeeding up to the age of two and beyond); and *complementary feeding* (introducing safe, age-appropriate soft and solid food starting at six months of age).[3] The *Lancet* 2016 Breastfeeding series confirms that appropriate breastfeeding practices provide major protection against child morbidity from diarrhea and respiratory infections in countries affected by infectious diseases.[4] One study estimates that improved breastfeeding practices worldwide could annually prevent the deaths of 823,000 children under five and the deaths of 20,000 mothers from breast cancer.[5] Breastfeeding is further associated with increased intelligence in children, and thus with enhanced human capital in adulthood.[6] A recent economic analysis estimates that present low global levels of breastfeeding at six months could account for a global loss of gross national income (GNI) amounting to US$302 billion—about 0.5 percent of world GNI.[7] Poor complementary feeding practices have also been identified as a risk factor associated directly with stunting.[8] Moreover, for the increasing number of countries now facing a double burden of malnutrition (both under- and overnutrition), optimal IYCF and early intervention are even more critical to ensure that investments are targeting children under two years to reduce their risk of becoming both stunted and obese.[9]

Developing a Global Strategy

For most of the past century, initiation and duration of breastfeeding have declined globally as a result of rapid social and economic change, including increased urbanization, increased women's employment, and marketing of breast-milk substitutes.[10] In the 1970s, a global coalition formed by civil society and other stakeholders campaigned against the unethical marketing strategies of infant formula companies that resulted in many infants' becoming malnourished or dying from contaminated or diluted breast-milk substitutes (Box 3.1).[11] Key developments include the following:

- 1981: *International Code of Marketing of Breast-milk Substitutes*[12] (hereafter "the Code") and subsequent relevant resolutions adopted by the World Health Assembly.
- 1990: *Innocenti Declaration on the Protection, Promotion, and Support of Breastfeeding*[13] (developed by WHO and UNICEF policy makers) recommended establishment of national breastfeeding committees, national legislation to protect the breastfeeding rights of employed women, and implementation of the Code.
- 1991: *Baby Friendly Hospital Initiative*[14] launched to scale up "10 Steps to Successful Breastfeeding." Maternity facilities achieve baby-friendly status when they adopt a policy of not accepting free or low-cost breast-milk substitutes and have implemented the 10 steps. There are now more than 15,000 baby-friendly facilities in 134 countries.
- 2002: WHO/UNICEF *Global Strategy for Infant and Young Child Feeding*[15] galvanized world attention around the importance of IYCF for child survival, growth, and development. It also emphasized the need to strengthen breastfeeding support at the community level and addressed the needs of children living in difficult circumstances, such as infants of mothers living with HIV, low birth-weight infants, and infants in emergency situations.

BOX 3.1 Marketing of infant formula

Since its inception in 1981, enforcement of the International Code of Marketing of Breast-milk Substitutes has been undermined by the active and aggressive marketing of substitutes by their manufacturers and distributors.[16] Clear evidence of negative impact on breastfeeding is found when breast-milk substitutes are provided for free in health facilities and promoted by health workers and in the media—practices in direct contravention of the Code.[17] Less than a quarter of 199 countries have a robust implementation and monitoring system in place.[18] Brazil's breastfeeding success is due in part to its rigorous monitoring of compliance.[19] Despite its progress, Brazil is the 10th-largest market for infant formula, a market expected to reach US$951 million by 2019.[20]

- 2003: Pan American Health Organization/WHO *Guiding Principles for Complementary Feeding of the Breastfed Child*[21] proposes 10 guiding principles for complementary feeding, which cover areas such as meal frequency, energy density, and feeding during and after illness. Similar guiding principles are available for feeding of non-breastfed children.[22]

Breastfeeding initiatives have been the most successful aspect of IYCF programs at scale to date. Stories of intervention effectiveness in improving complementary feeding come mainly from small-scale programs. In Madagascar, a project to improve maternal nutrition and IYCF in a target population of 6 million implemented a combination of health-worker training, community mobilization, and mass media to great effect. Results showed an increase in EBF in infants under six months from 42 to 70 percent between 2000 and 2006.[23] More widely, evidence indicates that countries with policies and programs most closely aligned to recommendations from the WHO/UNICEF global strategy—a multipronged approach with both cross-cutting and targeted strategies at community, health system, and national levels (Box 3.2)—achieve the greatest impact.[24]

BOX 3.2 Key components and interventions of IYCF strategy

Legislation

» Marketing of breast-milk substitutes
» Maternity protection

Skilled support by the health system

» Curriculum development for IYCF
» IYCF counseling and other support services
» Capacity development for health providers
» Institutionalization of the Baby-Friendly Hospital Initiative

Community-based counseling and support

» Established community-based integrated IYCF counseling services
» Mother support groups

Communication

» Community for behavior and social change

Additional complementary feeding options

» Improving the quality of complementary foods through locally available ingredients
» Increasing agricultural production
» Provision of nutrition supplements and foods
» Social protection schemes

IYCF in difficult circumstances

» HIV and infant feeding
» IYCF in emergencies

Source: Adapted from UNICEF, *Programming Guide: Infant and Young Child Feeding* (New York, 2011).

Breastfeeding—Best Progress in Developing Countries

Findings from the *Lancet* 2016 Breastfeeding series confirm that breastfeeding is one of the few positive health behaviors that is more prevalent in poor countries than in rich ones.[25] Moreover, poor women breastfeed for longer than rich women in low- and middle-income countries. The reverse is true in high-income countries, suggesting that in low- and middle-income countries, breastfeeding contributes to reducing health inequalities between rich and poor children.[26] Yet global progress has still been slow to date. In 2000, 37 percent of infants under six months were exclusively breastfed—by 2012 this had increased to just 41 percent.[27] However, 25 countries increased their rates of EBF by 20 percentage points or more after 1995; this puts these countries on track to achieve the World Health Assembly global nutrition target of increasing the rate of EBF to at least 50 percent in the first six months by 2025.[28] Although less than half of all infants worldwide (44 percent) were put to the

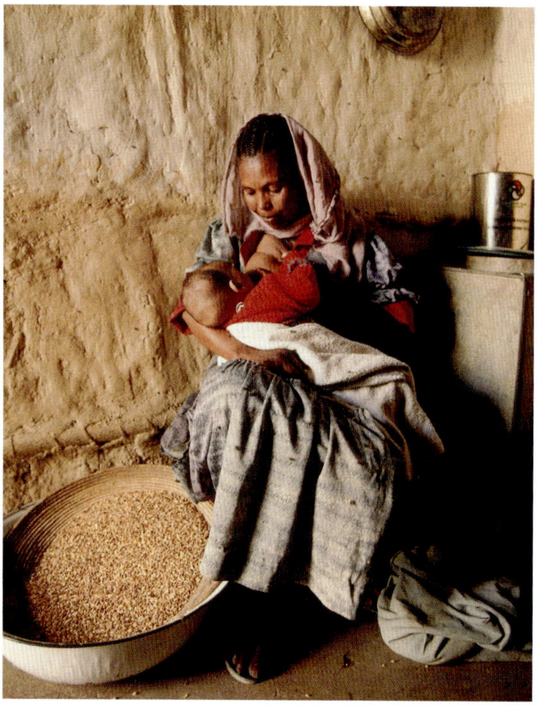

Panos/B. Press

Exclusive breastfeeding—giving an infant only breast milk and no other food and water—for the first 6 months is linked with lower mortality of children and mothers.

breast within the first hour after birth (first milk, or colostrum, is rich in antibodies and important for the baby's immune system), 68 percent of infants were still being breastfed at 12–15 months.[29]

Key to success are national plans that create an enabling environment through elements such as the adoption of legislation on the marketing of breastmilk substitutes (Box 3.1), baby-friendly maternity facilities, and skilled support by health providers and community workers. Education interventions increased EBF by 43 percent at day one, by 30 percent at one month, and by 90 percent from one to five months, with a combination of individual and group counseling found to be more effective than either intervention on its own.[30] However, more progress needs to be made in addressing the barriers presented by work environments. Nearly all countries have maternity protection legislation, but only half (98 out of 185 countries) provide the recommended 14 weeks of maternity leave.[31] Moreover, hundreds of millions of working women in informal work sectors, mostly in Africa and Asia, have either no maternity protection or inadequate protection.[32]

Success Stories in Boosting Breastfeeding

Brazil made impressive strides in improving breastfeeding practices beginning in the mid-1970s.[33] Between 1974/1975 and 2006/2007, the median duration of breastfeeding increased from about 2.5 months to 14 months.[34] There was also a steep rise in EBF rates from a low of about 4 percent in 1986 to 48 percent by 2006/2007.[35] Brazil launched its National Program for the Promotion of Breastfeeding in 1981 through a mass media campaign to sensitize decision makers and the public about the urgent need to improve breastfeeding rates.[36] Targeted communication strategies were developed, using multiple channels and messages tailored to the local context and to the specific barriers to breastfeeding, such as the belief that women do not produce enough milk for EBF.[37]

Brazil's success was not instant. There was a time lag of approximately six years before significant increases in breastfeeding duration began to be detected. Analysis of the program identifies a number of threats to breastfeeding, including free formula distribution, unethical advertising by infant formula companies, and medical education biases. For the first three to four years of the program, these negative influences were much stronger than breastfeeding promotion and advocacy efforts. But barriers declined over time as Brazil's institutional capacity increased and the country reduced its reliance on foreign aid to sustain the program.[38] Brazil's achievements in improved breastfeeding do not exist in isolation—they are part of a broader expansion in access to maternal and child health and nutrition services and pro-poor policies such as targeted cash transfer programs.[39] The Brazilian government has also shown regional leadership through its support of human-milk banks in neonatal intensive care units in nearly all countries in Latin America, which not only provide human milk for critically ill newborns but also foster a culture of breastfeeding in the hospital.[40]

Bangladesh was motivated to re-evaluate its breastfeeding promotion efforts when EBF rates remained static. From 1994 to 2007 the EBF rate hovered between 42 and 46 percent.[41] The Bangladeshi program included successful implementation of the Code, the introduction of maternity leave legislation, and promotion of major investment in Baby Friendly Hospital Initiative efforts, but it had failed to engage a key target audience, namely women who still had little contact with health sector maternity services.[42] Lessons learned led to the piloting of innovative community-based breastfeeding promotion approaches, such as community nutrition promoters and mother-to-mother support groups. Subsequent scale-up of these new IYCF practices through Alive & Thrive's program (2010–2014) paid huge dividends—an increase in EBF from 48 percent to 88 percent in intervention areas.

In contrast, Sri Lanka is a country where 95 percent of women attend prenatal care and give birth in healthcare facilities. Between 1995 and 2007, the average rate of EBF among infants up to six months of age increased from 17 percent to 76 percent, an annual increase of roughly 6 percentage points a year.[43] The country's breastfeeding program was characterized by extensive training in lactation support both for the vast majority of health workers based in hospitals and field clinics and for public health midwives making home visits within the first 10 days after delivery.[44] The Sri Lankan experience underlines the need to engage women at both health-facility and community levels, with outreach to extend breastfeeding into the community.[45]

Complementary Feeding

Feeding with appropriate, adequate, and safe complementary foods from six months onward contributes to better health and growth outcomes, although breast milk remains an important source of nutrients until children reach two years of age.[46] Complementary feeding is the period of transition from breast milk (or breast-milk substitutes) to the gradual introduction of new foods until a baby is eating the same foods as the rest of the family.[47] The timing of complementary feeding, usually between 6 and 23 months of age, is the most nutritionally vulnerable period for young children. And in developing countries, this period coincides with a rapid acceleration in the incidence of stunting, particularly among children age 6 to 12 months.[48] Inappropriate complementary feeding (such as poor-quality food, inadequate practices, and poor hygiene and food safety) has been strongly linked with undernutrition, growth faltering, diarrhea, increased rate of infections, vitamin-mineral deficiency, poor cognitive development, and increased mortality among children.[49]

Most examples of successful complementary feeding programs are at the community level rather than at scale (one exception is Alive & Thrive's multiple-country intervention).[50] This may be due to the fact that although complementary feeding is practiced worldwide, it is a complex set of behaviors, comprising food choices and preparation, active feeding or responsiveness to infant cues, and so on, and practices vary greatly across cultures, individuals, and socioeconomic classes.[51] Moreover, indicators for measuring complementary feeding (Box 3.3) were not in place until 2008.[52] In the Indian state of Maharashtra, one study suggests

BOX 3.3 Indicators for measuring complementary feeding

In 2008 the WHO issued the following indicators for measuring complementary feeding[53]:

- **Dietary diversity:** Proportion of children 6–23 months of age who receive foods from four or more food groups daily (out of the following seven food groups: (1) grains, roots, and tubers; (2) legumes and nuts; (3) dairy products (milk, yoghurt, cheese); (4) flesh foods (meat, fish, poultry, and liver/organ meats); (5) eggs; (6) vitamin A–rich fruits and vegetables; and (7) other fruits and vegetables).
- **Minimum meal frequency:** Proportion of breastfed and non-breastfed children 6–23 months of age who receive solid, semi-solid, or soft foods (but also including milk feeds for non-breastfed children) the minimum number of times per day: 2 for 6–8 months, 3 for 9–23 months, 4 for 6–23 months (if not breastfed).
- **Minimum acceptable diet (composite indicator):** Proportion of children 6–23 months of age who meet both minimum meal frequency and dietary diversity criteria (in both breastfed and non-breastfed children).
- **Consumption of iron-rich or iron-fortified foods:** Proportion of children 6–23 months of age who receive an iron-rich food or iron-fortified food that is especially designed for infants and young children or that is fortified in the home.

that improvement in child-feeding practices was one of the key determinants in reducing stunting, which declined from 36.5 percent to 24 percent between 2005/2006 and 2012.[54] Between these two surveys, the percentage of children 6 to 23 months old who were fed a required minimum number of times per day increased from 34 to 77 percent, although less than 7 percent received a minimum acceptable diet in 2012.[55]

High-quality counseling of mothers or caregivers and appropriate behavior change communication are essential for improving complementary feeding practices. In addition, provision of complementary foods offering extra energy (with or without added micronutrients) and fortification of complementary foods may be needed to fill nutrient gaps when locally available foods alone cannot satisfy nutritional requirements.[56]

Approaches to improve complementary feeding in different contexts may also encompass various social protection measures, such as cash transfers, and nutrition-sensitive measures in the agriculture sector. The Enhanced Homestead Food Production (E-HFP) model in Burkina Faso used an agricultural platform to improve nutrition during the first 1,000 days, combining home gardening and small animal production with behavior change communication over two years (see Chapter 6 for more on this intervention). An impact evaluation found that program beneficiaries showed a marginally statistically significant increase in dietary diversity and intake of nutrient-rich foods, with improvements in IYCF knowledge. Children (aged 3–12 months) showed statistically significant reductions in anemia (14.6 percent) and diarrhea (15.9 percent) and a marginally statistically significant reduction in wasting (8.8 percent) between 2010 and 2012.[57]

Alive & Thrive

The Alive & Thrive multistakeholder program (2009–2014) aimed to improve IYCF practices at scale in three very different contexts: Bangladesh, Ethiopia, and Vietnam. The initiative sought to address the dearth of field-tested, documented examples of large, multicomponent IYCF programs.[58]

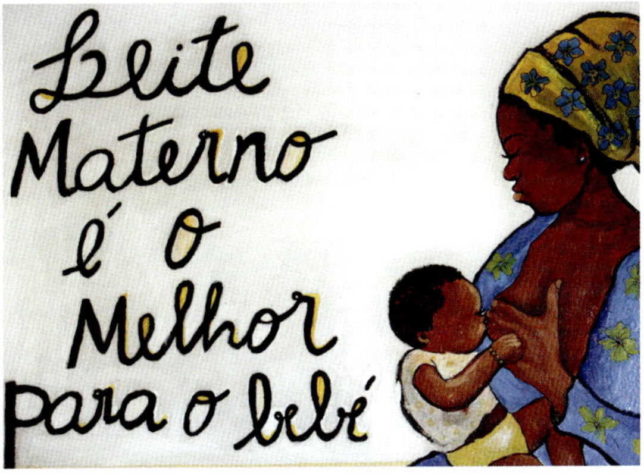

Panos/G. Pirozzi

A health education mural in Mozambique reads, "Mother's milk is best for baby."

Preliminary findings from the 2015 endline survey report impressive results in changing feeding behavior and diets (although no results were reported on stunting and wasting). This suggests that effective interventions can be delivered at scale to improve infant and young child nutrition. In Bangladesh, Alive & Thrive's program of advocacy, community mobilization, and mass media is reported to have led to rapid improvements in breastfeeding and complementary feeding behaviors. From 2010 to 2014, the percentage of infants under six months who were exclusively breastfed increased from 49 percent to 86 percent in places that received the comprehensive intervention package. Additionally, the proportion of children who consumed a diverse diet increased by 30 percentage points. In Vietnam, EBF prevalence (initially lower than 20 percent) nearly tripled in areas where Alive & Thrive initiated high-quality interpersonal counseling services in health facilities in addition to a mass media campaign. The Vietnam program introduced an innovative social franchise model for delivering infant and young child nutrition counseling services, which was successfully integrated into the health system. In the two countries (Bangladesh and Vietnam), Alive & Thrive conducted an estimated 3.3 million counseling sessions with mothers of children under two years of age, making it the first project of its kind to implement IYCF interventions at scale. National mass media campaigns allowed both countries to reach millions more mothers in a relatively short period of time.

Preliminary results from Alive & Thrive's Phase 1 (2009–2014) in Ethiopia suggest that is possible to effect change in complementary feeding practices. The proportion of children who met minimum dietary diversity and minimum adequate diet, while still extremely low, doubled in the program evaluation areas. In addition, minimum meal frequency increased by more than 20 percentage points (from 46 to 70 percent).[59] These gains were all achieved against a backdrop of high levels of food insecurity in Alive & Thrive's intervention areas.

In response to the continuing complementary feeding challenges in Ethiopia, Alive & Thrive's Phase 2 (2014–2017) is building on its learning from Phase 1. Data identified gaps between health-education workers trained by the program and community volunteers and mothers, highlighting the need for more frequent and better quality interactions with mothers and family members. To support and sustain behavior change at the household level, the new phase is emphasizing frequent interpersonal contacts between caregivers and frontline workers at critical points during a child's first two years, providing age-specific messages and counseling.[60]

Conclusion

IYCF interventions have a crucial role to play in successful nutrition programming, particularly in the critical first 1,000 days. Breastfeeding promotion has shown the most promise at scale to date in improving nutrition, but recent multi-component initiatives such as Alive & Thrive are breaking new barriers in addressing complementary feeding practices for millions of infants and young children.

CHAPTER 4

Hidden Hunger

Approaches to Tackling Micronutrient Deficiencies

JUDITH HODGE

AROUND THE WORLD, more than 2 billion people are thought to be affected by an often invisible form of malnutrition: micronutrient malnutrition, commonly known as hidden hunger.[1] Vitamin and mineral deficiencies—at least in mild to moderate forms—may not be as observable as wasting or obesity, but their effects are far-reaching. Globally, vitamin A deficiency (VAD) is the leading cause of blindness in children.[2] Iodine deficiency causes 18 million babies to be born mentally impaired each year.[3] And severe anemia caused by lack of iron is associated with the deaths of 115,000 women annually during childbirth.[4] Vitamin A, iodine, and iron are classified as "the big three," but deficiencies of other micronutrients, such as folate, zinc, vitamin B12, and vitamin D, are also important.

Many people in developing countries lack the means to grow or buy micronutrient-rich foods, such as animal-source foods (meat, fish, poultry, eggs, milk, and dairy products) and fruits and vegetables. Instead, they rely on nutrient-poor staples, such as rice and maize. Their lack of dietary diversity is exacerbated by poor access to healthcare and a high burden of disease. Certain deficiencies, such as those of iron, iodine, and vitamin D (due to low exposure to sunshine), are also public health issues in industrialized countries, despite their higher incomes and better health services. In those countries, food high in micronutrients is more expensive than the cheaper, processed foods consumed more frequently in poorer households.[5]

Strategies to combat micronutrient malnutrition generally focus on pregnant and lactating women, infants, and young children—those most at risk from micronutrient malnutrition because they have a relatively greater need for micronutrients. Targeting these populations achieves higher rates of return by improving health, nutritional status, and cognition later in life.[6] The main approaches to preventing and treating micronutrient malnutrition typically include exclusive breastfeeding (breast milk provides the main source of micronutrients during the first six months of life, apart from iron), dietary diversification to include foods with highly absorbable vitamins and minerals, fortification of staple and complementary foods, control

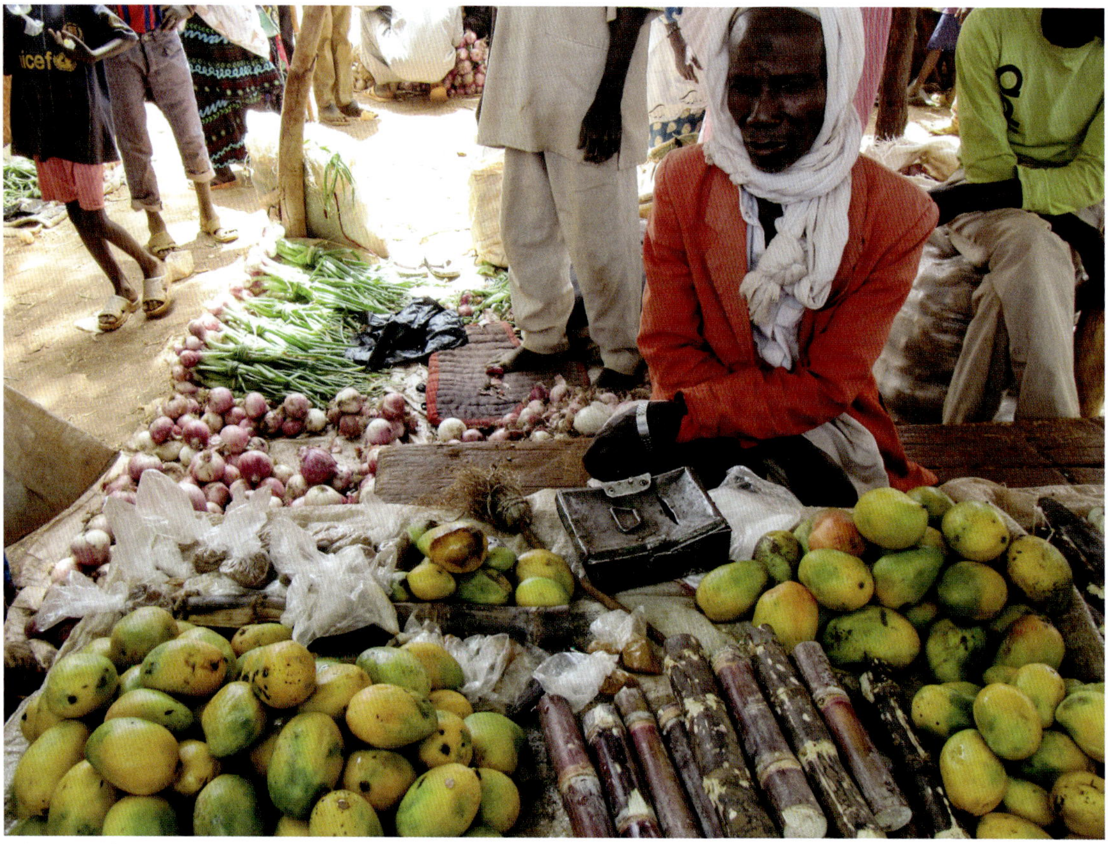

EU/ECHO/A. Delafortrie

Fruits and vegetables, like the ones being sold here at a market in Niger, supply essential vitamins and minerals.

of parasitic infections, and provision of nutritional supplements.[7] Because vitamin and mineral deficiencies often exist together, newer interventions have focused on multiple micronutrients.

This story focuses on three interventions: universal salt iodization in China, vitamin A programs, and the development of micronutrient powders or "Sprinkles." All of these interventions have experienced varying degrees of success and hold lessons for the future.

Success in a Pinch of Salt: Universal Salt Iodization in China

Humans require iodine for their health and their cognitive and physical development, and they can get it naturally in their diets if they eat enough seafood, or crops and livestock grown in areas with adequate iodine in the soils. But people whose diets do not contain enough iodine are susceptible to iodine deficiency disorders (IDDs). These can include goiter (a swelling of the thyroid glands in the neck) and cretinism (severely stunted physical and mental growth caused by maternal iodine deficiency).

Universal salt iodization (USI)—in which all salt for human and livestock consumption is fortified with iodine—is recognized as the most effective and cost-efficient strategy to eliminate iodine deficiency. Estimates for salt iodization suggest that every dollar invested generates up to US$81 in benefits.[8]

The spread of USI is widely viewed as a shining public health success. Before 1990, only a few countries—including Canada and the United States—were sufficient in iodine, and 130 countries were iodine deficient. Worldwide, fewer than one in five households used iodized salt. By 2011, thanks to global efforts to ensure access to iodized salt for more than two-thirds of the world's population, the number of iodine-deficient countries had plummeted to 32.[9]

China's experience is part of this larger story. The country's consumption of iodized salt climbed from 20 percent in 1990 to more than 97 percent of salt consumed in 2005.[10] How did the world's most populous country turn a patchy program of implementation into a successful scaling up of USI?

Threat to IQ Levels

Iodine deficiency is a longstanding and widespread problem in China. Goiter was first documented in Chinese medical literature as early as 3000 BCE. About 60 percent of China's land is low in iodine, especially mountainous areas where soil leaching occurs, and many communities in western China were affected by a high prevalence of goiter and cretinism. A national survey in 1970 estimated that 35 million people had visible goiter, there were 250,000 affected by cretinism, and 720 million people were at risk for severe or moderate IDD.[11] Subsequently the country's iodized salt program was expanded to all IDD-endemic areas, and by the 1980s rates of goiter had decreased and few cretins were being born. However, IDD was still not completely under control because of a combination of irregular salt iodization, ineffective monitoring systems, and lack of political will.[12] And studies in different parts of China showed that the effects of iodine deficiency went even further: IDD was associated with IQs that were significantly lower, by an average of 11 points. In many IDD-endemic areas, 5–15 percent of children had mild mental retardation, with an IQ of 50–69.[13]

This was the insight that made the difference. The recognition that iodine deficiency was damaging children's intelligence—and the implications for human and economic development—had an impact on China's political leadership at the highest level. Organized by the World Health Organization (WHO), UNICEF, the World Bank, and others, a high-level meeting in 1993 brought together national and provincial representatives from different sectors. Among the attendees was then–Vice Premier Zhu Rongji, an economist, who became convinced of the potential benefits of USI and stimulated action on this front. This meeting offered key lessons on advocacy: the importance of presenting a persuasive argument to policy makers—in this case, the high cost of lower intelligence rather than high rates of goiter—and of defining a clear and feasible solution such as USI.[14]

From 1993 onward, China showed leadership at both the international and the national level that would pave the way for USI's global uptake. In 1994 the State Council (the highest national policy-making body, headed by Madam Peng Peiyun, the premier's wife) approved a new National IDD Control Program, which introduced mandatory salt iodization and formed a working partnership with the Ministry of Health and the salt industry to make it happen.

Ramping Up Production

At the start of the program, China had the capacity to produce only 40 percent of the iodized salt needed for USI.[15] Much of the salt consumed by households was raw and unprocessed. To ensure an adequate supply of properly iodized salt, China needed substantial funding, technical assistance, and an industry commitment to iodization.

The State Council made two key moves. First, it set up a special fund for USI, with a total investment of US$125 million to upgrade production facilities. Second, it recentralized the salt industry as a state monopoly, reversing the move toward privatizing the salt industry that had started in the mid-1980s.[16]

These two moves set in motion a series of changes. With the establishment of the national monopoly—the China National Salt Industry Company—China prohibited the sale of non-iodized edible salt. It set up legal enforcement systems, and by 2000, 25,000 salt police were playing a major role in stopping the transport and sales of illegal salt.[17] It made substantial investments in technology and equipment, modernizing 115 salt plants. And it used health education and IDD Days to raise the public's awareness of the adverse effects of iodine deficiency (May 15 is national IDD Day in China).

Thanks to these steps, China's annual production and distribution rose from 5 million tons of salt—not all of it iodized—to 8 million tons of iodized salt in less than seven years.[18] By 2000, China had achieved USI (in other words, more than 90 percent of household salt consumption was iodized), and it had virtually eliminated IDD.[19] This remarkable feat confirmed the program's status as one of the most successful in the world.

Sustaining Success

Although China achieved consistent success on a national level, certain counties in Hainan, Qinghai, Tibet, and Xinjiang—particularly in rural areas with hard-to-reach populations—remained below 90 percent household consumption of iodized salt. International partners such as UNICEF were also raising concerns that China might not achieve complete coverage of iodized salt and might even regress. Their concerns were based on factors such as the country's large size, anticipated privatization of the salt sector, and the technical and behavioral challenges inherent in the USI effort, including ongoing issues with leakage of cheaper, non-iodized salt.[20]

Monitoring and evaluation are an integral part of China's national IDD surveillance plan: as they develop policies and implement programs, Chinese officials are guided by, for example, an annual survey on the household coverage of iodized salt and a survey of iodine status—measured through urinary iodine concentration in school-age children—every two to three years. New surveys in the 2000s highlighted areas at high risk of both iodine deficiency[21] *and* iodine excess, which has been linked with thyroid disease.[22] In 2005 an investigation identified regions in the former flood plain of the Yellow River with high levels of iodine in drinking water.[23] Two years later, a survey identified 249 new cases of cretinism and a more than 5 percent goiter prevalence in 40 counties caused by access to raw salt from local salt lakes.[24] Clearly, Chinese policy makers needed to adjust the country's USI program to meet these new and continuing challenges.

In response, China has developed a multipronged approach. Since 2007, central and local administrations have implemented both an iodized oil supplementation program for targeted populations in remote areas (including children and reproductive-age, pregnant, and lactating women) and subsidies for iodized salt, which has significantly increased consumption.[25] For areas at risk of *excessive* iodine intake, non-iodized salt has been made available. And in 2012 China introduced new standards that both lowered the amount of iodine in salt and reduced the range of salt allowed, and it instructed each province to choose its own iodine content (within the permitted range) to match the needs of the local population.[26] This move from national to provincial standards is designed to prevent the reemergence of both iodine deficiency and iodine excess.[27]

Challenges Ahead

The program context for USI has altered significantly in the last 25 years. China was able to chalk up early and rapid success in scaling up USI partly because of its focus, its vertical approach, and its state monopoly. For countries without this central control, strong political will and a flexible strategy are keys to success in tackling IDD. The Scaling Up Nutrition (SUN) Movement and other relevant movements have proposed a new, more integrated approach to addressing iodine deficiency, one in which iodine programs are embedded in micronutrient policies and strategies rather than serving as standalone interventions.[28]

Despite substantial progress, an estimated 1.88 billion people globally, including 241 million schoolchildren, still have inadequate iodine intakes.[29] Even countries with successful USI programs such as China struggle to reach disadvantaged and marginalized populations, and in industrialized countries mild to moderate iodine deficiency is a forgotten problem.[30]

Vitamin A: A Changing Story

For decades, vitamin A supplementation has been the recommended approach to treating and preventing vitamin A deficiency, but new thinking is now emerging about how best to reach various populations.

The Spread of Supplementation

Supplementation emerged as the most effective short-term measure for vitamin A deficiency in the mid-1980s to 1990s, when population-based trials in areas of endemic vitamin A deficiency showed impressive results in reducing child mortality by 23–34 percent.[31] For the past 25 years WHO has recommended universal supplementation programs of twice-yearly doses of vitamin A, striving to achieve more than 80 percent coverage of children aged 6–59 months. (Although the goal is universal coverage, a coverage threshold of at least 70 percent is needed to achieve reductions in child mortality comparable with large-scale vitamin A trials.) Despite its low cost, the intervention was facing poor coverage rates in the late 1990s. Global partners—including WHO, UNICEF, the Micronutrient Initiative, and the Canadian International Development Agency—focused attention on the issue, helping national governments to scale up vitamin A supplementation through a public-sector approach with free distribution.[32] The efforts paid off: global coverage rates of children improved from 16 percent in 1994 to 77 percent in 2009.[33]

Success stories from this era include countries such as Mozambique and Zambia with high vitamin A supplementation coverage (99 and 93 percent, respectively).[34] These countries succeeded at scaling up by integrating child survival interventions and linking vitamin A supplementation to people's other contacts with the health sector. In 2008, Mozambique introduced Child Health Weeks, which offered vitamin A supplements alongside other interventions such as deworming, mosquito net distribution, and measles vaccination. By offering services closer to people's homes, these events could serve hard-to-reach populations. Zambia was able to scale up combined vitamin A and deworming coverage to more than 80 percent in all but two provinces through similar child health events and innovations such as text messages encouraging parents and caregivers to participate.[35] These types of events need a large amount of planning and logistical support, but the pay-off is that they are effective in reaching the majority of children targeted.

Bihar—one of the India's poorest states—has achieved 95 percent coverage of vitamin A supplementation (in sharp contrast to India's 54 percent countrywide coverage) through a partnership between the Government of Bihar, UNICEF, and the Micronutrient Initiative. Bihar's program is designed to target children from scheduled castes and minority groups, who are traditionally excluded from services. The state has strengthened implementation through a combination of detailed district planning, training of frontline health and nutrition workers and community volunteers to administer vitamin A syrup and nutrition counseling on vitamin A–rich foods, and intensive social mobilization and communication. The program has mobilized more than 11,000 health centers; 80,000 *anganwadis,* or child development centers; and 3,400 temporary sites in isolated communities as distribution sites for vitamin A supplements.[36]

Looking at Alternatives

Recently, concerns have been expressed that since the 1990s, twice-yearly, high-dose vitamin A supplementation has largely displaced alternative ways of addressing vitamin A deficiency, including opportunities to deal with mild to moderate vitamin A deficiency in women and children.[37] Supplementation programs for vitamin A were originally intended to be a short-term solution to be phased out and replaced by more sustainable food-based or fortification measures. Moreover, changing disease patterns—particularly reductions in measles and diarrhea—may have made periodic high-dose vitamin A capsules less relevant today (vitamin A deficiency is a risk factor for measles-related mortality and diarrhea-related mortality).[38] Critics claim that only one large-scale program evaluation—the DEVTA trial, ending in 2003, in Uttar Pradesh, India[39]—has ever been published, and it showed no impact on the mortality of children aged 1–6 years (although inclusion of the DEVTA data with results from previous trials still showed a significant effect on mortality from vitamin A supplementation, albeit reduced from 20–30 percent to 11 percent).[40] An analysis of recent randomized controlled trials suggests that high-dose vitamin A supplementation may even have harmful effects in some subgroups.[41] Options are now being sought to both expand on the current "one-size-fits-all" supplementation approach and reduce disparity in vitamin A status using creative local solutions that directly confront nutrition and dietary conditions.[42] For example, unlike high-dose vitamin A capsules, daily or weekly supplements are safe for reproductive-age women.

Supplementation is probably the most widespread intervention, but other successful strategies for increasing people's vitamin A intake, particularly food-based approaches, are now coming to the forefront. Dietary diversity programs such as Bihar's combine supplementation with counseling on vitamin A–rich foods. A number of countries have implemented mass fortification of staple foods with vitamin A at the national level, including edible oil (Morocco), wheat flour (Philippines), and sugar (Guatemala and Zambia).[43] Some studies have found fortification to be cost-effective but lacking sufficient coverage since it left "too many" micronutrient-deficient people.[44] Biofortification programs promoting consumption of crops high in vitamin A, including orange-fleshed sweet potatoes, are being scaled up in countries such as Mozambique and Uganda (see Chapter 6 on agriculture).

A Sprinkle of Success

Iron-deficiency anemia (IDA) is the most prevalent form of micronutrient deficiency: WHO estimates that IDA affects about 47 percent of preschool-aged children and 42 percent of pregnant women, mostly in Africa and Asia.[45] Young children are particularly vulnerable because they have high iron needs (their fetal iron stores are depleted four to six months after birth) and the cereal-based diets they are typically weaned on are low in iron.[46] Historically, children at risk for anemia were given iron syrups and drops, but they often do not adhere to these because these supplements can have a strong metallic taste and lead to teeth staining and

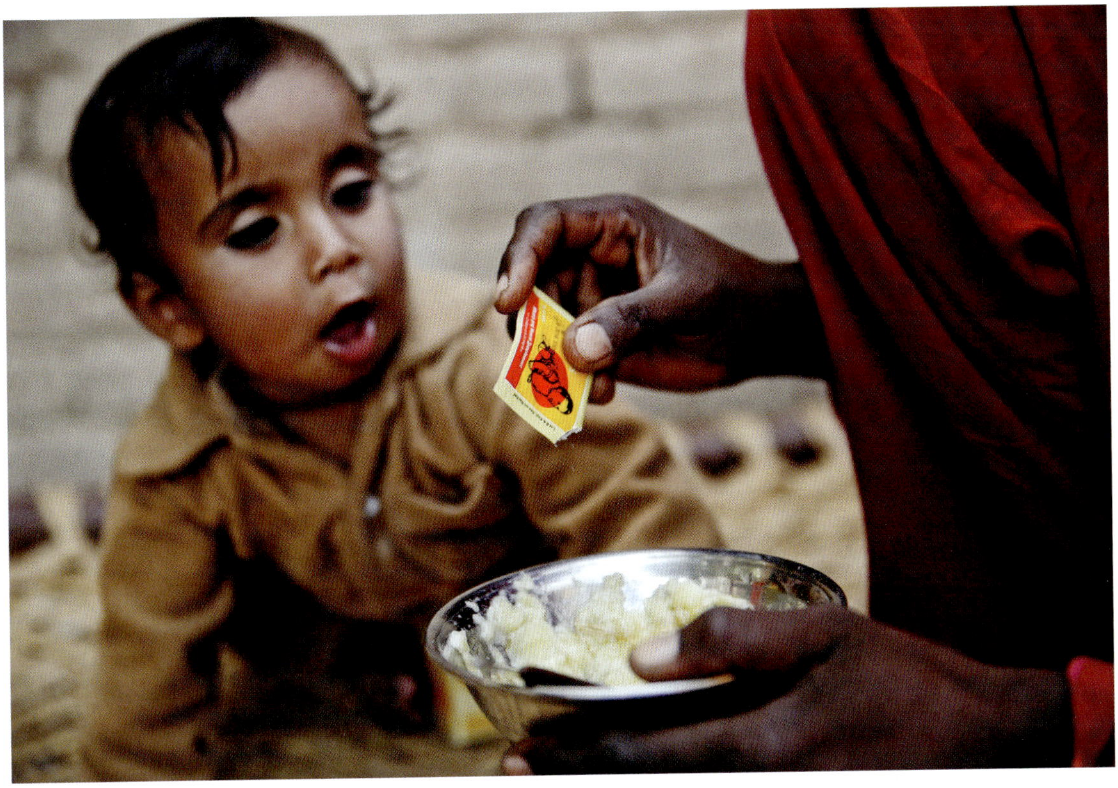

Micronutrient Initiative

A Pakistani mother pours micronutrient powder, commonly known as Sprinkles, onto her child's food to help prevent micronutrient deficiencies.

abdominal discomfort.[47] Moreover, the supplements have a short shelf life and, because they are heavy, high transportation costs.

Inventing Sprinkles

In the late 1990s, the search for a more palatable alternative led a Canadian doctor, Stanley Zlotkin, to invent micronutrient powders (MNPs), frequently referred to by the brand name Sprinkles. MNPs come in single-serving, one-gram packets—inspired by ketchup sachets—containing premeasured vitamins and minerals, including specially coated iron. These powders can be mixed into a child's usual foods at home for instant fortification. They require minimal behavior change and no additional work for women. Two common product formulations are currently in use: one contains 5 micronutrients (initially called "anemia formulation"), and the other has 15 micronutrients (considered optimal for complementary feeding). A standard course of treatment is 60 sachets.[48] A review of eight trials found Sprinkles to be effective—home use of MNPs was associated with a reduced risk of anemia and iron deficiency in children under two.[49]

MNPs were first endorsed by WHO in 2007 to improve the iron and anemia status of populations affected by emergencies and strongly recommended in 2011 as a public health intervention.[50] Mongolia was the first country to pilot Sprinkles, and it scaled up their use to the national level in three phases over a 10-year period. The country's story and the challenges it faced are both generic to the intervention and context-specific, but all of them provide food for thought on how to tackle hidden hunger, and IDA in particular.

Mongolia's interest in the intervention began in 1997, when a national survey of iron and vitamin D deficiency in Mongolia generated alarming findings: among children 6–59 months old, 46 percent had anemia and 28 percent had rickets—a painful, bone-deforming disease caused by lack of vitamin D (one symptom is bowed legs).[51] In response, the Ministry of Health collaborated with World Vision to deliver an integrated nutrition package targeted to pregnant and breastfeeding women and children under age five in underdeveloped areas. As part of this package, Sprinkles were distributed free of charge to more than 14,000 children 6–36 months old.[52] The sachets contained powders specially formulated to address the high levels of anemia and rickets in Mongolia, wrapped in culturally acceptable packaging bearing local-language instructions and artwork.

Success in Addressing Anemia: The Mongolia MNP Pilot

The pilot phase of Mongolia's Sprinkles project in 2002–2004 faced several obstacles. Advocates had gained the support of a key Ministry of Health secretary, but otherwise the project had little political support. The country's public health care system had limited capacity, so the delivery system relied on World Vision's resources, undermining the project's sustainability. And the Sprinkles were originally more expensive than supplementation.[53]

But the pilot phase achieved promising results. Sprinkles were distributed to more than 88 percent of children 6–36 months old in the program areas, and the prevalence of anemia fell from 55 percent in 2002 to 33 percent in 2004 (although rickets did not decline). The program had other components, such as prenatal iron supplements and activities encouraging consumption of iron-rich foods, that may have contributed to this result. But an evaluation showed that 93 percent of children 6–36 months old who used Sprinkles did so at least three times a week, and this group had a lower prevalence of anemia (31 percent) than those who used Sprinkles less often (52 percent).[54]

The success of this pilot approach proved to be a powerful advocacy tool, winning new supporters and paving the way for scaling up from scattered communities to an entire province. From 2005 to 2010 the intervention was scaled up in Selenge province in northeast Mongolia, with funding secured from a Canadian mining company with operations in the province. The project partners—the Ministry of Health and World Vision—incorporated lessons learned from the pilot phase. They sought technical expertise to help adjust the amount of vitamin D in the Sprinkles, provided vitamin D supplements, and launched additional behavior change initiatives. They also found ways to produce the Sprinkles more cheaply. There was still no network of community nutrition workers in this phase, so the partners raised awareness through leaflets and televised educational messages and improved delivery by distributing Sprinkles at health posts during immunizations. Finally, they recruited volunteer mothers to help mobilize communities and monitor the use of Sprinkles.[55]

Again, the results for this phase were convincing: the intervention reached 7,000 children under 5 years old and 1,300 pregnant women and new mothers in the province. The prevalence of rickets fell the most, from 62 to 25 percent between 2005 and 2010, but the prevalence of anemia in children also declined from 26 percent to 22 percent, and stunting levels fell from 26 percent to 9 percent in the same period.

Part of National Health Policy

The phased approach allowed Mongolians to determine that the innovation was appropriate and successful in their own context,[56] and the government accepted Sprinkles as an effective tool in its battle against childhood anemia. In 2009, the Ministry of Health launched Phase III, a national program targeting 50,000 children 6–24 months old in certain provinces based on poverty levels, health indicators, and geographical access. Ongoing technical and financial support was provided by the Asian Development Bank, World Vision, and UNICEF.[57] The establishment of Micronutrient Working Groups at national, provincial, and district levels was essential to both the provincial and national scale-up.[58] The partners have worked to build the capacity of existing systems and programs to ensure that Sprinkles are delivered through the public health care system and integrated within current mother and child health programs.[59] The Mongolian story shows that scale-up is feasible: the government went from being a detached observer at the pilot stage to taking ownership of the intervention, and Sprinkles have now become part of Mongolia's national health policy.

Despite the evidence on impact[60] and cost effectiveness (MNPs cost about US$0.03 per sachet, or US$1.80 per 60-sachet course, to public sector buyers),[61] just a handful of countries to date have implemented large-scale distribution. These include Bangladesh, Bolivia, Dominican Republic, Kyrgyzstan, and Mongolia. There are pilot programs in about 55 other countries,[62] and Afghanistan, Cambodia, and Tanzania are using MNPs in pilot school-feeding programs targeting children and adolescents.[63] The number of sachets distributed by UNICEF and the World Food Programme (WFP) rose from 50 million in 2008 to about 350 million in 2010,[64] but this intervention reaches only about 13.6 million children—less than 5 percent of anemic children globally. The role played by Sprinkles in tackling Mongolia's micronutrient deficiencies offers a success story from which other countries can take inspiration.

Lessons Learned

While it is not possible to generalize about what works in scaling up micronutrient interventions from a few case studies, the experiences described here share some common elements. Both universal salt iodization in China and the Sprinkles intervention in Mongolia relied on a staged approach—from pilot to district to national level—that afforded opportunities to iron out issues such as the levels of micronutrients required by different populations. In both countries, nutrition champions in influential positions, secured through effective advocacy, ensured support and government buy-in for the interventions. Micronutrient programs such as vitamin A supplementation and Sprinkles are often led by donors initially, but integrating these interventions into existing broader health programs and training community volunteers can help make them more sustainable. This shift occurred in the merging of vitamin A supplementation with Child Health Weeks in Mozambique and Zambia and the adoption of micronutrient powders into Mongolia's national health policy. Ongoing monitoring and evaluation of such programs are crucial for gauging whether interventions are still relevant: today's micronutrient success stories such as universal salt iodization and vitamin A supplementation may be eclipsed by other strategies in the near future, such as fortification or food-based initiatives.

CHAPTER 5

Addressing a Neglected Problem

Community-based Management of Acute Malnutrition

JUDITH HODGE AND JESSICA WHITE

SEVERE ACUTE MALNUTRITION (SAM)—extremely low weight for one's height—is a life-threatening condition affecting mostly children under five years of age. It is caused by a combination of infection, such as diarrheal disease, and poor diets that are inadequate for nutritional needs.[1] SAM is one of the top three nutrition-related causes of death in children under five, according to the *Lancet* 2008 Maternal and Child Nutrition Series.[2] A child with SAM is 11 times more likely to die than a well-nourished child.[3]

Recent global estimates suggest that 52 million children suffer from moderate to severe malnutrition, and 17 million of those are estimated to be severely malnourished or wasted, based on national prevalence data (see Box 5.1 for definitions).[4] Africa is home to 5.6 million children with SAM, but the majority of all moderately (69 percent) and severely (71 percent) wasted children live in Asia: India alone has more than 8 million children with SAM—nearly half of the world's wasted children.[5] Moreover, current global estimates may well underestimate the actual annual burden, because they may miss a sizable proportion of new cases of wasting occurring over time. Depending on the timing of the survey on which they are based, estimates may also miss seasonal peaks.[6]

Despite the size of the problem, until the early 2000s SAM appeared to be a so-called neglected condition: little support went to large-scale treatment programs targeted toward children with SAM. Few countries—even among those with a high prevalence of malnutrition—had a clear national policy for detecting and treating SAM children.[7] The development and adoption of a new approach—the community-based management of acute malnutrition (CMAM)—was to change the public health nutrition landscape by bringing treatment out of hospitals and into the community.

Dramatic improvements in identifying, rehabilitating, and curing children with SAM have been made in recent years—and CMAM lies at the heart of this story. Although accurate coverage data on the proportion of SAM children receiving treatment are difficult to obtain, global treatment of SAM is estimated to have more than doubled from

1 million children in 2009 to more than 2 million in 2011.[8] Moreover, policy formulation at the country level has progressed rapidly; by 2012, 95 percent of countries had national guidelines and protocols for acute malnutrition, with 60 countries implementing CMAM programs, and an additional seven countries in the planning stages.[9] Still, although certain countries have made progress, coverage levels of treatment programs remain low. In the 2013 *Lancet* series, Bhutta et al.[10] estimated that scaling up SAM management to 90 percent coverage through a package of key interventions could save 285,000–482,000 lives annually.

Birth of the CMAM Approach

Until the early 2000s, case-fatality rates for SAM in developing countries had remained unchanged for more than 50 years. About 20–30 percent of children with marasmus (wasting malnutrition) and up to 50–60 percent of children with kwashiorkor (malnutrition with edema) died.[11] Children were treated as inpatients in district hospitals or clinics, often based in towns far from where families lived. Treatment involved long stays of between five and eight weeks for both child and carer—difficult for mothers who had other children at home and whose labor may have been vital to the household's economic survival.[12] These high costs of obtaining transport to treatment centers and being away from home for long periods were barriers to access to care, leading to low coverage.[13] Admission for treatment was also limited by bed availability, with each center typically treating fewer than 30 cases at a time. Unsurprisingly these centers served only 4–10 percent of the affected population.[14]

Over the past 50 years, humanitarian agencies had been scaling up SAM treatment during emergencies (such as Ethiopia's famines in the mid-1970s and mid-1980s) with inpatient feeding centers to care for large numbers of children. While these centers reduced mortality rates among those treated to less than 10 percent, coverage rates were still low, and the infrastructure costs were not sustainable beyond the crisis situation.[15] In addition, given that the majority of acutely malnourished children live outside of the emergency context, this inpatient model, while successful in improving recovery rates, failed to tackle SAM as a public health problem in the wider development context.

Emergencies—A Chance for Change

In the early 2000s, the relief agencies tried a radically new approach, working with national

BOX 5.1 What is acute malnutrition?

The World Health Organization (WHO) classifies acute malnutrition (also known as wasting) in children as severe or moderate, according to WHO growth standards[16]:

- Severe acute malnutrition (SAM) is visible severe wasting—that is, very low weight-for-height—in children 6–60 months old. It may or may not occur with nutritional edema (a form of swelling caused by insufficient intake of certain nutrients). One way of measuring it is mid-upper-arm circumference (MUAC); a MUAC of less than 115 millimeters indicates SAM.[17]
- Moderate acute malnutrition (MAM) is moderate wasting, indicated by a MUAC greater than or equal to 115 millimeters and less than 125 millimeters.[18]
- Global acute malnutrition (GAM) is the combined prevalence of severe and moderate acute malnutrition in a population. A prevalence of 10–14 percent is classified as serious, and a rate of more than 15 percent is considered an emergency.

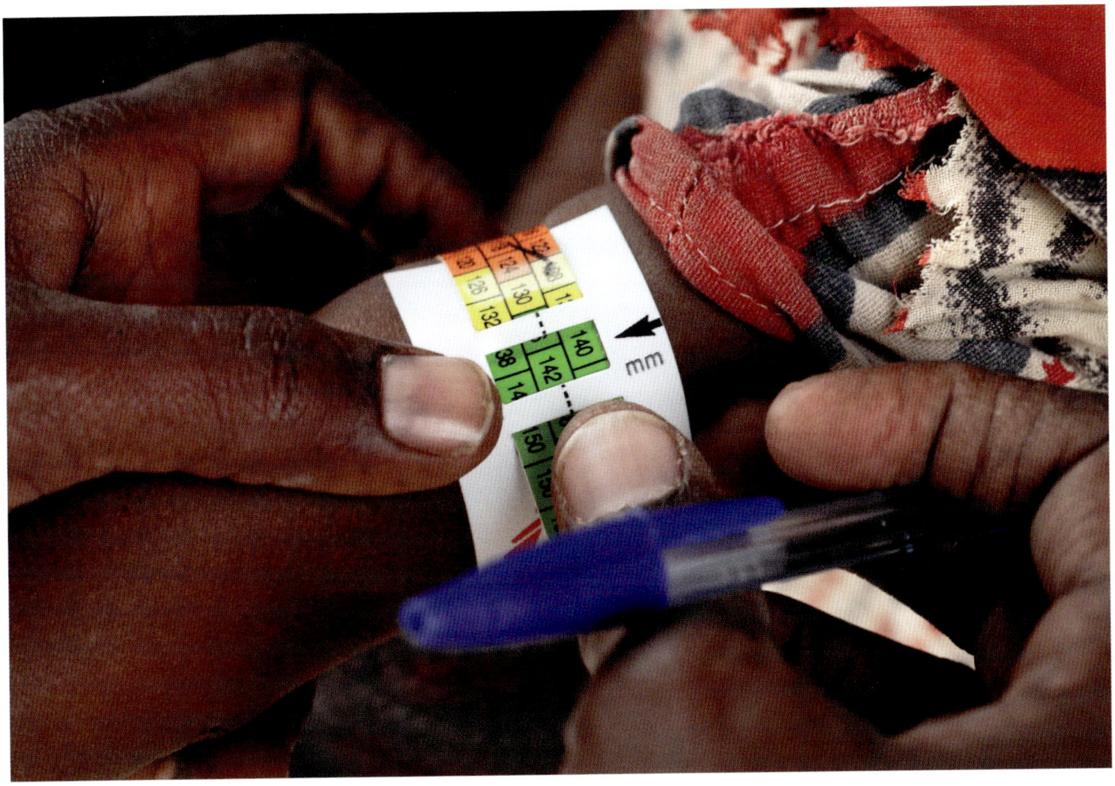

Panos/D. Telemans

Training community members to measure a child's mid-upper-arm circumference improves timely identification of children at risk of acute malnutrition.

governments in Ethiopia and Malawi to move treatment of SAM from inpatient hospitals and feeding centers into community-based programs in resource-poor settings.[19] NGOs, donors, and governments, in collaboration with other relevant authorities, were willing to depart from existing protocols, often because of the urgency of the situation and the inadequacy of existing approaches.[20]

The community-based approach, or CMAM, trained volunteers and mothers to detect SAM early by using plastic strips to measure children's mid-upper-arm circumference (MUAC). By actively finding cases and training community members to refer themselves, CMAM allowed for more timely presentation of cases at new, more decentralized outpatient clinics. More serious cases were referred to inpatient care (see Box 5.2 for more detail on the CMAM model). Evidence suggests that most children with SAM—more than 85 percent in most settings—can be treated as outpatients through CMAM programs.[21] The other key innovation underpinning CMAM was the development of ready-to-use therapeutic foods (RUTFs) for use in treatment in the community (see Box 5.3 for more information). As a result of this approach, people presented for treatment at a time when their condition was still treatable at home.

The outcomes for CMAM were impressive. The Sphere project, a joint project of the International Red Cross and Red Crescent Movement and other nongovernmental organizations, specifies internationally recognized standards for humanitarian responses related to food and nutrition. It calls for a recovery rate of more than 75 percent, a death

BOX 5.2 The CMAM model

The CMAM approach has three main components[22]:

1. **Community outreach and mobilization:** Community members screen and actively find cases of children with SAM by measuring mid-upper-arm circumference (MUAC).
2. **Outpatient therapeutic program (OTP):** Children with SAM who have no medical complications are referred to an OTP. The program monitors the child's response to treatment and provides additional medical treatment as required before sending children home with enough ready-to-use therapeutic food to last until the following visit, allowing recovery to take place in the community.
3. **Inpatient care:** Children with SAM who have medical complications and/or poor appetite are referred for inpatient treatment at a health facility. These children are also linked to an OTP to allow them to be discharged and undergo continued treatment within the community when possible.

In some countries, there is a fourth CMAM component: supplementary feeding for children with moderate acute malnutrition (MAM). Children identified with MAM during community outreach and mobilization are referred to a supplementary feeding program where the family receives food rations.

rate of less than 5 percent, and a default rate of less than 15 percent (default occurs when a beneficiary is admitted to a program but leaves without being formally discharged).[23] Among 23,511 severely malnourished children treated from 2001 to 2005 in 21 community-based programs in Ethiopia, Malawi, and Sudan, death rates were 4.1 percent, recovery rates were 79.4 percent, and default rates were 11.0 percent. Moreover, 74 percent of these children were treated solely as outpatients.[24]

Global Endorsement

In 2007, based on evidence from operational research, CMAM was officially endorsed by the United Nations and the World Health Organization.[25] Global endorsement paved the way for international agencies, donors, and governments to begin scaling up CMAM programming at the national level and to start viewing community-based management of SAM as integral to routine health activities.[26] While direct action by NGOs remains critical in a number of humanitarian contexts, a child suffering from SAM today is more likely to be treated by national health staff in a government health facility than by any other service provider.[27]

The transition to a community-based approach continues to deliver success: a recent review found that the CMAM model performed consistently well in a variety of contexts, achieving high recovery rates (more than 90 percent) and low rates of death (less than 2 percent) and default (less than 10 percent).[28] Despite increased treatment in Africa south of the Sahara (which accounts for 80 percent of all children treated for SAM),[29] less than 15 percent of the global SAM population is currently receiving treatment.[30] Reducing the overall burden of wasting globally will require that key high-burden countries in South Asia—particularly India—commit to launching CMAM services at scale and that current and future CMAM programs strengthen their links with wider stunting-reduction efforts.[31]

A Story of Three Countries: CMAM in Ethiopia, Malawi, and Niger

In Ethiopia, Malawi, and Niger, it was the onset of a large-scale nutrition emergency—when programs identified large numbers of children with SAM—that provided an opportunity to introduce CMAM pilots or to scale up existing ones. These three early adopters of the community-based approach have all achieved high geographic coverage of SAM treatment: in Malawi, an estimated 84 percent of health care facilities deliver SAM treatment; in Niger, 78 percent; and in Ethiopia, 75 percent.[32] Each country has charted a different path to success, facing challenges in attempting to scale up while addressing issues of cost and capacity.[33]

From Start-up to National Level: CMAM's Beginnings and Scale-up

Both Ethiopia and Niger have a long history of recurrent droughts and frequent food insecurity, but Malawi's food crisis of 2001/2002 took policy makers by surprise. The country had been considered food secure for a number of years and was even exporting agricultural products, such as beans and maize.[34] A sharp shortfall in the maize harvest in 2001/2002 led to widespread hunger and a food emergency. Initiated in response to the 2001 crisis, CMAM was driven from the start by champions within the Ministry of Health who had been convinced of its potential impact by NGOs and international experts.[35] Although NGOs played a major role in supporting CMAM scale-up in Malawi, it was the district health officers who demanded CMAM programs in their districts following a 2004 Ministry of Health workshop presenting successful results from two district pilots, including death rates of 1.7 percent.[36]

Further impetus for expanded CMAM coverage in Malawi was provided by another food emergency in 2005. Rates of global acute malnutrition reached 6.2 percent in the country and surpassed 10 percent in four districts.[37] In 2006 the community-based model was adopted as a national strategy. Between 2004 and 2013, program performance rates exceeded the recommended Sphere standard of 75 percent of treated children recovered from acute malnutrition.[38] Today, Malawi has achieved the highest level of CMAM scale-up of any country. Following a process of gradual scale-up and integration into the primary-health-care system, Malawi now has programs in all 28 districts and health facilities, 98 percent of hospitals provide inpatient care (100 of 102), and 82 percent of health centers act as OTPs (512 of 624).[39] This scale-up likely contributed to the dramatic declines in under-five mortality rates in Malawi, from 174 deaths per 1,000 live births in 2000 to 71 deaths per 1,000 live births in 2012.[40]

In Ethiopia, CMAM programs started relatively slowly. They were first piloted in 2000 in two sites, but a drought and food crisis in 2002–2003

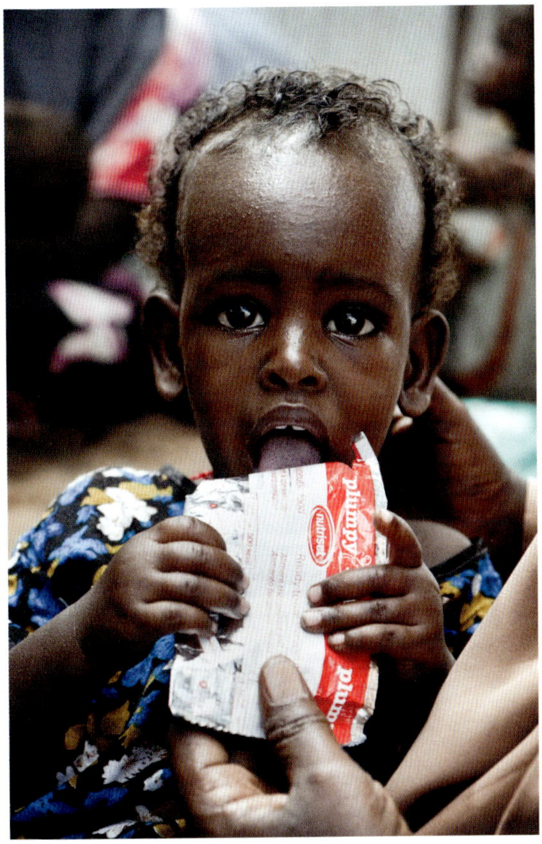

Panos/S. Torfinn

A child at a refugee camp in Kenya eats Plumpy'Nut, a nutritious peanut-based paste that has revolutionized care for acutely malnourished children.

served as a catalyst for scale-up. NGOs shifted from therapeutic feeding centers for treatment of SAM into community-based management of wasting.[41] Initially, coverage was low, with a maximum number of 24,600 admissions in 44 inpatient units.[42] Between 2004 and 2008, inpatient facilities and OTPs in Ethiopia were scaled up to 165 hospitals and health centers. Until 2008, there was a period of slow expansion when OTPs were established and ran parallel to the national health system rather than integrated, in contrast to Malawi, although both countries depended heavily on external resources and expertise.[43]

In 2008, though, a sea change in Ethiopia's policy environment led to a period of rapid expansion. Another drought, compounded by increases in food prices, caused a spike in SAM cases. The Federal Ministry of Health decided to rapidly scale up CMAM, making it a key component of the country's National Nutrition Strategy and its Health Sector Development Plan, which guides investment in the health sector.[44] After 2008, the government, with support from development partners, extensively decentralized treatment services to trained health extension workers (frontline health workers) based in health posts to ensure wider access to, and coverage of, services to treat SAM.[45] In the four years between 2008 and 2011, the number of children treated for SAM rose 12-fold to 230,000. During 2013—a year of good harvest—a total of 267,500 children were admitted for therapeutic care (250,000 to OTPs and 17,500 to inpatient care). Results continually exceed Sphere standards, with a recovery rate of 86 percent reported for 2014. As of 2013, more than 10,000 facilities offered CMAM services.[46] This mass decentralization of treatment services may well have contributed to Ethiopia's dramatic decline in child mortality: between 2000 and 2012, mortality rates for children under five fell by more than half, from 146 to 68 deaths per 1,000 live births.[47]

Niger, which ranked 187th out of 187 countries in the 2014 UN Human Development Index,[48] has been plagued for years by high levels of malnutrition due to drought, recurring food crises, poor feeding practices, and inadequate access to health services. In 2005, nutrition surveys showed that in several regions the prevalence of global acute malnutrition was above the emergency threshold of 15 percent, triggering a major emergency response by the government and the international community.[49] Before this, treatment of SAM had been restricted mainly to NGO programs outside of Ministry of Health facilities.[50] The 2005 emergency catalyzed the development of national CMAM guidelines by the government. The CMAM approach in Niger included treatment of children not only with SAM but also with MAM, in contrast to Ethiopia and Malawi, which used CMAM to treat SAM exclusively. Once the guidelines had been developed, many NGOs rapidly expanded community-based services, but the result was a patchwork of CMAM programs with varying degrees of quality and staff training.[51] Government-run facilities continued to operate using the traditional approach, treating all cases as inpatients. However, the CMAM approach gained momentum in Niger following a government directive calling for all stakeholders involved in managing SAM to integrate their operations into the national health system and waiving health service fees for children under five and pregnant women.[52] In 2011, the launch of the newly elected president's "3N" initiative (Nigeriens Nourish Nigeriens) heralded a new era for nutrition—and was a far cry from the days when aid agencies were expelled from the country for daring to admit the existence of a food crisis.[53]

Niger has moved from a position of negligible nutrition programming in 2005, when the whole country had only one therapeutic feeding center, to treating 1 million children with acute malnutrition—both SAM and MAM—in 2014.[54] In 2010, Niger was again faced with food insecurity following a poor 2009 rainy season, adding further impetus for scale-up. During this crisis, 330,000 children aged 6–59 months were treated for SAM (with a further 257,000 treated for MAM). By 2011, inpatient care for SAM was available in all 50 national, regional, and district hospitals, 772 of the 850 integrated health centers offered OTP services, and both inpatient and OTP treatment exceeded the minimum Sphere standard for recovery.[55] These centers also offer treatment for children with MAM with a range of products, including traditional fortified blended flour. Although the country's under-five mortality rate halved from 227 to 114 deaths per 1,000 live births between 2000 and 2012,[56] and significant progress has been made in Niger's ability to treat acutely malnourished children, prevalence of acute malnutrition remains high.

Success Factors and Challenges to Sustainability

In all three countries, increased political commitment to tackling malnutrition has galvanized adoption of the CMAM model. For both Malawi and Niger, this commitment is linked to initiatives at the very top level. In Malawi, the Office of the President/Cabinet assumed responsibility for coordinating nutrition in 2005, and in Niger, the Prime Minister's Office took over leadership of emergency nutrition response in 2011, although the Ministry of Health retains responsibility for managing acute malnutrition (both SAM and MAM). In Ethiopia, the government ensured that nutrition became a cross-cutting issue with its multisectoral approach and National Nutrition Strategy (2008), in which CMAM was embedded. It was, however, Ethiopia's push to decentralize treatment services to health extension workers at the community level that facilitated the rapid scale-up of the community-based approach to SAM.[57]

Ministry of Health Support

In Malawi, the push to scale up came from advocates of CMAM within the Ministry of Health from the outset, whereas in Ethiopia and Niger adoption by the health ministries was more gradual. In Niger, the Ministry of Health has taken the lead in managing the expansion of CMAM through the work of its Nutrition Directorate, with NGOs supporting the program in terms of surge capacity and quality assurance.[58] All three countries have benefited from dedicated services underpinning CMAM delivery, though this is most developed in Malawi, whose CMAM Advisory Service provides advice on scale-up, integration, and quality service delivery. NGOs have played a crucial role by offering technical support and helping expand CMAM services, but the extent of their combined coverage is unlikely to ever match that of a government health service—even an underresourced one—over time.[59]

Yet only Malawi's government has committed to take over the financing of the CMAM program by developing a costed CMAM operational plan for integrating the approach into Ministry of Health services—a stand-out success compared with other countries.[60] Niger's Ministry of Health has yet to integrate nutrition into its annual planning or budgeting, leaving NGOs to fund doctors and nurses who work in the field, and UNICEF picks up the bill for 80 percent of RUTFs.[61] Like many other countries, Ethiopia has relied on short-term funding from donors in "non-emergency" periods. As a result, it has scaled up CMAM and integrated it into the national health system without a central plan.[62] Costed plans like Malawi's are particularly important because treatment of SAM is often relegated to emergency budgets rather than being seen as part of routine health care.

Reducing CMAM Costs

Local production of RUTF is one way governments can reduce the cost of CMAM programs, although there are caveats to this approach (see Box 5.3 on RUTF). Both Malawi and Ethiopia have established facilities to produce therapeutic food locally in conjunction with NGOs. Two companies in Malawi produce RUTF locally and even supply Zambia's CMAM program.[63] Ethiopia produces less, and it also faces challenges related to its lack of logistical capacity to store and transport large quantities of RUTF and difficulties forecasting the need for therapeutic food. During the 2009 food emergency, stock-outs were a serious problem, with a wait of up to eight weeks for supplies from France.[64] Niger has established in-country RUTF production, but the Ministry of Health reports that a key threat to the sustainability of the program is the difficulty of sustaining adequate supplies of expensive therapeutic products.[65]

Weak Health Systems

All three countries face challenges in supervising and monitoring CMAM treatment because of their generally weak health systems. This weakness is especially pronounced in the community component, where outreach to identify those most at risk of malnutrition remains limited, particularly in Niger. Unlike Ethiopia, Malawi and Niger rely on a network of volunteers that is often undermined by retention problems. CMAM programs struggle to maintain high-quality care in all treatment centers; in Niger, the decentralization of services is hindered by the limited capacity of the health system at the health-post level.[66] Even with Ethiopia's measures to extend its health services, NGOs have raised concerns about supervision structures; monitoring has revealed quality issues and a need to give health extension workers more training to ensure that they are fully competent with CMAM protocols.[67] However, better use of data from monthly CMAM reporting at both the district and federal level in Ethiopia enabled organizations to detect an increasing trend in CMAM admissions and to distribute CMAM supplies to the most affected areas during the 2010/2011 emergency in a timely response.[68]

Lessons Learned and Looking Forward

The move from centralized, inpatient care for SAM to a community-based model was arguably one of the most important paradigm shifts in public health nutrition within the past decade.[69] Countries such as Ethiopia, Malawi, and Niger that have adopted the CMAM approach have all relied on political will to enable scale-up. Engaging the ministries of health in these countries was critical to success, particularly in the handover from NGO-run pilots to national programs, and so was the recognition that SAM is a broad problem outside of emergencies that needs to be built into health and nutrition plans. But until governments are able to incorporate the cost of the program into their health budgets, CMAM sustainability remains vulnerable to changes in donor priorities. To date, Malawi is the only case study country to address this. In countries with high caseloads like Ethiopia and Niger, this goal may remain out of reach until the incidence of wasting declines countrywide.

Progress on reducing wasting depends not only on scaling up interventions to treat SAM, but also on the strength and effectiveness of prevention strategies, such as promotion of improved infant and young child feeding, promotion of good hygiene and sanitation, and better social protection policies and programs (for more information on these interventions, see Chapters 3, 7, and 8). Looking forward, one priority is to better integrate activities for preventing wasting with treatment of MAM, particularly through incorporating MAM treatment within the community-based approach.

BOX 5.3 Ready-to-use therapeutic foods: The Plumpy'Nut debate

Ready-to-use therapeutic foods (RUTFs) are energy-dense, micronutrient-enhanced pastes made from peanuts, milk powder, oil, sugar, and vitamin and mineral supplements. Developed for therapeutic feeding of children suffering from SAM, RUTFs contain the necessary nutrients for recovery, have a long shelf-life, are safe to use without refrigeration (there is limited risk of bacterial growth since the product is oil-based with low water activity), and can be used in combination with breastfeeding and other appropriate infant and child feeding practices.[70] By providing a therapeutic food that is safe to use in outpatient settings, RUTFs revolutionized the treatment of SAM, but their production and use are also subject to controversy.[71]

Before the development of RUTFs, children with SAM were admitted to inpatient facilities and treated with a strict regimen of specialized therapeutic milk. However, it was difficult for children in areas with limited health infrastructure—often in the most marginalized populations—to reach these treatment facilities and remain there for the entire treatment period, which was often several weeks. When RUTFs were adopted for treating SAM, outpatient care expanded and coverage of CMAM increased dramatically: in 2011, about 1.96 million SAM children (10 percent of the estimated 20 million suffering globally) were treated with RUTFs.[72]

The predominant RUTF product, Plumpy'Nut, was invented by scientist André Briend and is produced by the France-based company Nutriset. Until 2002, Nutriset was the only producer of Plumpy'Nut, at a cost of approximately US$3,500 per ton, not including the cost of transporting the product from Europe.[73] The high cost of Plumpy'Nut—which accounts for about half of all CMAM costs—resulted in a push for local production, not only to reduce costs but also to contribute to the local economy. But this move has been challenging. So far, Nutriset has patented Plumpy'Nut in about 35 countries, where local producers must essentially operate as local franchises for the French company. The development community has argued that these patents keep the cost of production prohibitively high. Nutriset claims that the patents protect the quality of the product and the interests of local producers because if more advanced economies were to produce RUTFs, they risk flooding the market and pushing local producers out of business.[74]

Moreover, producing RUTFs locally is not always cheaper than purchasing imports. In addition to facing patent difficulties, local producers can find it hard to source ingredients. Milk powder is expensive and often not locally available; for local producers in Malawi, for example, imported milk powder represents more than half of the cost of the product.[75] And peanuts can be contaminated with aflatoxin. In turn, the quality control procedures necessary to ensure a safe product can drive up the cost of production.[76]

Despite these challenges, local production of RUTFs is increasing. In 2012, local production met 27 percent of need, and African-produced RUTFs represented 45 percent of the total RUTFs purchased by UNICEF, the world's largest RUTF purchaser and distributer.[77] Nevertheless, the procurement of commercially or locally produced RUTFs is still almost exclusively financed by development agencies. In fact, in 73 percent of countries operating CMAM programs, UNICEF still provides 100 percent of the RUTFs. This overreliance on development partners raises questions about the sustainability of scaled-up support.[78]

In addition to criticism surrounding the cost and production of RUTFs, there are also concerns about the use of RUTFs over traditional local foods. For example, India banned the import of Plumpy'Nut in 2009 over concerns that importing packaged foreign foods could result in dependence on a "product"—rather than locally available foods—for treatment. Alternative RUTF recipes produced from locally available foods could greatly reduce the cost of production and make local production, even

(Box 5.3 continued)

at a subnational level, more feasible.[79] Recent evidence has also found no discernable difference in treatment outcomes between RUTFs and local foods (in this instance, flour porridge).[80]

Despite the ongoing controversy over production, cost, and appropriateness of RUTFs, the product has undeniably contributed immensely to the scaling up of CMAM and the treatment of millions of children worldwide.

Part II: Transforming Sectoral Actions

CHAPTER 6

From the Ground Up

Cultivating Agriculture for Nutrition

SIVAN YOSEF

FEW SECTORS HAVE clearer links to nutrition than agriculture. Most simply, of course, agriculture is a source of food. Because many poor households around the world grow food that they both consume and sell for income, agricultural interventions can have a massive effect on the lives of people in developing countries. Through the decades, and most famously in Asia's Green Revolution, development projects have sought to boost agricultural production of staple foods as a way of improving people's nutrition.[1] Yet, while consuming a sufficient quantity of calories is important, especially among undernourished populations, quality matters too. Thus, the traditional focus on producing enough food to meet people's calorie needs has evolved into a deeper understanding that to improve nutrition, we also need people to consume balanced, high-quality, and diverse diets that contain enough essential nutrients to meet their daily requirements.

Beyond food production, agriculture is linked to nutrition in a host of other ways, both positive and negative. Agriculture employs the majority of the world's rural poor people, who can use the income they earn to purchase more nutritious and diverse foods or to invest in education, health, or water and sanitation—all of which are crucial for improving nutrition. National and global agricultural policies also affect nutrition. Policies on subsidies, taxes, and trade determine the prices of food and nonfood crops, which in turn affect the income of net sellers and the purchasing power of poor consumers. Growth in agriculture as a sector has been projected to have benefits for nutrition: a simulation model suggests that an additional US$8 billion invested annually in agriculture would, by the year 2050, reduce the number of hungry people in the world by 210 million and the number of underweight children by 10 million.[2] At the same time, agriculture can expose farming households to hazards that can harm people's nutrition, such as vector-borne diseases from irrigation or zoonotic diseases from animal husbandry.[3]

Gender roles also link agriculture and nutrition. Women play a pivotal role in agricultural livelihoods and in most regions of the world make up the majority of agricultural laborers—up to 80 percent in Africa, for example.[4] Agricultural investments, when implemented in a gender-sensitive way, can improve female farmers' control over resources and assets and increase their power to make decisions about household investments in food, health, and education. Research has shown that women's control of resources is linked to a larger share of the household budget allocated to food as well as greater height-for-age Z-scores (reduced stunting). It has also found that greater female empowerment in agriculture (defined as having decision-making power over agricultural production and productive resources, control over use of income, leadership in the community, and time for work and leisure) is linked to higher per capita calorie availability and household dietary diversity and overall better maternal nutrition.[5] On the flip side, however, the time women spend on agriculture is also time they cannot spend feeding and caring for their children and themselves.

These many links between agriculture and nutrition are complex, and research is currently under way to build up and improve the evidence base so that we can gain a better understanding of them, especially in developing countries. Even so, a number of experiences offer lessons that can already be gleaned. This chapter focuses on two promising stories in the world of agriculture and nutrition. The first is homestead food production—an approach that combines home gardens and animal husbandry with information to help people adopt better agriculture, health, nutrition, and hygiene practices, as well as with actions that give women more control over resources and decision-making authority in their households. This case

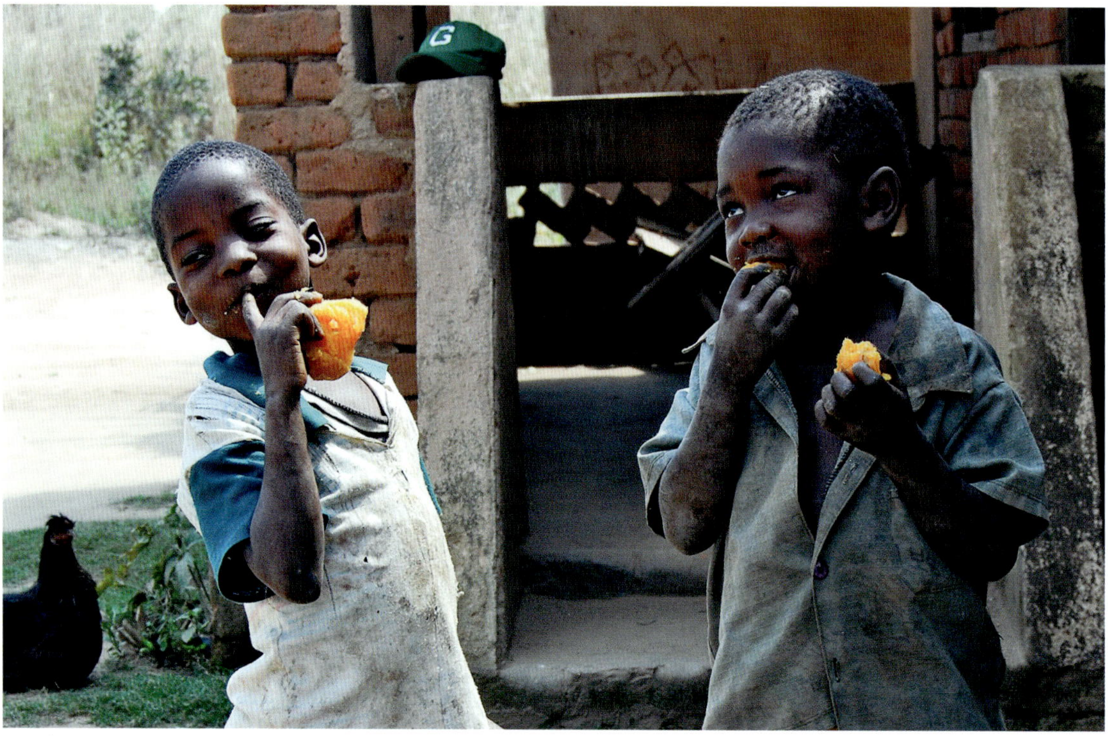

HarvestPlus

Children in Mozambique enjoy beta-carotene-rich orange sweet potatoes that can improve their vitamin A status.

study was first highlighted in the book *Millions Fed: Proven Successes in Agricultural Development* and is updated here with emphasis on its potential when implemented alongside interventions that emphasize behavior change communication and gender. The second is biofortification, in which plant scientists breed micronutrients into the staple crops that poor people commonly eat. The chapter also touches on the potential of another new way of thinking about agriculture and nutrition: the value-chain approach, which involves finding ways to maintain or boost the nutritional value of foods as they move along the different stages of the value chain from farmers' fields to consumers' tables. While these stories focus on big, scaled-up initiatives, they also illustrate the potential of agricultural interventions, both small and large, to address malnutrition in all its forms.

Roots at Home: Enhanced Homestead Food Production

In the early 1980s, two national nutrition surveys in Bangladesh revealed a worrying trend: 3.6 percent of preschool-age children, or 1 million children, suffered from night blindness.[6] Caused by severe vitamin A deficiency, the night blindness was higher in households without home gardens. In response, Helen Keller International (HKI), an international nonprofit organization, decided to test a new concept: homestead food production (HFP). The HFP model encouraged women to grow gardens of vitamin A–rich fruits and green leafy vegetables for their households, building on existing local practices and using local varieties. The focus on women was not a coincidence: rural Bangladeshi women have historically been responsible for homestead food production and distribution in households.[7]

In 1990 HKI launched two small pilots covering 1,000 households.[8] The pilots aimed to increase households' consumption of home-grown vegetables and fruits rich in vitamin A, provide nutrition education, and improve the health and nutritional status of women and children. As the project expanded over time to address deficiencies of multiple micronutrients, including iron and zinc, it integrated animal husbandry into the model, since the iron and zinc in animal-source foods are more bioavailable, or easily absorbed by the human body. By 2003, the project was reaching more than 870,000 households, or half of the country's subdistricts, and partnering with more than 70 local nongovernmental organizations and the government of Bangladesh.[9]

In the late 1990s and early 2000s, researchers began documenting the impact of home gardens and homestead food production, which had now expanded to other countries.[10] Research suggested that these programs were generally successful in increasing households' production of beneficial foods, such as vegetables, eggs, lentils, and animal products. Poorly designed evaluations, however, meant that it was impossible to determine whether HFP improved the participants' consumption of nutritious foods and micronutrients and contributed to dietary diversity.[11] Additionally, no one studied the cost-effectiveness of the approach compared with other interventions.[12] Just as important, there was little evidence that these programs affected mothers' or children's nutrition status (anthropometry or micronutrient status).[13] Vitamin A intake and status was a possible exception, with a review showing a serum retinol (the predominant form of vitamin A in the blood) improvement of 2.42 micrograms per deciliter (μg/dl) in young children (a serum retinol level of less than 20 [μg/dl] is usually used to determine vitamin A deficiency among preschool-aged children).[14]

HKI responded to these findings by collaborating with researchers to improve the intervention model. It combined the gardening and animal husbandry intervention with better communication about optimal agriculture, health, nutrition, and hygiene practices as well as a stronger emphasis on the role of women, by providing them with training on best HFP practices, and enlisting other women to impart knowledge on health and nutrition.[15] A 2012 evaluation of this Enhanced HFP (E-HFP) model in nearly 30 villages in Burkina Faso suggested that the combined model was more promising, leading to reported increases in vegetable production and intake among participants. Results also suggested improvements in women's status: women gained control over the gardens and profits from surplus sales. More work was needed to address looming challenges, such as scarce water for gardening, lack of home visits for beneficiaries, sparse knowledge in some areas of nutrition, and limited adoption of nutrition-related practices.[16]

Another recent evaluation of a variation of the model in Burkina Faso showed a wide array of results. This E-HFP model was targeted solely to women and children in the first 1,000 days of life, and it integrated strong health behavior change communication and women's empowerment activities, such as building up assets and knowledge of optimal agriculture, health, nutrition, and hygiene practices. Among children, researchers found a marginally statistically significant 0.5–0.7 g/dL increase in mean hemoglobin levels (levels less than 11 g/dL in children aged 6 months to 6 years indicate anemia) and an 8.8 percentage-point reduction in wasting (low weight-for-height), as well as a statistically significant 15.9 percentage-point decrease in diarrhea and a 14.6 percentage-point decrease in anemia.[17] New findings also suggest that the program decreased the prevalence of underweight among mothers by 8.6 percentage points and increased their intake of fruits, as well as raising their meat intake and dietary diversity by marginally statistically significant amounts.[18] Results suggest that beneficiary mothers gained control over their produce, agricultural assets, small animals, and profits from surplus sales and expanded their power in healthcare and purchasing decisions. There were also potentially positive spillover effects on indicators for other members of the household two years after the end of the program, including children's weight-for-height Z-scores and prevalence of wasting and mothers' body mass index and prevalence of underweight.[19] There were no significant impacts on the prevalence of stunting or underweight among children.[20] This evaluation represents one of the first studies to provide rigorous evidence that agriculture, coupled with behavior change communications and women's empowerment activities, can improve maternal and child nutrition during the first 1,000 days. Given the importance of this 1,000-day window for lifelong health,[21] this model of HFP shows potential.

Around the world, the HKI model has inspired countless interventions based on home gardening, either used alone or combined with education or behavior change communication initiatives around the world. The Sustainable Cocoa Production Program in Indonesia, for example, has provided 21,000 cocoa farmers, 80 percent of whom are women, with nutrition education and gardening skills, setting up more than 1,000 vegetable demonstration plots.[22] The project has self-reported modest increases in dietary diversity. More research is needed to document nutritional impacts from these and other similar initiatives, to generate more lessons, and to help improve the design of future enhanced homestead food production models. Furthermore, ultimate judgment on the viability of the home garden model of intervention will depend on proving the cost-effectiveness of this approach relative to other kinds of nutrition interventions and on documenting sustainability over time. These aspects have not been extensively studied so far.

Breeding for Nutrition: Biofortification

What if an extra boost of much-needed minerals and vitamins could be bred into widely consumed food crops, without negatively affecting their appearance, taste, or smell? What if, for example, rice and wheat seeds could be bred to contain extra iron and zinc that were undetectable to farmers or consumers but able to improve public health in a big way?

In 1993, this idea was posed by a group of scientists from CGIAR (then the Consultative Group on International Agricultural Research). At the time, many economists held firmly to the idea that global malnutrition could best be addressed by ensuring that people consume adequate calories. But burgeoning research showed otherwise—it suggested that good nutrition, as reflected by greater height and less illness, requires not only energy, but also vitamins and minerals. These extra vitamins and minerals could come from a diverse diet, rich in more nutritious staple and nonstaple foods and animal products.

Initially, the development community was skeptical. The prevailing thought was that a crop with higher levels of vitamins and minerals would also be lower yielding, making it unappealing to farmers.[23] Researchers soon showed that wheat seeds with higher levels of zinc actually used that zinc to improve their productivity and yields. Armed with this new evidence, CGIAR scientists secured initial funding to screen germplasm and prove that high-yielding and high-nutrient crop varieties could be achieved through conventional breeding.[24] A few years later, other donors came on board with major funding, and the Biofortification Challenge Program, later renamed HarvestPlus, was born in 2004.

Biofortification must go through a number of steps before it can be considered successful in reducing micronutrient malnutrition. An acceptable level of micronutrients must be bred into and retained by the crop, and it must be bioavailable. The biofortified crop must then be accepted and adopted by farmers on a large scale, as well as accepted and consumed by target populations.[25] HarvestPlus and its alliance of more than 70 partner organizations have applied some of these steps to three micronutrients (vitamin A, zinc, and iron) in seven crops (cassava, maize, sweet potato, bean, pearl millet, rice, and wheat). In Brazil, China, and India, where these targeted crops are produced and eaten in significant amounts, the alliance sponsors country programs.

Two decades after the initial idea, there is convincing evidence that breeding biofortified crops is possible and that the micronutrients are retained and bioavailable. People who consume iron-biofortified rice and beans, for example, have shown improved iron status. A study in the Philippines showed a 20 percent increase in serum ferritin and body iron among women consuming high-iron rice.[26]

And researchers have begun to probe the effectiveness of biofortified crops—that is, the extent to which farmers and consumers actually adopt or consume them. Effectiveness trials on the pilot distribution of biofortified orange sweet potato to farmers and consumers in Mozambique and

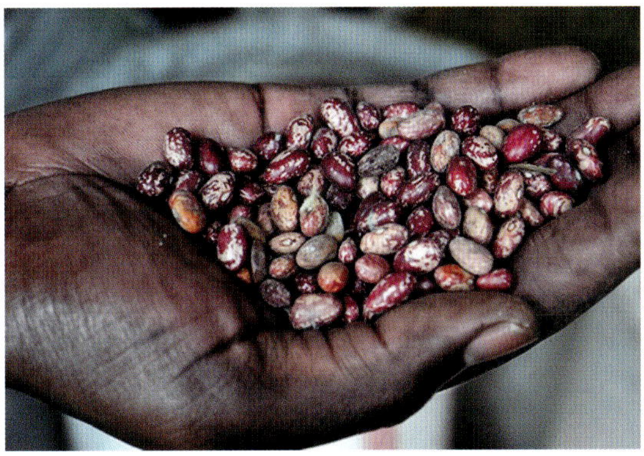

HarvestPlus, Neil Palmer (CIAT)

Some farmers in Rwanda now grow beans bred with high iron content.

Uganda have shown a great level of success, with farmers adopting the beneficial crop and consumers significantly increasing their vitamin A intake. In Uganda, vitamin A status among children improved.[27] In Mozambique, biofortification reduced the prevalence of diarrhea in children under age 5 by 11.4 percent and the duration of diarrhea by 10 percent.[28] As part of an integrated agriculture and nutrition intervention there, orange sweet potato reduced the prevalence of vitamin A deficiency among children by 15 percent.[29] Estimates of the cost-effectiveness of vitamin A–biofortified orange maize in Zambia suggest that it would save US$24 per DALY (disability-adjusted life year or the number of years lost due to ill-health, disability, or early death), with additional cost savings when biofortification was combined with fortification interventions.[30] Whether these successes can be scaled up remains to be seen as HarvestPlus embarks on the third phase of its program.

New Directions in Nutrition and Agriculture: Value Chains

A value chain refers to the path that a food takes from the farm to the table. The journey begins with production—and even the inputs that go into production, such as water, soil, and technologies—and continues through processing, distribution, retailing, promotion, labeling, and finally consumption. As the commodity goes through the various stages of the value chain, it gains value. This value has traditionally been defined in economic terms, but in recent years, nutritionists and development professionals have explored the idea of expanding the concept of value to mean enhancing or retaining the nutritional value of foods, especially micronutrient-rich foods that poor people find difficult to access because of their cost and perishability, such as fruits, vegetables, dairy, meat, and seafood.[31] A pro-nutrition value chain might find ways to improve the incentives and coordination among different actors along the chain to make foods more available, affordable, acceptable, nutritious, and safe.

The effectiveness of a value-chain approach to improving nutrition has not yet been studied extensively; research is currently limited to case studies.[32] One area where value chains could potentially make a contribution is through school-feeding programs, which have had some small nutrition wins. For example, a review of 18 studies suggests that children in school-feeding interventions in various low-income countries gained an average of 0.39 kilograms more than the control group over an average of 19 months when looking at higher-quality studies, or 0.71 kilograms over 11.3 months when looking at lower-quality studies.[33] Another meta-analysis found similar results: an average weight gain of 0.37 kilograms per school year but no significant effects on height.[34] A more integrated approach—homegrown school feeding—uses value chains to connect schools with local farmers and in turn boost the local economy and improve the nutritional status of school-age children and their families. This approach has been used by high- and middle-income countries such as Brazil (see Chapter 11), Chile, and the United Kingdom and is now at various stages of implementation in low-income countries such as Ghana and Nigeria.[35] The success of these initiatives will depend on many factors, including the ability to ensure a continuous supply of food throughout the year. If successful, these initiatives would fulfill two different policy objectives—child welfare and pro-poor agricultural development—while potentially increasing farm productivity in some cases, in regions such as Africa south of the Sahara, to effectively meet the demand from schools.[36]

Lessons Learned

The stories in this chapter highlight a few lessons and challenges. First, long-term impact is a challenge. While homestead food production, for example, had spillover effects on some indicators of children's and women's health two years after the end of the program, preliminary analyses suggest that it had no impacts on children's anemia or diarrhea, household assets and livestock ownership, dietary diversity, or food security.[37] To ensure a long-term impact on nutrition, homestead food production and biofortification programs will need to depend on many local partners around the world to help design, implement, and evaluate programs, to build up local capacity, and to share existing local tools and practices. This can also help ensure that agricultural projects and policies do no harm to people's health and nutritional status or to the environment.

Second, research is key. Enthusiasm for biofortification intensified after research showed that the concept was feasible and effective. Rounds of evaluation of the homestead food production model have underscored the finding that combining agricultural programs with behavior change communication and a focus on gender may have larger impacts than stand-alone home gardening initiatives. In general, the relationship between agriculture and nutrition deserves far more analysis and research to generate, for example, stronger program designs and in-depth analyses and understanding of program impact pathways. [38] Analyses of the cost-effectiveness of different approaches, which have so far been rather scarce, would also be useful for guiding public investment decisions. Large research partnerships such as the CGIAR Research Program on Agriculture for Nutrition and Health (A4NH) and the Leveraging Agriculture for Nutrition in South Asia (LANSA) consortium are making strides in these areas.

The intersection of nutrition and agriculture will certainly continue to yield even greater insights in the years to come. Research advances can be used to make programs and policies more nutrition sensitive and in some cases to overhaul entire food systems. Investments in agriculture have high economic returns compared with other economic investments.[39] That 75 percent of the world's poor people live in rural areas—and depend on agriculture[40]—means that integrated agriculture-nutrition interventions have the power to improve not only the nutrition and health, but also the livelihoods and overall well-being, of the poorest and most vulnerable populations living in the world today, a truly exciting prospect.

CHAPTER 7

Reducing Risk, Strengthening Resilience

Social Protection and Nutrition

SCOTT DRIMIE AND SIVAN YOSEF

IN THE MID-1990S, governments and researchers in three countries from very different parts of the world—Bangladesh, Brazil, and Mexico—began moving toward a new type of poverty alleviation program. Struggling to meet the needs of their poor populations through various poverty-reduction initiatives, they wondered whether attaching conditions to those programs would make a difference. What if in exchange for receiving a food basket or a cash voucher, program beneficiaries were asked, for example, to bring their infants to the local health clinic for growth monitoring, or enroll their older children in secondary school? Such a change could not only meet the immediate needs of citizens, but also help improve their longer-term welfare and development, all of which affect nutrition.

Social protection has been around for millennia, but this "conditional transfer" approach goes beyond welfare per se to address human development. Today, social protection is generally understood to encompass three types of public intervention: (1) social safety nets; (2) state-contingent insurance; and (3) social-sector policies.[1]

Social safety nets are targeted, noncontributory programs that transfer resources to poor households that are deprived owing to their income, social status, or nutritional status. These programs include cash transfers through welfare payments, in-kind transfers such as food aid or school feeding programs, allowances or pensions to aid children, subsidized products that are purchased or produced by poor populations, and public works or workfare schemes. In some regions, such as Latin America, cash and food transfers are increasingly linked with nutrition-, health-, or education-related conditionalities, such as requirements to take children for regular health checkups, attend nutrition education workshops, administer nutritional supplementation, or maintain children's attendance in primary or secondary schooling.

A second component of social protection is publicly provided state-contingent insurance that depends on the occurrence of an adverse event such as illness, drought, or loss of employment. Such

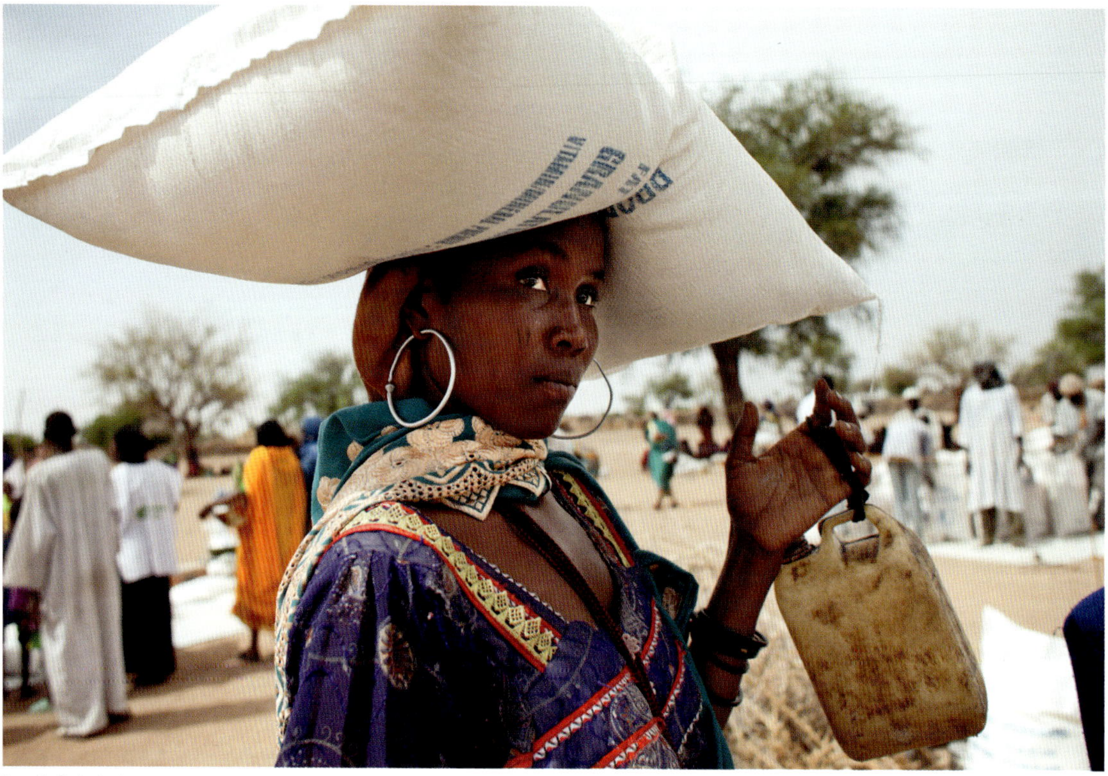

Panos/A. Trayler-Smith

A woman in the Guerra region of Chad carries a bag of food aid—a form of social protection that can be made more effective in improving people's nutrition.

insurance-based programs pool contributions from individuals or households to protect them against risk and include social insurance (for example, pensions and unemployment programs) or health insurance. These instruments are needed to fill the gaps left by missing insurance markets or market failures in savings and credit markets for the poor.

The third component consists of social-sector policies, including, for example, waived fees for health care facilities; free primary schooling; and preventative malnutrition interventions targeted to poor, pre-school-aged children. These policies originate in the health and education sectors while also complementing social safety net interventions, especially when they are means tested to ensure they provide assistance exclusively to low-income individuals and households.[2]

Although countries around the world use social protection programs, populations in industrialized countries have more comprehensive coverage, usually through social security. Seventy-three percent of the global population has only partial or no access to social protection coverage.[3]

There are many pathways through which social protection can have a positive impact on people's nutrition. Some pathways are direct, encompassing nutrition-specific interventions that address the immediate determinants of nutrition. For example, social protection instruments such as food transfers can raise people's overall food consumption and provide them with more diverse diets. If social protection is linked to conditionalities such as behavior change communication on nutrition or supplementation, it can also directly influence people's nutrition behaviors or knowledge.

Other critical pathways are more indirect, addressing the underlying determinants of malnutrition, such as poverty, through nutrition-sensitive interventions. Arguably, the goal of most social protection interventions is to increase income, enabling families to pay for everyday needs and services and allowing them to spend more money not only on more food and but also on nonstaple foods, including fruits, vegetables, and animal food products (see, for example, Box 7.1). Research suggests that cash, food vouchers, and food transfers significantly improve the quantity and quality of food people consume. The relative impact of cash and vouchers is context specific.

Social protection instruments can also help households become more resilient, and thus improve their nutrition, by building up assets, savings, or investments in human capital such as education that can help them weather future shocks.[4] When households are more food secure, they are better able to cope with seasonal fluctuations in food security or shocks due to natural or manmade disasters.[5] By strengthening income security and investing in rural livelihoods, social protection can also help improve agricultural productivity, stimulate local economic development, build resilience, encourage sustainable natural resource use, and promote social inclusion. It can help reduce child mortality, particularly deaths associated with poverty-related causes, such as malnutrition and diarrhea. Further, if properly designed, social protection can benefit women by promoting their economic and social empowerment.[6]

The evidence of the impact of social protection programs on nutrition is mixed. A 2013 systematic review of 15 conditional cash transfer (CCT) programs around the world found on average nominally positive but insignificant effects on nutritional status, in particular on children's height-for-age, verifying previous researchers' observation that such programs have inconsistent effects on child nutritional status.[7] These programs have achieved success on many other fronts such as improving education, decreasing child labor, and increasing access to health care (such as vaccinations). Another systematic review of 16 studies of CCT programs, mostly in Latin America, found that such programs can have a positive impact on access to health care, child and maternal nutrition, morbidity risk, immunization rates, and household poverty, particularly in middle-income countries.[8] These results should be interpreted with some caution, however. Another review, for example, found mixed results on whether cash transfers have a positive impact on growth-related outcomes among children, particularly in Africa south of the Sahara: some studies in the review had small but positive effects on child weight and height, while several others were found to have no significant impacts on child nutritional status.[9]

This chapter focuses on two interventions: PROGRESA/Oportunidades/Prospera in Mexico and various initiatives in Bangladesh that have made measurable improvements in people's nutrition. These stories illustrate how social protection can be part of a multisectoral effort to address both nutrition directly and the key underlying determinants of malnutrition.[10] The PROGRESA results and the Bangladesh experience suggest that social protection may work effectively when twinned with nutrition behavior change communication.

PROGRESA/Oportunidades/Prospera in Mexico

The Programa de Educación, Salud y Alimentación (PROGRESA)—the Education, Health, and Nutrition Program—is a social protection and poverty alleviation program initiated in 1997 by the Mexican federal government.[11] In 2002, the name of the program was changed to Oportunidades, and it was later changed again to Prospera. This program forms part of an integrated, multisectoral poverty alleviation plan aiming to increase the health, nutritional, and educational status of the country's poorest households by helping parents invest in their children in order to break the intergenerational transmission of poverty.[12]

The program intervenes at each of the three core levels of determinants of malnutrition—basic, underlying, and immediate—as outlined by UNICEF's conceptual framework of malnutrition. It does so by addressing household financial resources and food security, maternal and child care and education, child feeding practices, and maternal and child undernutrition. The nutrition-specific intervention consists of a CCT targeting mothers, because research shows that when resources are given to mothers rather than fathers a higher percentage of investments goes toward the health and nutrition of children.[13] The program aims to increase the nutritional quality and diversity of children's food intake by providing food supplements, as well as by using cash transfers to boost families' ability to buy more nutritious foods, such as meat, eggs, dairy, fruit, and vegetables. This pathway was enhanced by early intervention in cases of child growth faltering as well as continued health and nutrition education for parents. This education component may be key; new research from Bangladesh suggests that social protection may work best when combined with nutrition-oriented behavior-change communication.

Eligible households, selected from rural areas in most states of Mexico, were those considered most marginalized owing to socioeconomic factors or remoteness, although the communities had to have primary and secondary schools and a health clinic to maintain eligibility. The initial program covered 140,500 households in 3,400 areas. In 2000, the program expanded to urban areas, covering 2.6 million households in 72,300 areas in all states. By 2008, the program covered approximately one-quarter of the Mexican population.[14] Since its inception, the model has been replicated in 52 countries around the world.

After the initial phase of the PROGRESA program, a 2001 evaluation established that after just one full year, the program had a significantly positive impact on nutritional status for those children who also received supplementary food.[15] This result was demonstrated by a one-sixth increase in average annual growth in children between the ages of 12 and 36 months; for children who received the supplements, the probability of stunting was one-third that of children in control groups. The effect was larger for children from poorer communities whose mothers were literate. This result alone has been estimated as increasing subsequent adult lifetime earnings by 2.9 percent.[16] Another study found no significant impact on growth outcomes on children aged 6 to 24 months. It did, however, find that children younger than 6 months at baseline grew a statistically significant 1.5 centimeters taller and gained a significant 0.76 kilogram more than their nonbeneficiary peers after two years.[17] The researchers could not isolate which component of the program caused this effect but concluded that the provision of fortified food was not the main determining factor because the level of food provided was too low.

Other studies also documented nutritional benefits. One compared a group that had benefited from PROGRESA for two years with a group that had participated for only one year. Children ages 0 to 6 months from the first group were taller (with a 1.1 centimeter greater height-for-age) and had a lower prevalence of anemia (44.3 percent compared with 54.9 percent).[18] Another assessment found that PROGRESA boosted intake of iron, zinc, and vitamin A among beneficiary children who consumed a program-provided micronutrient-fortified

BOX 7.1 Ethiopia's Productive Safety Net Programme

The Productive Safety Net Programme (PSNP) is one of the largest social protection interventions in Africa, reaching 8 million food-insecure Ethiopians in 2011 through two components: public works (temporary employment) for households with labor capacity and direct support (unconditional cash or food transfers) to labor-constrained households (see Chapter 16). The overarching objective is to reduce Ethiopia's dependency on annual emergency food aid appeals by building community assets such as roads through public works and providing predictable transfers to households over multiple years. A recent evaluation uses a generalized propensity score method to examine the impact of the duration of PSNP participation. When the program began in 2006, participating households reported, on average, 3.6 months of food insecurity; that number fell to 2.2 months in 2008, representing an improvement of 39 percent. Further, PSNP protected food security and asset levels in the presence of repeated shocks.[19] One study tentatively concluded that the program improved the diet of 75 percent of participants in both quantity and quality; beneficiaries were more likely to consume the required 1,800 calories per day than nonbeneficiaries.[20] Preliminary findings show that PSNP improves diet quantity, quality, and diversity by providing additional resources for families to pay for everyday needs and services, allowing them to spend more money on nonstaple foods, including fruits, vegetables, and animal food products.[21]

food, but the rate of use of the fortified food was not high enough to have more than a small effect on the children's mean hemoglobin levels or rates of anemia reduction.[22]

Doubling cash transfers to mothers was associated with a substantial 0.20 higher height-for-age Z-score among their children and a lower prevalence of both child stunting and overweight. Citing insufficient data, the researchers recommended future research to explore the pathways by which additional income positively affects child development. The same study found that mothers spent 70 percent of the cash transfer they had received on a higher-quality diet for their children consisting of meat, fruits, and vegetables.[23]

According to other studies, mostly non-refereed, there were other nutrition-related health impacts, which provide tentative results. After six months of implementation of Oportunidades, coverage of vaccines against tuberculosis among children less than 12 months old may have increased by 4 percentage points (88 to 92 percent) compared with 2 percentage points among the control groups (91 to 93 percent).[24] During the first six months of implementation of PROGRESA, measles vaccination coverage may have increased from 92 to 96 percent and in low-coverage communities from 75 to 92 percent after 12 months of implementation.[25] Findings also suggest that PROGRESA reduced the morbidity, or the rate of illness, among children under 5 years of age by 12 percent, though with no impact on older children.[26] After one year of PROGRESA, beneficiary children under 5 years of age were estimated to be 32 percent less likely to be sick with diarrhea than their control peers.[27] Finally, PROGRESA may have also affected the use of health services, increasing growth monitoring and promotion visits by 30 to 60 percent for children up to 2 years of age and 25 to 45 percent for children between the ages of 3 and 5.[28]

Social Protection in Bangladesh

Bangladesh has been home to many social protection initiatives. The SHOUHARDO (Strengthen Household Ability to Respond to Development

Opportunities) program, for example, is one of the world's largest nonemergency food security programs. During its first phase from 2006 to 2010, it served 2 million people (see Chapter 2 on community nutrition and Chapter 12 on Bangladesh). Another example is the Food for Asset Creation (FFA) program, a component of Bangladesh's Integrated Food Security program. FFA pays beneficiaries a daily wage in food plus cash (2 kilograms of wheat plus 20 taka) in exchange for labor on public works.[29] Aligned with the Rural Maintenance Programme (RMP), these programs have contributed to the construction and maintenance of rural infrastructure, particularly feeder roads that connect remote villages to major highways. Because these roads were built at an elevation, they are not washed out by floods and rains, and the government and donors have used this road network to move food to needy communities during emergencies. Preliminary findings show that participation in FFA and RMP increased households' per capita food consumption by a statistically significant 194 and 271 kilocalories per person per day, respectively, relative to matched control groups. Yet another example of a social protection program with a potential for a positive impact on nutrition can be found in the Chars Livelihoods Programme, which works with ultra-poor households in northwestern Bangladesh, reaching more than 1 million people. Women who earned money from the program

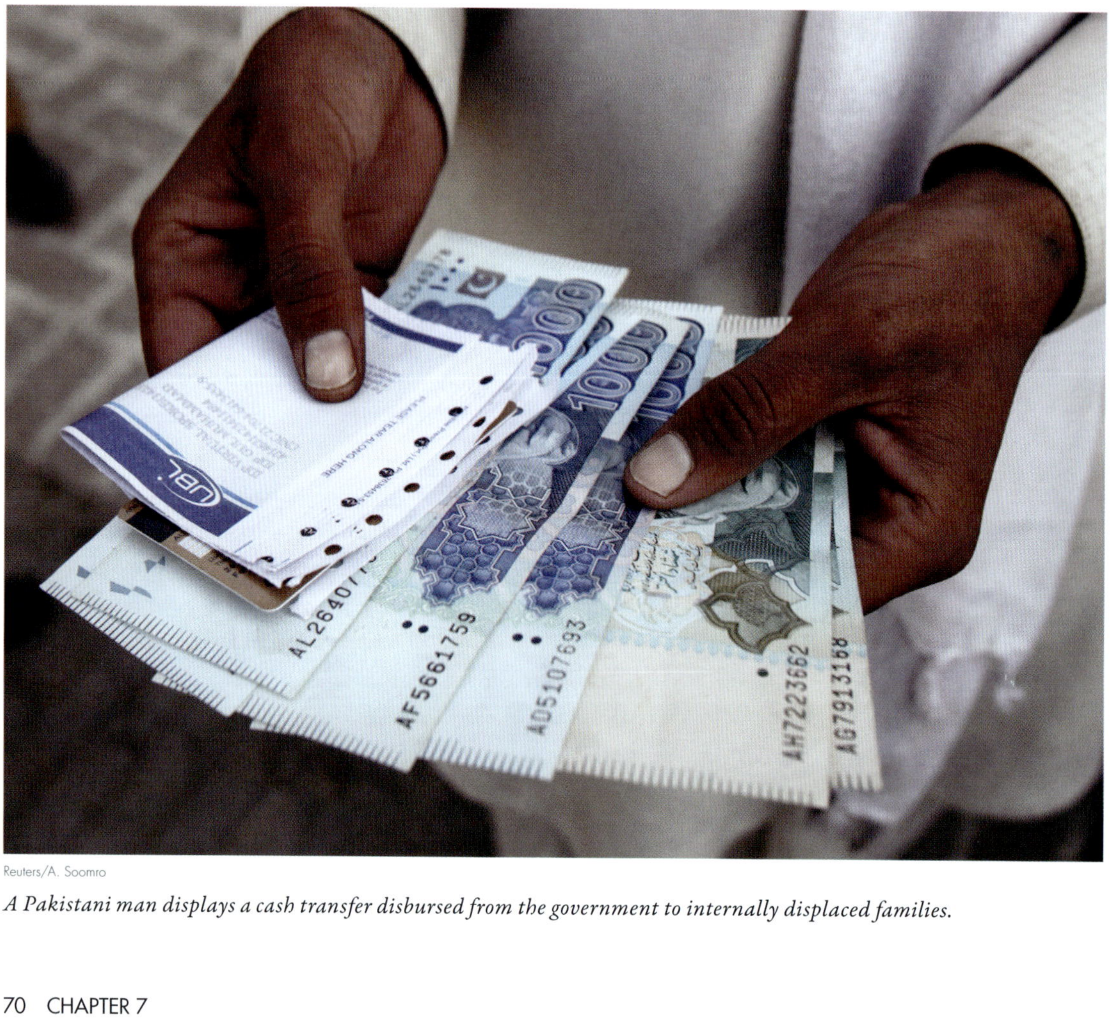

Reuters/A. Soomro

A Pakistani man displays a cash transfer disbursed from the government to internally displaced families.

reported spending it on nutrient-rich food such as eggs, meat, fish, pulses, green leafy vegetables, milk, and fruit. After 10 weeks, their children younger than 5 years were a statistically significant 0.7 millimeter taller on average than nonbeneficiaries, were 210 grams heavier, and had a 1.39-millimeter greater circumference of their mid-upper arm.[30]

One of the more recent social protection research projects coming out of Bangladesh ran in 2012–2014. The Transfer Modality Research Initiative (TMRI), undertaken by the International Food Policy Research Institute (IFPRI) and the United Nations World Food Programme (WFP), investigated how effective various forms of social protection intervention were in improving income, food security, and maternal and child nutrition status. Under the initiative, 4,000 ultra-poor women and their 21,600 family members in the northwestern and southern regions of Bangladesh received five modalities of social protection: cash transfers only, food transfers only, 50 percent food and 50 percent cash transfers, cash transfers and nutrition behavior change communication, and food transfers and nutrition behavior change communication. The nutrition behavior change communication consisted of conveying information to households on the importance of nutrition and diet diversity for health, hand-washing and hygiene, diversifying diets with micronutrients, infant and young child feeding practices, and maternal nutrition.

Preliminary results presented in 2015 suggested that all forms of transfer in both the northwestern and southern regions caused meaningful improvements in nearly all measures of consumption: spending on food and nonfood consumption, calorie intake, and diet quality. Adding nutrition behavior-change communication to transfers may have led to much larger improvements than transfers alone. In the northwest, cash transfers combined with nutrition behavior-change communication may have led to a decrease of 7.3 percentage points in child stunting over the two years of the study—an achievement almost three times the national average decline. Other forms of transfer had no impact on any measure of the anthropometric status of children.[31] These results suggest that social protection may be most effective at improving nutritional status when it is combined with behavior change communication.

Lessons Learned

The array of social protection programs around the world demonstrates the potential for great synergies between social protection and nutrition. Social protection interventions, perhaps when combined with behavior change communication, can not only improve food security but also go further to address dietary diversity, child growth and health, illness, and a plethora of other nutrition- and health-related indicators, such as the use of health services and nutrition education. Social protection interventions are especially useful in times of crisis and shocks, to which the poor are particularly vulnerable. They can help smooth volatility in food security throughout a crisis, ensuring that the nutritional and health status of vulnerable households is not compromised and thereby helping prevent a downward cycle of poverty and malnutrition.

One lesson that emerges clearly from these stories is that nutrition needs to be explicitly woven into social protection programs. This approach might mean "sensitizing" a program to add nutrition-related components such as supplementation, behavior-change communication, or nutrition education–related conditionalities. Or it might mean changing the entire focus of a program, such as looking beyond individuals engaged in productive labor—the target of many social protection programs—to ensure that young children are also protected. At the same time, it should also be noted that integrating nutrition into social protection programs can generate unintended consequences unless care is taken in their design. Mexico's Programa de Apoyo Alimentario (PAL), a CCT and in-kind transfer program, was found not only to improve household dietary quality, but also—owing to the food basket's provision of energy-dense staple and basic food products—to increase total energy consumption among populations that already had a high prevalence of female overweight and obesity.[32]

Social protection now features as one of the proposed targets of the Sustainable Development Goals (SDGs). Target 3.1 in SDG 1 calls for countries to "implement nationally appropriate social protection systems and measures for all, including floors, and by 2030 achieve substantial coverage of the poor and the vulnerable."[33] This inclusion underlines the growing importance of social protection in the post-2015 development agenda. It is now up to policy makers, researchers, program designers, and implementers to integrate nutrition into social protection, turning it into a transformative tool that can address both the immediate and underlying causes of malnutrition.

CHAPTER 8

Clean Is Nourished

The Links between WASH and Nutrition

SIVAN YOSEF

MORE THAN 660 million people lack access to an improved water source and 2.4 billion people lack access to improved sanitation.[1] Growing awareness of the global challenge we face in improving water, sanitation, and hygiene, widely known as WASH, has won the problem a prominent place on global nutrition and health agendas. And an expanding body of research points to the great potential of WASH, as a set of interventions, to improve nutrition and health. For example, systematic reviews have shown that improving water quality can reduce the risk of diarrhea by 17 percent[2]; and introducing hand hygiene interventions can reduce gastrointestinal illness by 31 percent and respiratory illness by 21 percent.[3]

WASH comprises three very different sets of interventions that address similar environmental barriers to good nutrition. The synergistic relationships between low quality or quantity of water, poor sanitation facilities (or lack thereof), and poor hygiene practices have complex links with nutrition. Aside from the indirect ways in which WASH affects nutrition, such as the time taken away from food production or childcare to collect clean water, there are at least three direct pathways between WASH and nutrition outcomes. The first is through diarrhea, the leading cause of mortality and morbidity among children under five. Diarrhea impairs appetite, the absorption of nutrients, the immune system, and physical and cognitive development.[4] In 2013, 578,000 children under five died from diarrhea globally, despite a 6.5 percent annual decline in these rates from 2000 to 2013.[5] Evidence shows some links between poor WASH conditions and diarrhea.[6] For example, research provides strong evidence that better water *quality* reduces reported diarrhea, but finds a lack of high-quality evidence on the effects of water *quantity,* especially on handwashing practices.[7] There is also substantial evidence of the association between diarrhea and nutrition. In 2010, children in low- and middle-income countries each experienced nearly three episodes of diarrhea annually, on average, increasing their risk of stunting during the first two years of life, the most critical window for development.[8] Every five diarrheal episodes puts a child of two years at a 13 percent greater risk of being stunted, and diarrheal illnesses during this period may lead to an average growth shortfall of 8.2 centimeters.[9] Nevertheless, more rigorous research is needed on the entire impact pathway, from water quality, access to sanitation, and hygiene practices, to the prevalence of diarrhea, to final impact on nutritional status. Recent estimates suggest that access to different WASH interventions, especially safe and reliable pipe water supply (improvements in water quality) and sewer connections, could prevent more than 360,000 diarrhea-related deaths among children under five in low- and middle-income settings, a 5.5 percent reduction in deaths in that age group.[10]

A second link is through other types of infection. Poor sanitation, for example, can increase the risk of infestation of soils by the eggs and larvae of helminth (parasitic worms). When humans ingest contaminated water and food or walk barefoot on contaminated soil, these helminth and fomites (objects or substances that can carry germs or parasites) can cause parasitic infections such as roundworm, whipworm, and hookworm.[11] Infections in turn impede the absorption of nutrients and impair growth.[12] Hookworm infections also cause anemia in children and pregnant women, which increases the risk of preterm delivery and low birth weight.[13] Again, there is substantial research on the impact of various WASH conditions on infections (for example, the availability and usage of sanitation facilities is associated with a 46–78 percent reduction in soil-transmitted helminth infections[14]), but not enough data on the entire WASH–infection–nutrition pathway.

A third possible link is through environmental enteropathy. Poor sanitary environments contain

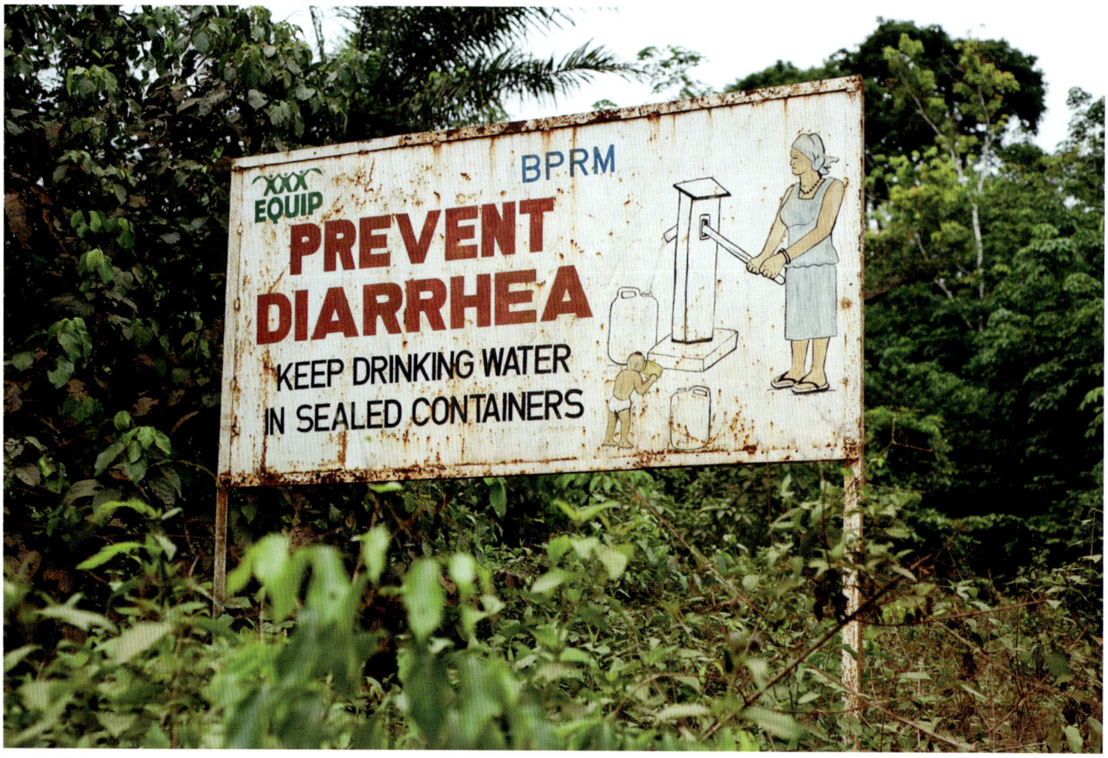
EQUIP
BPRM
PREVENT
DIARRHEA
KEEP DRINKING WATER
IN SEALED CONTAINERS

Panos/A. Wade

A billboard in Liberia suggests one way to prevent diarrhea, a leading cause of illness and death in children under five.

high levels of pathogens. When ingested by children, these may damage the gut and lead to poor absorption of nutrients, a condition known as environmental enteropathy or environmental enteric dysfunction (EED).[15] While diarrhea is episodic, EED can be a chronic condition: a study from the Gambia showed that while children had diarrhea 7.3 percent of their first two years of life, they had EED during 76 percent of that period.[16] Most research on the impact of improved WASH on EED is limited to animal-based studies; human-focused research is currently limited to observational studies that can only establish associations rather than attribution.[17] An observational study from Bangladesh, for example, found that children from physically clean households had less severe EED and higher height-for-age Z-scores (and 22 percent lower stunting prevalence) than their peers from contaminated households.[18]

What is the impact of WASH *conditions* on nutrition outcomes? While the literature on each condition—poor quality of water, poor sanitation, and poor hygiene—is vast, there are few studies that look at their impact on nutrition. An ecological study of 140 Demographic and Health Surveys suggested that over half, or 54 percent, of the variation in average child height in 65 poor and middle-income countries could be attributed to frequency of open defecation. When open defecation occurred in densely populated areas, it accounted for 65 percent of the variation in child height.[19] A study of 112 districts in India found that a 10 percent increase in open defecation was associated with a 0.7 percentage point increase in both stunting and severe stunting.[20]

Research on the impacts of WASH *interventions* on nutrition is also scarce. A systematic review of 14 studies with varying study designs produced a meta-analysis of five randomized controlled trials, the gold standard in research. The analysis found no evidence of an effect of WASH interventions on weight-for-age and weight-for-height Z-scores. It did find a borderline statistically significant effect of water quality and hygiene interventions on height-for-age, with the strongest effects in children under 24 months of age.[21] Research focusing on low- and middle-income countries showed that access to improved sanitation was associated with lower child mortality and lower diarrhea.[22] No study to date has looked at the impact of simultaneous water, sanitation, and hygiene interventions on nutrition, suggesting a need to probe the synergistic effect of these three types of interventions on nutrition (Box 8.1).[23]

Useful lessons can be drawn from two recent experiences in WASH: community-led total sanitation in Mali and an array of promising WASH interventions in Bangladesh. These cases offer a glimpse of the great potential of WASH interventions to change behaviors in target populations, and thus contribute to improvements in indicators of nutrition such as child growth.

Community-led Total Sanitation in Mali

Community-led total sanitation (CLTS) is a participatory approach, initiated in Bangladesh in 1999, aimed at the complete elimination of open defecation. In contrast to supply-driven sanitation programs, CLTS relies on communities, usually in rural, homogenous villages of less than 2,000 people or 200 households, to take the initiative in tackling open defecation, without financial or capital assistance.[24] Research has suggested that providing subsidies to construct in-home sanitation facilities is not effective as a stand-alone intervention for curbing open defecation and is best combined with behavioral change. This finding supports the tenets of CLTS.[25]

The CLTS process begins with a public community meeting, where education and awareness activities regarding open defecation are undertaken

BOX 8.1 WASH-nutrition research on the horizon

This is an exciting time to be studying the links among water, sanitation, and hygiene, and their synergistic effect on nutrition. A number of high-profile studies are underway that are helping to generate rigorous evidence on these relationships:

The WASH Benefits study is conducting trials in Bangladesh and Kenya with six different combinations of sanitation, water quality, handwashing, and nutrition treatments, looking at whether these interventions impact diarrhea, markers of environmental enteropathy, and growth and development in the first years of life.[26] The study is expected to be completed in 2016.

The MAL-ED Project (Interactions of Malnutrition & Enteric Infections: Consequences for Child Health and Development) is conducting WASH-nutrition research in eight countries that have especially high rates of undernutrition and diarrhea: Bangladesh, Brazil, India, Nepal, Pakistan, Peru, Tanzania, and South Africa. The project focuses on the impact of enteric infections on gut integrity, and subsequent physical and cognitive development during the first 1,000 days.[27] It is expected to be completed in 2017.

The SHINE Trial (Sanitation Hygiene Infant Nutrition Efficacy) is a Zimbabwe-based study investigating the effects of WASH and/or improved infant feeding on stunting and anemia among children 0–18 months of age who may have been exposed to high levels of mycotoxins, through possible ingestion of fecal microbes from, for example, open defecation or chicken droppings.[28] It is expected to be completed in 2017.

in an attempt to invoke disgust and shame, a controversial approach. Participants then commit to using proper defecation facilities. Monitoring is a key component of the CLTS approach, with follow-up visits conducted by program implementers. However, monitoring and evaluation need to be improved across many CLTS interventions. Reportedly, only one in ten organizations that promoted monitoring of CLTS worldwide has actually followed through.[29]

CLTS has been implemented in an estimated 66 countries but is extremely diverse in practice.[30] The approach also suffers from a lack of rigorous evidence, with purported problems in verifying the number of open-defecation-free (ODF) communities in countries such as Bangladesh and Indonesia, and corruption in certifying villages as ODF in India as a way of qualifying for awards.[31] With this disclaimer in mind, encouraging results have been reported from Ethiopia, Kenya, and Zambia, where sanitation coverage, defined as the ratio of number of toilets to number of households, in 12 pilot villages was reported to have increased from 23 percent to 88 percent in three months.[32]

One particular success with CLTS can be found in Mali. The country's CLTS campaign was spearheaded by the government with support from UNICEF and the Bill & Melinda Gates Foundation in 2009. The intervention followed the common practice of CLTS but went further to motivate participants to construct private latrines themselves. Follow-up visits were conducted for up to three months; once it was deemed that all households had properly-equipped latrines and had eliminated open defecation, a celebration event was held.[33] Following an apparently successful pilot in 15 villages (preliminary findings suggest that all pilot villages became fully ODF, bringing the percentage of families with latrines from 30 to 100 percent), Mali's National Directorate of Sanitation incorporated CLTS in its National Strategy for Rural Sanitation, leading the way for scaling up the initiative throughout the country.[34] The implementation of CLTS is ongoing and seems to have continued through political instability, including a military coup in 2012. The government is developing a national CLTS plan for 2015–2024, as well as a post-ODF strategy, CLTS implementation guide, and training manual. As of 2024, 1,400 villages had reportedly achieved ODF status, contributing to a 1 percent reduction in the national prevalence of open defecation.[35]

A cluster-randomized controlled trial among 121 villages conducted in 2011–2013 showed that the CLTS campaign in Mali had a positive impact on improving access to latrines and decreasing open defecation.[36] Participating villages enjoyed 65 percent coverage of private, household latrines, compared to 35 percent in control villages. Open defecation, as reported by participants, decreased by 71 percent among adults; 49 percent among children of 5–10 years of age; and 51 percent among children younger than 5.[37]

Impacts on health and growth outcomes were also positive. Young children (under five years) in participating villages had statistically significant 0.18 higher height-for-age Z-scores and were 13 percent less likely to be stunted. The effects were even larger (height-for-age Z-scores of 0.29) when restricting the sample to approximately 800 children younger than one year, signaling an impact within the critical 1,000-day window.[38] However, there were no significant impacts on the reduction of the proportion of children underweight or improvements in child weight.[39]

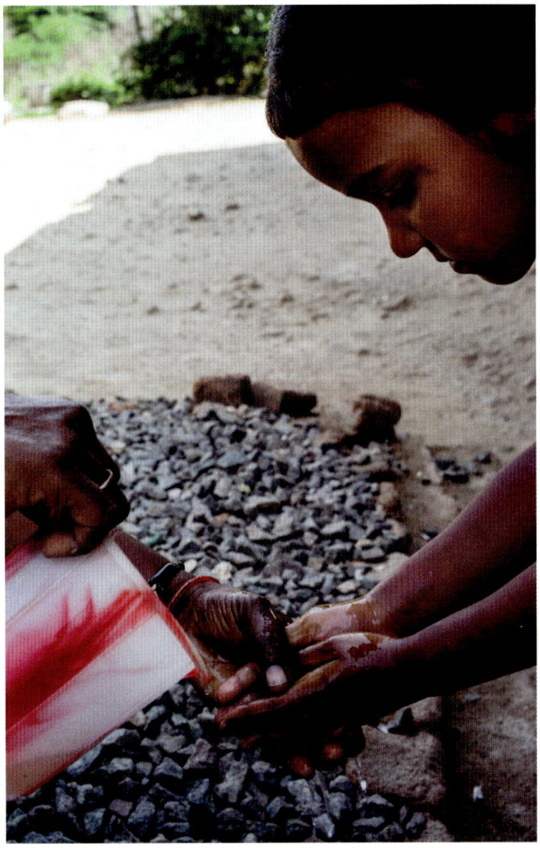

Panos/S. Das

An anganwadi worker helps a child properly wash her hands at a village center in Andhra Pradesh, India.

WASH in Bangladesh

In 1995, 35 percent of people in Bangladesh defecated in the open. By 2012, that number had dropped to 2.5 percent.[40] Many lessons can be derived from Bangladesh's experiences in tackling poor sanitation and hygiene, a journey that continues today. The Government of Bangladesh has passed a number of policies and plans directed at the water and sanitation sector, including the Water Act of 2013; the Sector Development Plan of 2010–2021, which calls for an integrated water and sanitation strategy; and, most notably, the National Water Supply and Sanitation Strategy 2014, which aims to increase WASH interventions and improve sector governance.[41] In 2003, the government launched a National Sanitation Campaign, which aimed to achieve 100 percent sanitation coverage by 2010, later revised to 2013. The campaign used many of the principles of CLTS and emphasized the containment of feces, rather than pressure to build a sanitary latrine. To implement the program at scale, the government earmarked 20 percent of local development funds, most of which was spent on procuring sanitation facilities and supplies for the ultra-poor, mostly in rural areas. (The intervention has failed to reach rural growth centers, urban slums, and remote areas.) An incentive scheme was also implemented: villages verified to have 100 percent household latrine coverage became eligible for cash grants of US$3,000.[42] Regional and local governments, as well as nongovernmental organizations, also joined the effort to mobilize communities to become ODF, as well as to help develop a decentralized sanitation model.[43] Sanitation coverage in the country increased by 9 percent annually, and by 2014, 57 percent of the population had access to improved sanitation facilities.[44] Research has suggested that the rapid reduction in open defecation is among the factors that are associated with long-term improvements in average child height, possibly through reduced incidence of EED.[45]

Evidence on the impact of other WASH interventions in Bangladesh is now being weighed. The first phase of the SHOUHARDO Project (Strengthening Household Ability to Respond to Development Opportunities, funded by the US Agency for International Development and designed and implemented by CARE and the Government of Bangladesh), for example, served 2 million people between 2006 and 2010 (see Chapters 2 and 12). SHOUHARDO promoted WASH actions such as handwashing, food preparation, latrine use, and hygiene practices, combined with health education, exclusive breastfeeding, and supplementation.[46] A mixed-methods non- and quasi-experimental study found that during this first phase, the percentage of households with access to a sanitary latrine increased from 13.8 percent to 54.6 percent.[47] Chronic malnutrition among children 6–24 months of age in project areas declined from 56 percent to 40 percent; in contrast, in rural Bangladesh as a whole during this period there was no decline in stunting, and even an increase in later years, although many confounding factors are possibly at play. For households in the project, dietary diversity also increased by 25.7 percent.[48] Isolating the effect of sanitation alone on children's height-for-age Z-scores revealed no significant difference between the participating and control groups. However, the impact on children's height seemed to double when sanitation was combined with other maternal and child health and nutrition interventions, suggesting that sanitation and direct nutrition interventions had strong synergistic impacts.[49] The project's second phase (2010–2015) is due to release its findings soon.

Lessons Learned

These experiences from Mali and Bangladesh highlight a few lessons. First, all levels of government and civil society, notably the communities themselves, played key roles in many of these initiatives. Both government and civil society are likely integral to success, with government providing strategic direction, funding, and coordination among multiple actors, and communities adapting models such as CLTS to their own unique environments, improving sustainability.

Second, behavior change is critical for the success of WASH (see Box 8.2). Improved hygiene and sanitation practices in particular (unlike water quality improvements) are difficult to achieve without appealing to individuals, households, and whole communities to change. Behavior change communication that can deliver WASH messages, while highlighting the positive impact of WASH on nutrition and health, is thus integral to better outcomes.

At the same time, there are some challenges. The fact that WASH depends on behavior change makes measuring its impact on nutrition difficult. Evaluations rely on the ability of interventions to change behavior, first and foremost—only after this

BOX 8.2 An unexpected entry point for WASH

The Alive & Thrive Project, which operated in Bangladesh in 2011–2014, aimed to reduce child stunting and anemia among 8.5 million households with children under 2 years of age. Initially, the project focused its intervention and media campaign on improved infant and young child feeding practices (see Chapter 3). But in light of research that uncovered high rates of child diarrhea and poor hygiene practices, it soon integrated handwashing with soap, training community workers to communicate the importance of WASH for health and nutrition. Project results suggested a 67 percentage point increase in improved handwashing behavior by mothers before food preparation and child feeding, with nearly two-thirds of participating households installing soap and water near food preparation and feeding areas.[50] However, participants were also observed using the handwashing materials for other purposes, making the long-term benefits of the project difficult to assess. Nevertheless, these results highlight the importance of behavior change communication to both WASH and nutrition.

has been achieved can interventions' specific impact on nutrition be measured.[51] Apart from a few recent exceptions, most large-scale WASH interventions have achieved only small improvements in sanitation behavior, making research conclusions difficult to derive.[52] Even when behavior has successfully been altered, nutrition and health outcomes are rarely the focus of WASH program evaluations.

The different objectives of WASH and nutrition interventions creates another challenge. WASH aims for universal application: universal access to water, sanitation, or hygiene. Nutrition interventions, on the other hand, are more varied. Some, such as exclusive breastfeeding or fortification, are universal; but others, such as supplementation in young children, are more targeted.[53] Development practitioners and local communities must take these differences into account when designing effective programs and interventions.

WASH and nutrition are both high on the global political agenda. The Rome Declaration on Nutrition and the Framework for Action, adopted at the second International Conference on Nutrition in November 2014, recommends "actions on water, sanitation and hygiene." And the Sustainable Development Goals, adopted by the United Nations in 2015, identify the clear goal of "ensur[ing] availability and sustainable management of water and sanitation for all."[54] The time is ripe to collaborate across sectors and bring past lessons to bear on future WASH-nutrition interventions.

CHAPTER 9

Malnutrition's New Frontier

The Challenge of Obesity

JUDITH HODGE, ROOS VERSTRAETEN, AND ANGÉLICA OCHOA-AVILÉS

OVERWEIGHT AND OBESITY prevalence has increased substantially over the past decades, affecting 2.1 billion people worldwide and causing 3.4 million deaths globally.[1] Currently, 42 million children are overweight or obese—the result of a staggering 47.1 percent rise in prevalence between 1980 and 2013.[2] No longer exclusive to affluent societies, obesity has reached alarmingly high levels in many low- and middle-income countries (LMICs).[3] In fact, the number of individuals who are overweight or obese has now surpassed the 794 million people who do not get enough calories.[4] Nearly half of all overweight children under 5 years of age now live in Asia, and a further 25 percent are found in Africa.[5]

Unhealthy body weight carries significant health risks for lifestyle-related noncommunicable diseases (NCDs), including type 2 diabetes, hypertension, dyslipidemia (defined as abnormal levels of lipids, such as triglycerides or cholesterol, in the blood), and various cancers. This unhealthy body weight is of particular concern in children, as it exacerbates risk factors for developing NCDs in adulthood,[6] especially in those who have poor linear growth.[7]

Although the rate of increase in overweight prevalence has apparently slowed in some high-income countries (HICs), it is expected to continue increasing in LMICs.[8] Obesity and diabetes are complex, multifactorial problems with genetic, lifestyle, cultural, medical, and social causes.[9] Their rise in LMICs has been fueled by rapid economic, societal, and cultural changes, including such factors as urbanization, altered food patterns, physical inactivity, and sedentary behaviors, previously described as a global "nutrition transition."[10] Furthermore, the complexity of the problem is reflected in its increase in both urban *and* rural settings and across all levels of socioeconomic groups, including the poorest.[11]

No country to date has reversed its obesity epidemic; therefore few, if any, success stories exist, and none has succeeded on a large scale. Isolated pockets of "progress" have stemmed mainly from the plateauing of childhood obesity levels in some cities and countries where prevalence was high.[12]

Even so, preventing obesity in LMICs is a challenging but not impossible problem. Analysis of population-based strategies employed in LMICs with a high burden of obesity and diabetes shows that multi-intervention packages (which include fiscal and regulatory measures and health information and communication strategies) can deliver large and cost-effective health gains.[13] Consensus is beginning to emerge about which actions can best promote healthy diets.[14] Promising interventions, such as targeted food taxes and subsidies, nutrition labeling, regulation of food nutritional quality and availability in schools, and mass media campaigns, are already being successfully implemented in some countries (see Box 9.1 on interventions and case studies).[15] However, despite official commitments to global action,[16] Lachat et al. reported that currently only 82 of 140 LMICs have policies in place to tackle at least one risk factor for NCDs[17] (see Box 9.2). LMICs could dramatically reduce illness

TABLE 9.1 World Cancer Research Fund International NOURISHING framework

Domain		Policy area	Examples of potential policy actions
Food environment	N	Nutrition label standards and regulations on the use of claims and implied claims on foods	Nutrient lists on food packages; clearly visible "interpretive" and calorie labels; menu, shelf labels; rules on nutrient and health claims
	O	Offer healthy foods and set standards in public institutions and other specific settings	Fruit and vegetable programs; standards in education, work, health facilities; award schemes; choice architecture
	U	Use economic tools to address food affordability and purchase incentives	Targeted subsidies; price promotions at point of sale; unit pricing; health-related food taxes
	R	Restrict food advertising and other forms of commercial promotion	Restrict advertising to children that promotes unhealthy diets in all forms of media; sales promotions; packaging; sponsorship
	I	Improve the nutritional quality of the whole food supply chain	Reformulation to reduce salt and fats; elimination of trans fats; reduce energy density of processed foods; portion size limits
	S	Set incentives and rules to create a healthy retail and food service environment	Incentives for shops to locate in underserved areas; planning restrictions on food outlets; in-store promotions
Food system	H	Harness the food supply chain and actions across sectors to ensure coherence with health	Supply-chain incentives for production; public procurement through "short" chains; health-in-all policies; governance structures for multisectoral engagement
Behavior-change communication	I	Inform people about food and nutrition through public awareness	Education about food-based dietary guidelines, mass media, social marketing; community and public information campaigns
	N	Nutrition advice and counseling in health-care settings	Nutrition advice for at-risk individuals; telephone advice and support; clinical guidelines for health professionals on effective interventions for nutrition
	G	Give nutrition education and skills	Nutrition, cooking/food production skills in education curricula; workplace health schemes; health literacy programs

Source: World Cancer Research Fund International. Reproduced with permission.

and death from NCDs by investing just US$1–3 per person per year—a global cost of $11.2 billion per year. Conversely, cumulative costs due to NCDs are estimated to reach $7 trillion between 2011 and 2025 if countries take no action.[18]

A "Systems Approach" to Preventing Obesity

It can be a challenge for programs and policies to address food insecurity and hunger without adding to the burdens of obesity and NCDs. In Egypt, for example, subsidies for bread, wheat flour, sugar, and cooking oil are thought to have contributed to excessive energy intake and to have been partly responsible for the country's high prevalence of overweight and obesity.[19] In contrast, a "systems approach" to tackling obesity requires the creation of wide-ranging and enabling environments—social, economic, and policy as well as physical environments.[20] The World Cancer Research Fund's NOURISHING framework draws together core policy actions to promote healthy diets using the consensus on "what works"' based on both research and practice (see Table 9.1).[21] (See Box 9.1 for examples of interventions in LMICs and case studies.) Furthermore, controlling nutrition policy and the food supply is important for preventing both stunting *and* obesity, in light of their coexistence within the same population or even in the same individual.[22] This type of control requires a coherent nutrition policy to address malnutrition

BOX 9.1 Some NOURISHING interventions in low- and middle-income countries

Monitoring and evaluation of these types of interventions in low- and middle-income countries (LMICs) are urgently needed to show evidence of impact.

Nutrition labeling: In 2014, Ecuador's Ministry of Public Health implemented "traffic-light" labeling on packaged foods to indicate levels of fats, sugar, and salt (red for high, orange for medium, and green for low).

Offer healthy foods in specific settings (for example, schools): Schools in Costa Rica are permitted to sell only food and drink that meet specific nutritional criteria (policy implemented in 2012 and upheld following a challenge from the Costa Rican Food Industry Association).[23]

Use economic tools: See the discussion of Mexico's soda tax in this chapter.

Restrict food advertising: Since 2003, 20 countries globally (including Malaysia and Thailand) have developed or are developing policies to restrict TV advertising of unhealthy foods to children.[24]

Improve nutritional quality of whole-food supply chain: Forty percent of manufacturers in Hungary changed their product formulas to reduce taxable ingredients, following a 2011 law taxing food and drink components that pose a high risk to health, such as sugar, salt, and caffeine. A year later, sales had fallen 27 percent and people consumed 25–35 percent fewer such products.[25]

Harness food supply chains across sectors (agriculture and food systems): Brazil's "home-grown" school feeding program legally stipulates that 30 percent of the national school meals budget be spent on healthy foods from family farms. Strong government leadership, an intersectoral decision-making process, and political pressure from civil society organizations were key factors in achieving this integrated approach. However, there is currently little evidence available on the specific impacts of school feeding on schoolchildren's diet and nutrition.[26]

Give nutrition education and skills: See the discussion of Ecuador's ACTIVITAL program in this chapter.

in all its forms, without too much emphasis on overweight but with a focus in the early years on healthy growth so that children do not become either stunted (low height-for-age) or overweight[27] (see Chapter 3 on infant and young child feeding).

Sweet Success for Mexico's Soda Tax

With one of the highest rates of diabetes, overweight, and obesity in the world, Mexico is in urgent need of strategies to tackle the obesity epidemic. Nearly 70 percent of the population is overweight (body mass index [BMI] ≥ 25 kg/m²), 9 percent of children are overweight, and approximately 1 in 3 adults are obese (BMI ≥ 30 kg/m²).[28] Each year, approximately 70,000 deaths in Mexico are attributed to diabetes (now the third leading cause of death), for which obesity is a significant risk factor.[29] One policy action is to use economic tools such as taxation to improve food environments.

Taxing sugary drinks in Mexico is an obvious policy choice, since the country's population drinks more than 160 liters per person per year (among the top global consumption levels), and 80 percent of teenagers and 71 percent of adults drink at least one full-calorie soda each day.[30] In 2013, the Mexican government passed an excise duty of 1 peso ($0.080) per liter on sugary drinks and a tax of 8 percent on foods with high caloric density. The sugar-sweetened beverage tax applies to any beverages with added sugar, such as sugar-sweetened carbonated drinks (soda or soft drinks), energy drinks, and bottled teas and coffees.

Raising Taxes Equals Lowering Consumption

The World Health Organization (WHO) claims that soda taxes are the most effective strategy for improving diet, along with subsidizing fruit and vegetables.[31] Evidence that taxing sugar-sweetened beverages can reduce obesity and chronic disease comes primarily from theoretical models, because it is difficult to isolate the taxes' effects since most countries tax a large number of foods. It is also difficult to determine the taxes' impact on obesity and disease, partly because so few sugar-sweetened-beverage taxes have been implemented.

When Mexico's sugar-sweetened-beverage tax went into effect on January 1, 2014, it increased the average price of a liter of soda by about 10 percent. During the first year, the average volume of taxed beverages purchased monthly was 6 percent lower than would have been expected without the tax.[32] The decline started slowly but accelerated; by December 2014 soda sales were down 12 percent from December 2013 levels. Moreover, the reduction was greatest among households of low socioeconomic status, which by December were buying 17 percent fewer sugary drinks. Purchases of untaxed beverages (mainly bottled water) rose by 4 percent, with households

BOX 9.2 Barriers to progress

Why has progress been so slow toward developing large-scale preventive policies and regulations to address global obesity and related NCDs? One of the greatest barriers is the increased access in LMICs to cheaper processed, energy-dense foods and beverages—also known as "junk food" or ultra-processed food.[33] Participants in a recent international symposium on obesity argued that this access is reinforced by concerted efforts by the large transnational food and drink manufacturers of these products (collectively known as "Big Food") to undermine and defeat many public policies to prevent obesity.[34] Other barriers include the restricted ability or unwillingness of governments to implement policies, lack of pressure from civil society for political action (particularly in LMICs), and too few evidence-based evaluations of the effects of many programs and policies that have been implemented.[35]

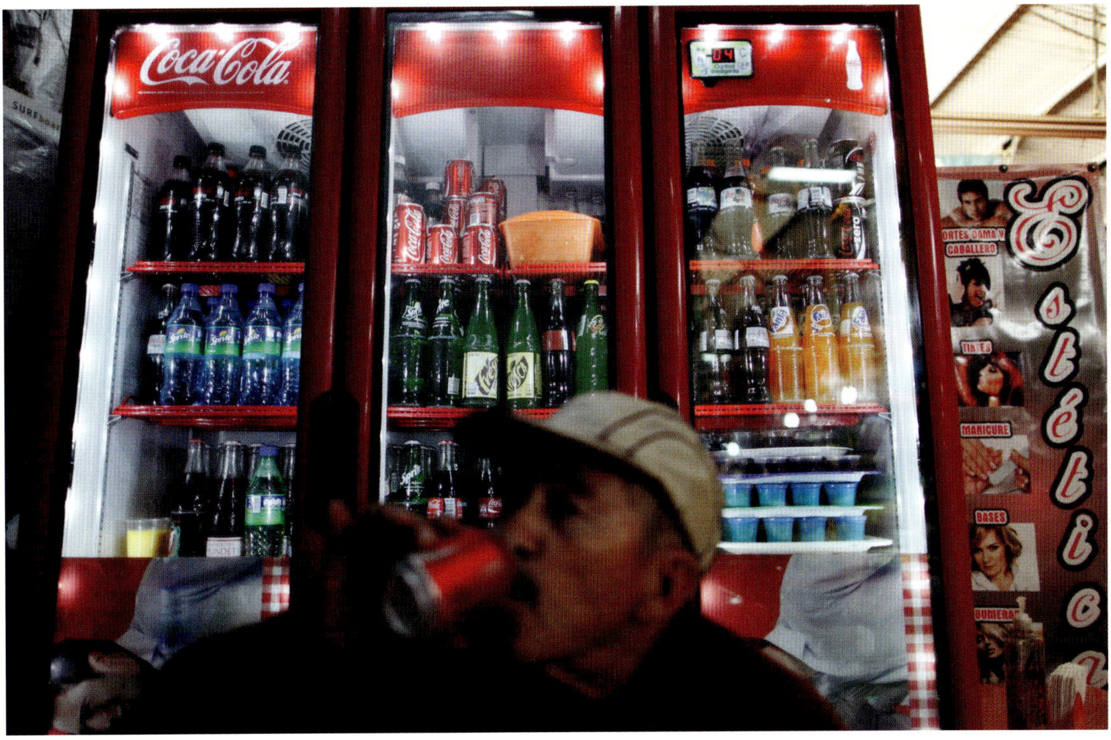

Reuters/E. Garrido

When Mexico, which has high rates of obesity and diabetes, initiated a soda tax in 2014, consumption of sweetened beverages started to fall.

of middle socioeconomic status increasing their purchases the most.[36]

The Road to Success

The release of the country's 2006 National Survey of Health and Nutrition was a wake-up call. Between 1999 and 2006, obesity in children aged 5–11 years rose by 40 percent—no other country in the world had experienced a rise in obesity of that magnitude within a similar time frame.[37] The health secretary at the time called on Juan Rivera, founding director of the Center for Research in Nutrition and Health at Mexico's Institute of Public Health, to come up with some urgent recommendations. Rivera responded with a comprehensive program to which the politician's pragmatic reply was, "It's too complicated; choose one thing!" Rivera chose reduction of soda consumption, but modest health promotion efforts (to put a poster in every health center of a jug illustrating the ideal balance for daily beverage intake) came to nothing in the face of overwhelming industry opposition.[38] With such formidable—and well-financed—opponents, how did the soda tax come into force less than 10 years later?

Passage of the sugar-sweetened beverage tax occurred quickly after President Enrique Peña included it within his September 2013 economic package, but the broad-based coalition proposing the bill had already developed a well-planned and coordinated strategy many years before the tax discussions. Each part of this alliance has played its role: researchers provided objective scientific evidence, lobbyists analyzed the political context and identified legislative allies, and consumer advocates fielded a strong media campaign.[39]

Twelve Spoonfuls of Sugar

One influential nutrition champion was Alejandro Calvillo (formerly of Greenpeace Mexico), who started the organization El Poder del Consumidor (Consumer Power), an informal network of groups working on health and environment issues (the Nutritional Alliance). The alliance succeeded in influencing government recommendations to keep junk food out of schools and to limit advertising on children's television. The soda tax (part of a broader policy agenda) was chosen as a high-priority goal, and a $10 million three-year fund from Bloomberg Philanthropies leveled the playing field against the food industry, enabling the alliance to create a high-impact media campaign and engage lobbyists.[40] The advertisement that came to symbolize the campaign was titled "12 spoonfuls of sugar" and drew attention to the amount in a bottle of soda, linking its consumption to diabetes. When television stations refused to carry the advertisements (citing concerns about loss of industry advertising revenue), advocates used social media, such as YouTube and Twitter, to highlight the censorship.[41]

Timing It Right

Political changes in 2013 (a newly elected president and legislature) presented the alliance with a window of opportunity, and its members knew that the government's priority of raising revenue had focused its interest on new taxes.[42] Initially, a 20 percent tax—the minimum recommended to theoretically have an effect on health outcomes—had been proposed,[43] with the expectation that this would be watered down. Efforts to tie some of the new revenue raised by the soda tax to installing water fountains in schools and public spaces garnered crucial public support; thanks to further advocacy, the senate passed a resolution to use part of the taxes to provide potable water to public schools, particularly in low-income areas.[44]

Key Lessons from Mexico

Although success depends on the social and political context of different countries, some features of Mexico's sugar-sweetened-beverage advocacy campaign could be adapted to other settings[45]:

1. engage organizations that have a strong background in media advocacy and strategic campaign development and that are recognized as legitimate defenders of the public's interest;
2. develop an understanding of the scientific literature and focus on how evidence can be used to defend policy measures and craft messages for media advocacy and lobbying;
3. understand and use the political context to effectively influence policy at opportune moments (seize the right window of opportunity).

ACTIVITAL: Evidence for Success in Promoting Child Health in Ecuador

An estimated 25 percent (51.8 million) of Latin American children and adolescents are overweight or obese, with adverse consequences for their health and their lives.[46] The rapid increase in unhealthy body weight has been fueled by poor diets (such as diets low in fruits and vegetables) and low levels of physical activity.[47] Ecuador—where 26 percent of adolescents aged 12–19 years are overweight or obese and have other equally worrisome risk factors[48]—is no exception to this general trend in Latin America.[49] Despite the high burden of childhood obesity in Ecuador, it remains mostly underappreciated as a public health issue, as shown by the absence of adequate intervention strategies and multisectoral public health policies. Preventive school-based interventions promoting a healthy diet and an active lifestyle are a promising means of improving child and adolescent health and curbing the rise of the obesity burden.[50] Most of the evidence on effective, well-documented, and properly evaluated interventions, however, originates from HICs.[51] Strong evaluation designs, documented pathways through which such interventions have their effect, and process evaluations are urgently needed to strengthen the evidence base in LMICs.[52]

A School-Based Health Promotion Program

This case study describes the participatory theory- and evidence-based ACTIVITAL program (Health Promotion Intervention in Ecuadorian Adolescents to Promote Healthy Dietary and Physical Activity Patterns), a school-based health promotion program aimed at improving dietary and physical activity behaviors among Ecuadorian adolescents aged 11–15 years. The intervention was implemented among 1,430 school-going adolescents in 20 schools in the urban area of Cuenca over three years from 2009 to 2012.

The intervention consisted of two components: one directed toward changing individual behavior and the other aimed at changing the environment. The individual strategy consisted of an interactive toolkit taught by schoolteachers on healthy eating and physical activity. The environmental strategy comprised participatory workshops with parents and food service staff (on topics such

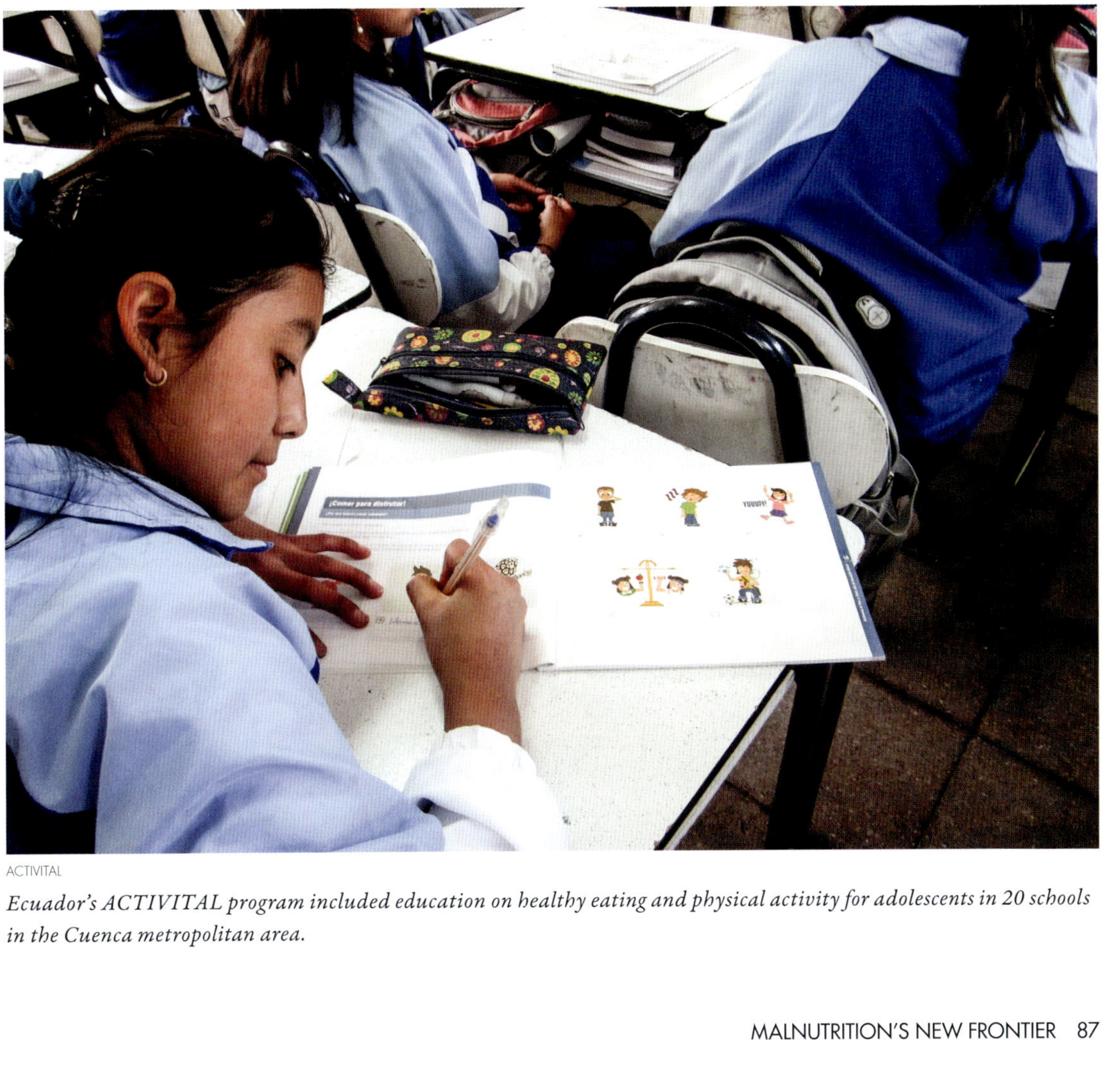

ACTIVITAL

Ecuador's ACTIVITAL program included education on healthy eating and physical activity for adolescents in 20 schools in the Cuenca metropolitan area.

as healthy eating, physical activity, portion sizes, and food safety), social events such as preparing healthy breakfasts, motivational talks by famous local athletes, and the creation of walking trails in the schools. These strategies were implemented in 10 intervention schools, while the normal curriculum was maintained in the remaining 10 schools. The primary indicators used to measure program performance were the nutritional value of dietary intake, physical activity, physical fitness, and screen time. Body mass index (BMI), waist circumference, and blood pressure were among the secondary indicators. An in-depth process evaluation was also carried out.

The program effectively decreased added sugar and processed food intake during snacks, waist circumference, and blood pressure among members of the intervention group. The intervention also weakened the trends toward lower fruit and vegetable intake, less physical activity, and more sedentary behavior.[53] Furthermore, the intervention had no adverse effects, did not result in stigmatization, did not increase undernourishment, and benefited socioeconomic groups equally.

Lessons Learned

The results of ACTIVITAL add to the available evidence on the effectiveness of school-based health promotion interventions in the wider context of obesity prevention in LMICs. One key lesson of ACTIVITAL was the importance of integrating this health promotion intervention within a broader structural platform to amplify its success. Recommendations for future studies include:

1. incorporating these types of programs into the standard educational curriculum (no support from government was obtained for ACTIVITAL);
2. integrating health education activities with environmental changes (for example, changing food offerings at school needs to go hand in hand with regulating food vendors in the immediate area of the school; see the NOURISHING framework); and
3. contextualizing intervention strategies.

On a positive note, political processes prioritizing chronic diseases and the obesity crisis in Ecuador are beginning to emerge, resulting in changes in nutrition labeling (see Box 9.1). Discussions have been initiated with the government to scale up the ACTIVITAL intervention to the national level.

Looking Ahead

Obesity and related NCDs are complex, multifaceted problems facing all countries. Although individual behavioral changes are important, individuals have little influence over factors such as globalization that have profoundly altered food systems. Success in addressing the "obesogenic environment" created by these changes requires a whole-society approach and the involvement of multiple actors. These include different government departments (not just health, but agriculture, education, food production, trade, taxation, and urban development), civil society organizations, the media, the food industry, healthcare providers, transport providers, and urban planners.[54] Much can be learnt from the well-documented story of the battle against the tobacco industry, such as the need to use the power of the media and to make data politically relevant, as well as the importance of community action in galvanizing the political will to intervene in market practices.[55]

Part III: Transforming National Policy and Programming

CHAPTER 10

Local to National

Thailand's Integrated Nutrition Program

STUART GILLESPIE, KRAISID TONTISIRIN, AND LAURA ZSELECZKY

THAILAND REDUCED CHILD undernutrition by more than half within one decade—an achievement recognized by the nutrition community as one of the best examples of a successful national nutrition program.[1] Underweight rates among children under five decreased from more than 50 percent to less than 20 percent from 1982 to 1991, and severe and moderate underweight rates were nearly eliminated.[2] The underweight rate was further reduced to 10 percent by 1996[3] and to 9 percent[4] by 2012. Maternal care interventions were also successful. Thailand improved the reach of antenatal care—coverage increased from 35 percent in 1981 to near 95 percent in 2006.[5] And iron-deficiency anemia prevalence among pregnant women was reduced from nearly 60 percent in the 1960s to 10 percent in 2005.[6]

Thailand's gains in nutrition were driven in large part by strong political will, clear goals, effective strategic and program planning, and sustained integrated action and systematic monitoring. Most notably, this success was fueled by widespread mobilization of volunteers and by community ownership. Nutrition was recognized as a fundamental element of development at all levels of society and across sectors ranging from health and agriculture to education and rural development. Communities were supported by government officials and professional experts in assessing their basic needs and creating development plans based on their priorities. Ongoing monitoring increased community awareness about the importance of nutrition and fed back to policies and programs at district and national levels.

This chapter explores the evolution of Thailand's approach to nutrition programming in the 1970s and 1980s, examining the factors that made it a success and lessons learned from the country's experience.

Tackling Undernutrition as a Symptom of Poverty

Nutrition was first integrated into Thailand's five-year national development plans in the 1970s and gained increasing importance in the country's

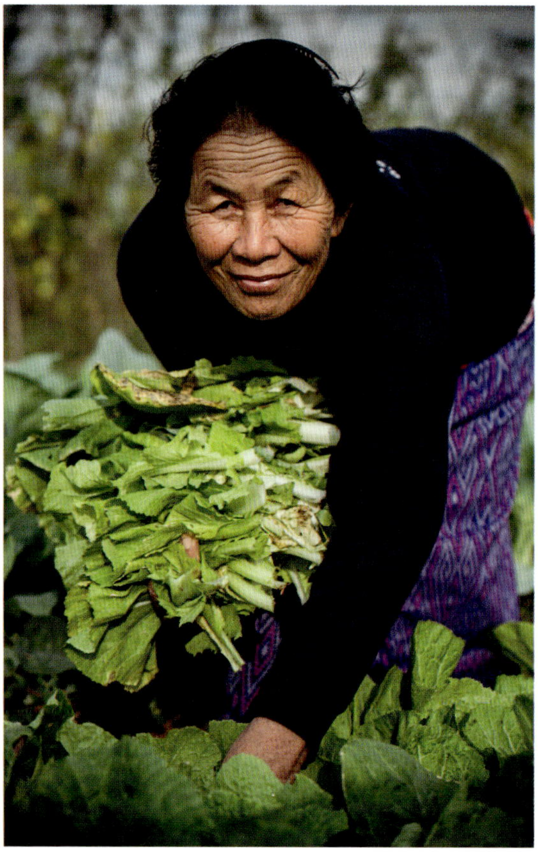

Asian Development Bank

Thailand adopted an integrated approach to nutrition policy that included a range of sectors, including agriculture.

efforts to address poverty in subsequent plans. In the 1960s and early 1970s, Thailand's National Development Plans focused primarily on expanding agricultural area to increase production, not on nutritional challenges.[7] Yet a Department of Health survey from 1960 revealed a 57 percent rate of anemia in pregnant women, national deficiencies in vitamin B1 (23 percent) and vitamin B2 (47 percent), and 29 percent of school children experiencing goiter.[8] At the time, nutrition was considered the purview of the health sector. While an Applied Nutrition Program with a focus on production and consumption of protein-rich foods was piloted in the poorest region of the country, nutrition was not viewed as a major development issue in terms of national planning.[9]

By the late 1970s, understanding of the role of nutrition had increased, and experts recognized the need to combat and prevent undernutrition through a multisectoral approach. The fourth National Development Plan in 1977 included the country's first Food and Nutrition Plan, which sought to provide health services and address key nutrition issues, including protein-energy malnutrition, iron deficiency anemia, iodine deficiency, bladder stones, and vitamin A, B1, and B2 deficiencies.[10] Interventions were targeted to pregnant women and young children, especially those under five, as well as economically disadvantaged groups.[11]

As undernutrition persisted, Thailand's approach evolved to meet the challenge. With the fifth national plan in 1982, undernutrition was not only recognized as a development issue but also as a symptom of poverty. A Poverty Alleviation Program (PAP) was introduced to improve nutrition and promote development. The PAP targeted 288 districts and sub-districts in 38 of the poorest provinces, covering about half of the country.[12] A National Nutrition Committee was established, with members from health, agriculture, education, rural administration, planning, and academic sectors, to support the PAP with input on nutrition indicators and actions. The multisectoral political commitment to nutrition at the national level was complemented by planning and implementation at province, district, and local community levels. Village health volunteers, 80 percent of whom were women, were trained to provide primary healthcare, especially to mothers and children, and communicate important nutrition messages.[13] With one volunteer for every 10–20 households at the program's outset, and eventually one for every 10 households, the most vulnerable members of the community could be reached. By 1989, more than 500,000 volunteers had been trained, covering most of the country's rural areas.[14] The PAP also incorporated the Food and Nutrition Plan, which emphasized local production of supplementary foods for pregnant women and complementary foods for infants and young children.[15]

Thailand also introduced the basic minimum needs (BMN) approach as part of the PAP. Communities conducted BMN surveys to identify priority areas for development, such as adequate food and nutrition, safety and security, basic health and education, efficient food production, and participation in community development. Each community then identified a set of actions to address the local issues. The central government ensured convergence of supportive multisectoral programs for job creation, agricultural production, and provision of services and basic sanitation at the community level. Nutrition indicators were included in the BMN indicators used to monitor progress and set goals. Under this system, growth monitoring and promotion coverage increased from approximately 1 million to 2.6 million children. The BMN approach promoted multisector development activities, as well as community ownership of assessment and monitoring processes. The major successes of the approach were the generation of local-level data that fed into district-, province-, and ministry-level monitoring and the prominence given to nutrition that led policy makers and communities to recognize its key role in development.[16]

Factors Contributing to Success

Thailand's nutrition program provides a clear example of how prioritized, effective, and explicit nutrition-relevant action on the part of governments can transform the nutritional status of a nation within a decade. Four key factors contributed to the rapid decline in undernutrition in Thailand: planning, integration, social mobilization, and local action-oriented surveillance.

Planning

Planning at micro and macro levels was facilitated through the BMN approach, whereby communities identified development priorities based on a survey measuring 32 indicators in eight areas; adequate food and nutrition was the first category on the list of indicators that communities considered in the prioritization process. Nutrition-relevant indicators included outcome indicators such as child malnutrition, low birth-weight, and micronutrient deficiencies, as well as process indicators such as immunization coverage, antenatal care coverage, availability of potable water, and sanitary services. At the micro level, teams of community leaders, nutrition and health experts, midlevel government officials, nongovernmental organization (NGO) representatives, and district and sub-district sector chiefs undertook community planning to assess community needs. They agreed upon a set of BMN indicators which would translate into goals reflecting local priorities and would then be monitored for progress. Working together, service providers and community leaders established plans for a set of nutrition-relevant actions targeted to vulnerable and disadvantaged groups in order to address the problems revealed by the indicators. At the macro level, a core group of representatives from the nutrition and health professions, government, and international agencies supported these community processes by promoting collaboration among the health, agriculture, education, and rural development sectors. Training and workshops on community-based nutrition programming were organized for district chiefs and reinforced through field visits to communities. Training workshops and seed money were also provided by international agencies.

Integration

Nutrition was understood to be a multifaceted issue, requiring change not only in the health sector but also in agriculture and education. The PAP cut across multiple sectors, facilitating coordination and integration of minimum basic services at all levels—national, regional, local, and community. Health components focused primarily on antenatal care for pregnant women, growth monitoring and promotion for infants and young children, and promotion and support of breastfeeding and appropriate complementary feeding. Program activities also covered other basic health services such as immunization, oral rehydration therapy, deworming, treatment of local endemic diseases, and the provision of potable water and sanitary latrines. In addition, individuals, families, and communities were involved in agricultural and education activities designed to build self-reliance through improved food security, income generation, and behavior change for long-term gains in nutrition.

Projects in the education sector, such as school meal programs and micronutrient supplementation, sought to improve child nutrition. Curricula were updated with nutrition and health education materials, and nutritious food production and consumption were promoted through investments in school gardens and kitchens. Outside of formal education activities, efforts were made to better coordinate health and agriculture extension services, develop information systems to monitor the nutritional status of vulnerable groups, and educate consumers to select, prepare, and store food in healthy and safe ways. Under the Poverty Alleviation Program, investments in agriculture included horticultural and animal husbandry programs to strengthen subsistence food production as well as support for home gardening to produce locally sourced supplementary foods for pregnant women and adolescent girls and complementary foods for young children. Community agricultural research through collaboration with universities and research entities, such as Chiang Mai University's Center for Community-Based Research, helped identify and address local agricultural challenges.[17]

Social Mobilization

Service delivery was supported by a cadre of community health and nutrition volunteers or "mobilizers" who were selected by their communities. These mobilizers were trained to work with service providers or "facilitators"—usually paid healthcare workers, NGO employees, or university or research staff—to implement nutrition programming. A ratio of one mobilizer to 10–20 households was sought for optimal program reach and effectiveness (see discussion of "intensity" in Chapter 2). These positions were unpaid, but mobilizers received free medical services for themselves and their families and public recognition of their work with awards and certificates.

Training and support formed a critical part of the program. Mobilizers participated in an initial two-week training focused on the theory and practical application of basic nutrition and health facts, especially antenatal and postnatal care, maternal and childcare practices, birth spacing, breastfeeding, immunization, complementary feeding, and growth monitoring and promotion. The training also emphasized communication skills to effectively provide information on nutrition and care of women and children, and to build interest in self-help activities, particularly among women's groups. Supervision at all levels was also key to the success of the mobilizer program. Facilitators visited mobilizers every one to two months to provide support—rather than policing—through on-the-spot training and problem-solving along with technical and managerial information-sharing. This form of regular supervision was most effective, but was supplemented with monthly or bimonthly review meetings and communication through social events and printed media. Key elements of the mobilizers' work were tracking and evaluating impact indicators and using growth charts to discuss and support child growth within communities.

Local Monitoring

Regular weighing and health checks of all preschool children every three months served as a screening, educational, remedial, and integrative tool for both mobilizers and mothers. This growth monitoring and promotion was designed to shift responsibility from health workers to the community by enabling mothers to visualize their children's growth and take responsibility for their nutrition improvement. An evaluation by the Ministry of Public Health (MOPH) and key informant interviews with senior MOPH staff involved in the program suggest that the program did a better job of weighing and charting than of analysis of the causes of undernutrition and subsequent counseling. The MOPH made an effort to improve growth monitoring and promotion in the late 1980s. Subsequent evaluation results revealed a reduction in child refusals to be weighed (from 31 percent to 8 percent) and an increase in the proportion of accurate weighings (from 79 percent to 92 percent), but analysis of the causes of undernutrition still remained low at 46 percent of cases and nutrition education was only provided to 64 percent of caretakers.[18] Communities also used the other BMN indicators to monitor progress and guide development activities. By the mid-1990s, these indicators were used in over 95 percent of villages. In areas with rapid improvement, modifications were made to add new indicators or raise the criteria for success to a higher level.[19]

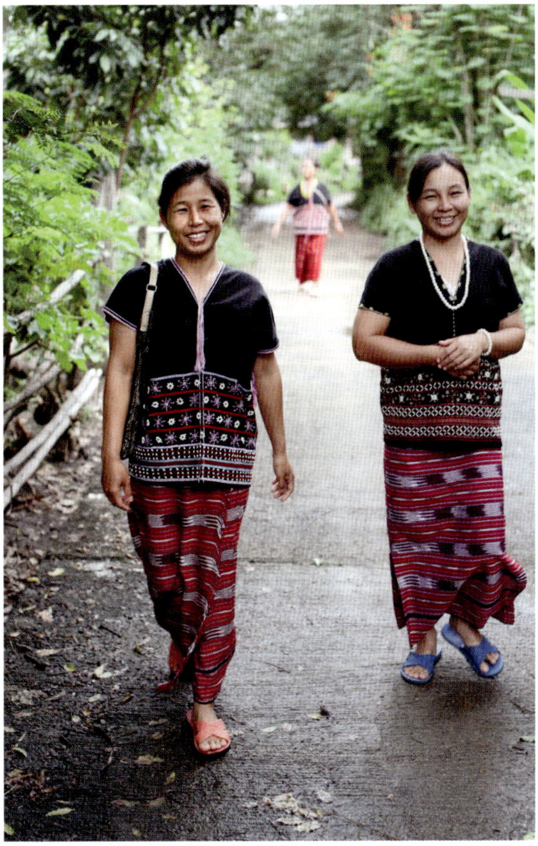

Thomas Fuller/ The New York Times/Redux

Widespread mobilization of community health volunteers like these helped Thailand make gains in nutrition.

Lessons Learned

Thailand's national nutrition development was accomplished through a process with nine key components: (1) recognizing nutrition problems, (2) assessing nutrition status, (3) using experience from successful nutrition programs to build critical mass around key influencers, (4) cultivating political and social commitment, (5) increasing collaboration and planning between sectors, (6) building awareness and initiating action, (7) integrating nutrition into social and health development, (8) improving quality of life through community participation, and (9) targeting services and resources to the areas and individuals with greatest need. The country's success in reducing undernutrition nationwide in such a short time span offers a number of lessons.

First, recognition of the importance of nutrition at the highest levels of the political system and by all sectors ensured the central role of nutrition programming in the nation's development efforts. Nearly 20 percent of total government expenditure was invested in health, alongside similar investments in education.[20] Undernutrition was understood not only as a health issue but also as a multisectoral problem to be addressed by agriculture, education, and income-generation schemes. Moreover, the country recognized the need for action at the level of the national planning committee as well as at district, sub-district, and local levels. Awareness at the community level increased in large part as a result of the growth monitoring and promotion and BMN programs and educational campaigns.[21]

Second, the nutrition program was the result of strategic planning and coordination at all levels, combined with government support for community priorities. The use of simple indicators for village-based social planning served to set locally valid program objectives and provide a framework for evaluation as well as empowering community members to participate in development activities with support and guidance from the government. The BMN approach offered a standard set of indicators, with backing from policy makers and experts at the national and district levels, which could be tailored to the needs of communities. Once priority areas were identified, communities were able to select from a menu of nutrition-relevant actions to develop a plan based on their needs. This menu of actions was supported and coordinated at national and district levels to ensure that standard approaches were used throughout the country while still allowing for flexibility based on local needs. Through this process, the role of local officers shifted from that of active agents to facilitators and advisers. Community-government partnership was strengthened as top-down and bottom-up approaches were integrated (Figure 10.1). With a wide range of sectors and issues represented by the indicators, this approach promoted the integration of multisectoral services at the community level and the targeting of resources to areas of greatest need.

FIGURE 10.1 **Nexus of community-government partnership for nutrition in Thailand**

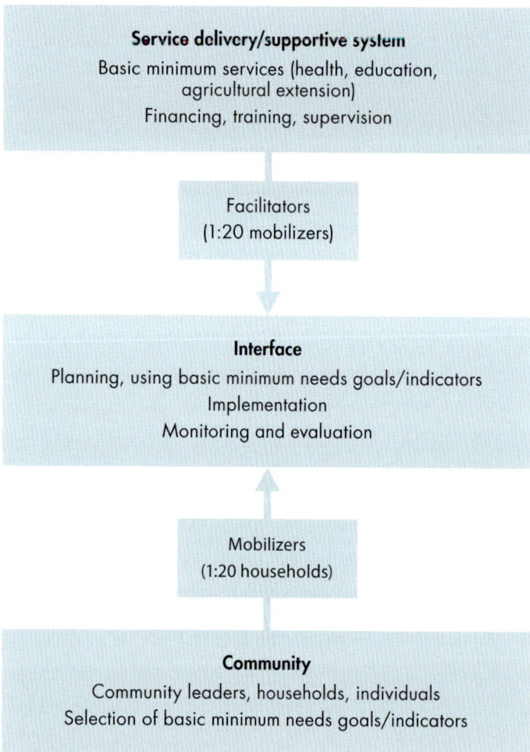

Source: K. Tontisirin and S. Gillespie, "Linking Community-based Programs and Service Delivery for Improving Maternal and Child Nutrition," *Asian Development Review* 17, no. 1–2 (1999): 50. Courtesy of MIT Press Journals.

A third lesson from the Thai experience is the need for adequate ratios of community workers or volunteers to the population for effective implementation of the national nutrition program. The involvement of community volunteers at such a large scale helped cut costs, empower local people, and build self-reliance.[22] Since mobilizers in Thailand were only responsible for 10–20 households, they were able to regularly monitor the nutrition and health needs of community members. This also enabled mobilizers to easily identify the most vulnerable individuals and target resources more effectively. Further, since the mobilizers were volunteers, this ratio prevented overburdening these community leaders.

Thailand's experience provides one of the best examples of national policies and strategies designed to be integrated with local decision making and responsive to the experience of community-based nutrition programs and projects.[23] Strong political will, multisector coordination, integration of macro- and micro-level planning, and the widespread mobilization and support of community volunteers were essential to the country's successful nutrition program.

Nutrition in Thailand: Present and Future

In the years since Thailand's success in driving down rates of undernutrition, new challenges have emerged. Some segments of the population continue to grapple with undernutrition, while the prevalence of overweight, obesity, and risk factors for noncommunicable diseases (NCDs) are cause for concern.

According to the *2015 Global Nutrition Report,* Thailand continues to face a number of malnutrition challenges and the country is off course for all World Health Assembly nutrition targets.[24] The report found that stunting still affects 16 percent of children under five (some 604,000 children), reflecting little improvement since 2006. Seven percent of children under five are affected by wasting, and 2 percent suffer from severe wasting. The rate of exclusive breastfeeding of infants under six months old is 12 percent, and 24 percent of women of reproductive age are anemic. At the same time, overweight, obesity, and NCDs are growing problems. Eleven percent of children under five are overweight; nearly a third of adults are overweight and 9 percent are obese. Adult females experience higher rates of both overweight and obesity than adult males. Risk factors for diet-related NCDs also present potential challenges.

A number of factors may be at work behind these numbers. The persistence of undernutrition among the poorest members of the population, as well as certain subpopulations such as the hill tribes, suggests that undernutrition is linked to broader issues of extreme poverty and social dislocation not addressed by the country's nutrition program.[25] The growing incidence of overweight, obesity, and NCDs may have diverted policy-maker attention from undernutrition issues.[26] Community health workers continue to be recruited, but mobilization is now focused on preventing and controlling obesity and NCDs. Rising incomes and lifestyle changes have contributed to reduced physical activity and increased access to processed foods among much of the population. And increased accessibility of supermarkets as well as fast food restaurants, particularly in urban areas, has changed where people buy food and how often they cook at home. These lifestyle changes have also decreased consumption of traditional Thai food that contains a number of nutritious ingredients.[27]

The Government of Thailand has committed to addressing its present nutrition challenges with plans that draw on the lessons learned two decades ago. In 2008, the government enacted the National Food Committee Act with the aim of developing food policies and strategies across sectors and at all levels throughout the country. The act integrates activities from more than 10 agencies and over 30 other acts. The prime minister (or designated deputy) chairs the committee; committee members include experts as well as representatives from 11 ministries.[28] In 2010, the Cabinet approved a Strategic Framework for Food Management for 2012–2016 comprising four themes that cover the food chain from the household to the national level: food security; food quality and safety; food education; and food management.[29] Thematic committees were appointed to facilitate and coordinate the framework at the national level, while implementation takes place at the local and workplace levels.

Similar to the Poverty Alleviation Program, the Strategic Framework identifies community actions to address the double burden of malnutrition and NCDs, including the provision of basic health, education, agriculture, and other social services, through the mobilization of volunteers.[30] Nutrition indicators now go beyond undernutrition to measure overweight, obesity, and other factors contributing to NCDs. The framework integrates a number of fragmented programs, including efforts to promote production and marketing of nutritious food; reduce sugar consumption, salt consumption, and obesity; improve labeling and food safety; and promote physical activity, exercise, and nutrition education. For example, programs to control overweight and obesity among students through monitoring, nutritious food promotion, and physical exercise are being tested in 27 schools in Bangkok and 600 schools throughout the country.

As recent studies indicate that Thailand's success in reducing child undernutrition has stagnated and that new challenges in terms of overweight and NCDs are on the rise, the country is committed to learning from past experiences. The set of nutrition challenges may be different today, but Thailand is striving to build on the lessons learned about the power of community-government partnerships that are aligned with well-monitored, multisectoral efforts to yield notable results.

CHAPTER 11

Nutrition and Equality

Brazil's Success in Reducing Stunting among the Poorest

MEAGAN KEEFE

RAPID ADVANCES IN economic development and healthcare in Brazil have contributed to significant improvements in child health and nutrition in recent decades. Brazil met Millennium Development Goal 1—halving the proportion of people whose income is less than $1 a day and halving the proportion of people who suffer from hunger, and Goal 4—reducing by two-thirds the under-five mortality rate. Beyond significant advances in reducing poverty and improving food and nutrition security throughout the country, Brazil has also been successful in reducing socioeconomic inequality in malnutrition.[1] What lies behind this success? This case study examines the policies, approaches, and process that contributed to the reduction in child stunting and other key indicators of malnutrition.

Child stunting levels provide dramatic evidence of Brazil's progress toward eradicating hunger. The overall prevalence of child stunting was reduced by more than 80 percent between 1974/1975 and 2006/2007 (from 37.1 to 7.1 percent). This decline accelerated over time from 4.2 percent per year between 1974/1975 and 1989, to 5.4 percent between 1989 and 1996, to 6.0 percent between 1996 and 2006/2007.[2] Brazil has demonstrated similar success in breastfeeding. In Brazil's 27 state capitals, the prevalence of exclusive breastfeeding in infants under six months of age (as recommended by UNICEF) increased from 26.7 to 41.0 percent between 1999 and 2008.[3] In addition, partial breastfeeding practices also improved from a median duration of 2.5 months in the 1970s to 7 months in 1996, and reached 14 months in 2006/2007.[4]

At the same time, Brazil also has made great strides in reducing the socioeconomic and geographic inequalities in child stunting across the country. Children from families in the lowest wealth quintile were 7.7 times more likely than children in the highest quintile to have stunted growth in 1989. By 2007/2008, they were only 2.6 times as likely to suffer stunting.[5] Historically, stunting prevalence has been much higher in Brazil's poorest region, the northeast, than in the wealthier southeast region. In 1996, stunting was four times more common in the northeast than in the southeast. But with the reduction in prevalence of stunting in the northeast from 22.2 percent in 1995 to 5.9 percent in 2006/07, little difference remained between the northeast and wealthier regions.[6]

A Multisectoral Approach

The 2013 *Lancet* Maternal and Child Nutrition Series provided a new framework for understanding how to achieve optimal fetal and child growth and development. Positive changes to enhance growth and development can be understood by examining the dietary, behavioral, and health determinants of optimum nutrition, growth, and development and how they are affected by food security, caregiving resources, and environmental conditions. This framework highlights the potential effects of nutrition-sensitive interventions that address the underlying determinants of malnutrition and shows how to build an enabling environment to support interventions that enhance health and nutrition outcomes.[7] Brazil's multisectoral approach to reducing poverty, inequality, and food insecurity targeted income redistribution and universal access to education, health, and sanitation services. Using the *Lancet*'s framework, we examine the policies and programs likely associated with improvements in several nutrition-relevant domains: maternal schooling, family purchasing power, maternal and child healthcare, and water supply and sanitation services. Brazil has made significant progress in these underlying determinants. However, their precise contribution to reductions in stunting cannot be directly measured.

Improvements in Women's Educational Status

The single most important factor associated with the decline in child undernutrition was the transformation in women's education that took place between 1996 and 2007.[8] Brazil implemented a range of policies designed to ensure universal access to primary education and to improve the quality of primary and secondary schools across all municipalities. Brazilian mothers became more educated than ever before.[9] In addition to substantial investments in public education, Brazilian policies also sought to reduce the significant disparities between poor and rich municipalities.[10] Starting in 1996, Brazil modified the way it was funding primary education. Moving from a formula based on population density to a system based on minimum per-pupil allocations helped reduce the bias toward large cities and made funding for education more equitable. A set percentage of revenue from federal, state, and municipal taxes was dedicated to basic and secondary education. In order to raise all elementary schools to the minimum per-pupil funding allocation, the government provided additional federal funding to states with fewer resources.[11]

At the same time, Brazil took steps to encourage parents to send their children to school and reduce child labor. In 2001, Brazil established Bolsa Escola, a conditional cash transfer program that provided income subsidies to parents who sent their children to school and took them for regular health checkups. Although the program didn't succeed in increasing enrollment in schools, it did raise the poorest families above subsistence level and improved school attendance rates among the children who were enrolled.[12]

Increased Purchasing Power in the Poorest Populations

Although Brazil experienced significant economic growth in the 1970s under the military regime, socioeconomic and geographic inequalities widened and the poor benefited little. Democracy was restored in the mid-1980s, during a period of economic instability, but it wasn't until the late 1990s and early 2000s that economic growth resumed and Brazil began to improve social protection.[13] Recent trends toward improved income distribution and

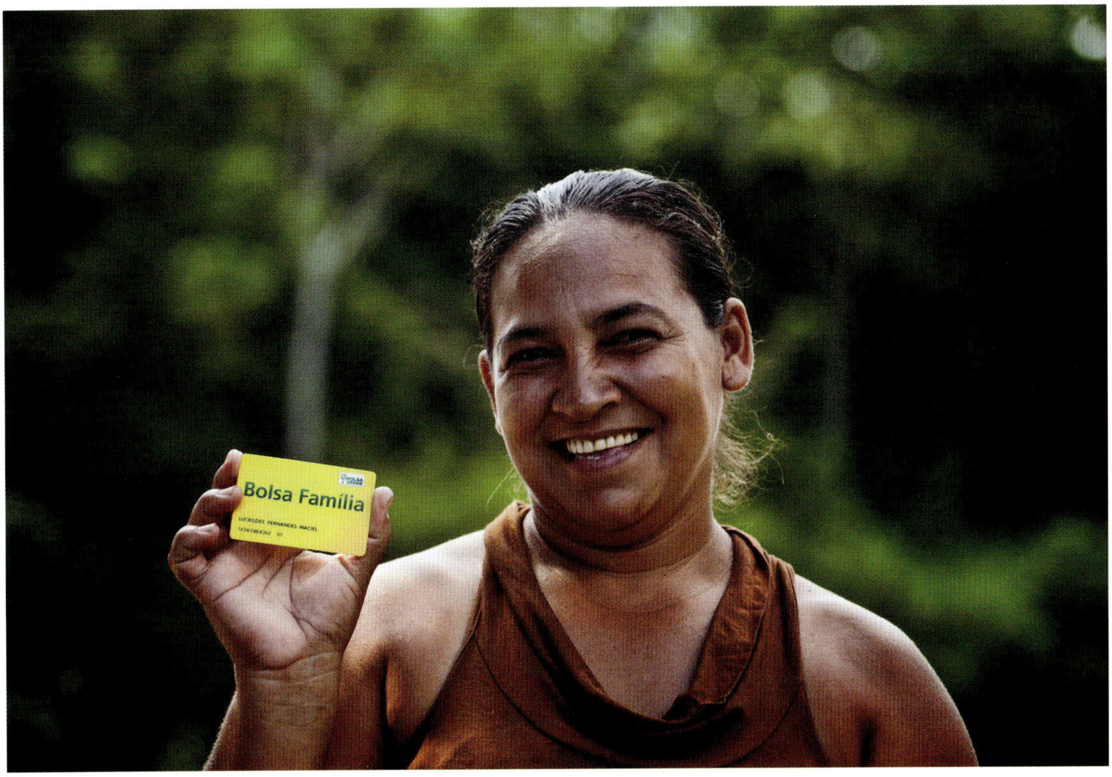

Ministério do Desenvolvimento social e Combate à Fome/S. Amaral

A woman holds up her Bolsa Família card, which gives families cash if their children go to school and get regular medical checkups.

reduced poverty in Brazil are reflected in a significant increase in purchasing power of Brazilian families between 1996 and 2007.[14] Gains in family incomes—resulting from the reactivation of economic growth in the country, as well as a decline in unemployment, increases in the official minimum wage for unskilled workers, and expanded coverage of cash transfer programs for poor families—were especially evident in poorer households.[15]

The initiation of Brazil's national food security policy framework, Fome Zero ("zero hunger"), in 2003 marked an important shift toward the integration of economic and social policies to fight hunger and poverty. In 2004, the government consolidated its cash transfers for health and nutrition, including Bolsa Escola, to create a broader social protection program, Bolsa Família, which encompassed up to 54 different instruments, programs, and initiatives under the umbrella of Fome Zero.[16] As the largest conditional cash transfer program in the world, Bolsa Família is a key element of the country's food security strategy. The program reached approximately 46 million people (25 percent of the Brazilian population) in all 5,564 municipalities in Brazil in 2006.[17]

In the agriculture sector, Brazil has been successful in linking supply from smallholder farmers to demand from food-based social protection programs through its Food Acquisition Program and National School Feeding Program. Because smallholder farmers typically have low incomes, the integration of programs that increase their purchasing power with health and nutrition programs likely has helped Brazil increase food and nutritional security, expand agricultural production, and raise rural incomes. With the development of the Food Acquisition Program in 2003, Brazil began to purchase food for stockpiling, price regulation, and food assistance for vulnerable groups, while providing market access for farmers' food crops. Although the National School Feeding Program had been established in the 1950s, it was only in 2009 that the Brazilian government began to integrate its investments in school meals with its smallholder agricultural policies, aiming to simultaneously promote food and nutrition security, improve attendance and performance in school, and strengthen smallholder agriculture.[18] Alongside these programs to support demand, Brazil also redefined its National Program for the Strengthening of Family Farms (PRONAF) to improve production through technical assistance, increased access to credit, marketing support, and improved infrastructure to assist smallholder farmers and improve the quantity and quality of food produced.

Expanded Coverage of Maternal and Child Health Services

Brazil's strong civil society movement campaigned for health reform in the 1980s, ultimately leading to the creation of a universal tax-funded national health service in 1988.[19] Real reform of the healthcare system, however, did not begin until 1994 when a new administration strengthened decentralization and community participation at all administrative levels and launched the Family Health Program. The health sector embarked on a radical decentralization process in the country, allowing for greater stakeholder participation in the decision making process and guaranteeing that each level of government supports national health policy implementation.[20]

The Family Health Program established family healthcare teams of doctors, nurses, and community health workers in specific geographical areas with the goal of reaching the poorest areas of the country. By 2006, over 26,000 family health teams working in over 90 percent of municipalities were able to provide coverage to 86 million individuals, most of whom were from low-income families.[21] The program was successful both in its targeting of the poorest rural municipalities and peri-urban slums as well as in its contribution to reducing child mortality.[22] Although the health system still struggles to ensure equitable and universal access, it has significantly increased access to healthcare, achieved universal coverage of vaccination and prenatal care, and invested in the expansion of human resources and technology across the country.[23]

Brazil also took significant action to promote optimal breastfeeding practices during this time. In 1981, it established the National Program for the Promotion of Breastfeeding, which included needs assessments, advocacy campaigns to sensitize decision makers and the general public about the relationship between breastfeeding and maternal and child health, training for health workers on lactation, and the engagement of civil society organizations, such as the International Baby Food Action Network, to increase community awareness.[24] Brazil enacted laws in 1988 that led to the enforcement of the International Code of Marketing of Breast-milk Substitutes.[25] Maternity leave was extended from two months to four months in 1998 and eventually to six months in 2006, enabling working mothers to choose breastfeeding. The exclusive breastfeeding rate increased from 4 percent in 1986 to 48 percent by 2006/2007. And between 1974/1975 and 2006/2007, the median duration of breastfeeding also increased from 2.5 months to 14 months.[26]

Expanded Public Water Supply and Sewage Services

Although Brazil has met the water and sanitation target of Millennium Development Goal 7 (halving the population without sustainable access to safe drinking water and basic sanitation), public investments in the water supply and sewage systems have been consistently inadequate. Access to improved sources of drinking water increased from 83 to 92 percent of the population between 1990 and 2012, while access to improved sanitation facilities increased from 71 to 81 percent over the same period.[27] These coverage improvements are likely to have contributed to reductions in child mortality from diarrhea over this time period.[28] In addition, expansion of sanitation services in the last decade has benefited the poor more than the more affluent, despite remaining gaps in coverage.[29]

Rising Obesity Levels: A New Challenge

Although Brazil has had tremendous success in reducing undernutrition and stunting, new nutrition challenges have recently emerged in the form of overweight and obesity. Consumption of foods rich in salt, fat, and sugar, sweetened beverages, and ready-to-eat meals are all increasing, while consumption of traditional food items such as rice, beans, fruits, and vegetables declines.[30] Although obesity rates have remained low and relatively stable among children under five, they have been increasing rapidly among older children, adolescents, and adults.[31] As the risk of obesity overtakes that of undernutrition in adults, lower-income women, in particular, are significantly more exposed than their higher-income counterparts to both undernutrition and obesity, indicating a critical risk for maternal health.[32]

Regulatory policies to restrict food advertisements in Brazil have only targeted food products manufactured to replace human milk, leaving the aggressive marketing of soft drinks, high-energy snacks, and other food and drink products of limited nutritional value unregulated. Despite several government and legislative attempts to regulate marketing of less nutritious foods, particularly those aimed at infants and children, heavy food industry lobbying has prevented any additional regulations.[33] Faced with a steadily increasing prevalence of obesity, Brazil did launch new dietary guidelines in November 2014 that provided its citizens with strong, clear recommendations that diets be based on freshly prepared and minimally processed foods and that people should avoid ultra-processed food and drink products.[34]

Key Factors in Brazil's Success

Brazil has successfully framed the country's nutrition challenges in terms of a national poverty reduction agenda and integration of its economic and social policies. Between 1996 and 2006, Brazil's food security framework was transformed into national law, complete with institutional structures designed to facilitate the realization of the human right to adequate food. The current government's Brasil sem Miséria initiative builds on this inclusive development model with the ultimate goal of eliminating extreme poverty throughout the country.[35] In addition to the strong and consistent political will to combat malnutrition, Brazil's success has been driven by its pro-poor policies, multisectoral approach, and active civil society involvement.

Pro-Poor Policies

While reducing child stunting across the country, Brazil also significantly reduced the inequality in malnutrition that existed across regions and income levels. By expanding and better targeting the country's pro-poor social assistance programs, Brazil helped accelerate the country's progress in reducing poverty.[36] This spending likely contributed to the reduction in malnutrition. The extensive social protection programs also promoted more inclusive growth throughout the country by helping people build assets, reducing inequality, facilitating economic reform, and more effectively allocating public resources.[37]

Multisectoral Approach

Brazil's success in alleviating poverty and reducing undernutrition was also supported by the multisectoral approach to program delivery that focused on income redistribution as well as improving access to education, healthcare, and sanitation services. Minimum wage increases and cash transfers were introduced alongside smallholder farmer credit and agricultural input procurement programs. And access to public services was improved across the country. Brazil's multisectoral approach, however, went beyond just implementing policies and programs across the education, health, agriculture, social development, and finance sectors. Programs also were funded in such a way that they promoted intersectoral cooperation among the different ministries *at the local level*. Under Bolsa Família, for example, to ensure that conditions were being met for the cash transfers, the health and education ministries had to share data on school attendance and health checks and coordinate their actions with the Ministry of Social Development, responsible for administrating the program. The school lunch program, Programa de Alimentação Escolar, was similarly designed to promote intersectoral coordination. Because the Ministry of Social Development was responsible for allocating money to food supply companies that bought from local producers, it needed to work with both the Ministry of Agriculture, which oversees food production, and the Ministry of Education, which eventually provided the school lunches.[38] The Food

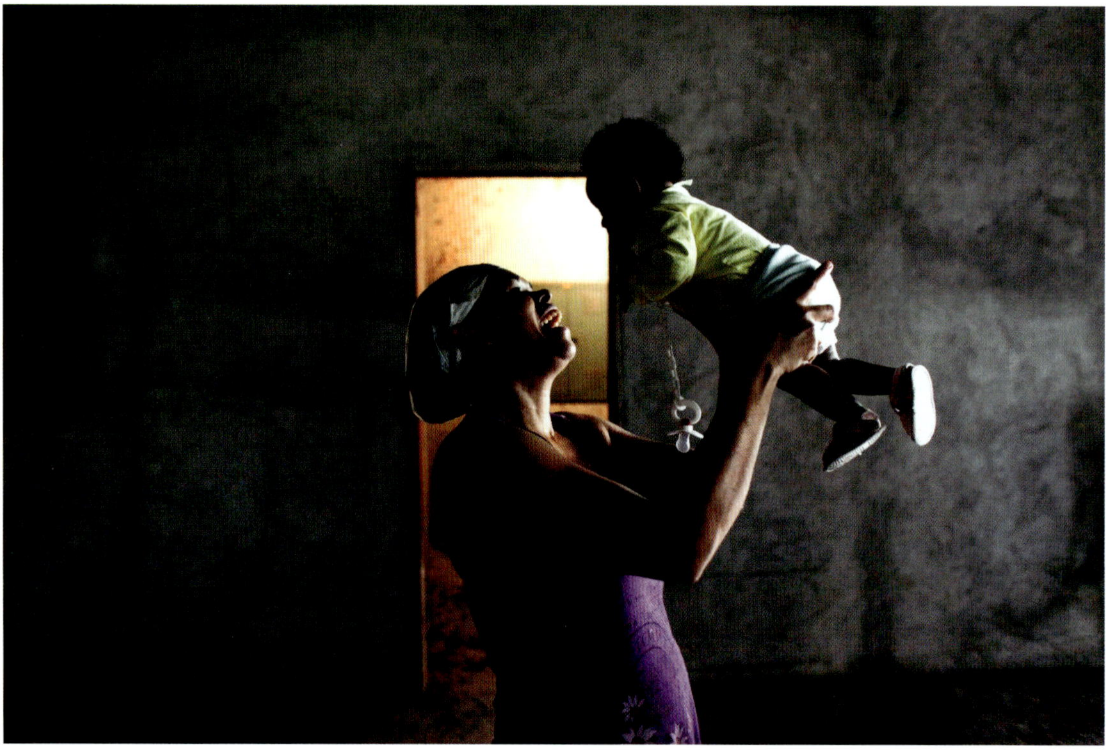

Reuters/N. Doce

Expanded health services for mothers and children played a large role in Brazil's approach.

Security and Nutrition Law, which strengthened Brazil's legal framework for food security and nutrition, institutionalized this cooperation in 2010 by establishing institutions to facilitate collaboration among ministries and within the different levels of government.

Civil Society Support

Brazil's strong civil society and social movements played a proactive role first in bringing food and nutrition security to the national agenda in the 1990s and later in the design and implementation of the country's nutrition policies. With two-thirds of its members representing civil society and one-third from the government, the National Food and Nutrition Security Council (CONSEA) provided a mechanism for civil society involvement in the policy process.[39] CONSEA is highly institutionalized, with an explicit multisectoral mandate and its own budget allocation, formal structure, and legal standing.[40] The government has worked closely with CONSEA to implement an information system to monitor food security and nutrition, guide policy decisions, and document progress. The information system includes over 50 indicators across six key dimensions of food security: food production; food availability; income and living conditions; access to adequate food and water; health, nutrition and access to related services; and education.[41]

Conclusion

Brazil's significant reduction of both stunting and geographic and socioeconomic inequality in malnutrition can serve as a powerful example for other countries in the region and around the world. The country has demonstrated the power of investing in human and social capital through its conditional cash transfers and health and nutrition programs.[42] Sustaining the gains in nutrition security now depends on maintaining economic growth and income redistribution policies, universalizing access to elementary and secondary education, and ensuring adequate healthcare and sanitation services while simultaneously addressing new challenges, including rising obesity.

CHAPTER 12

Getting to Specifics

Bangladesh's Evolving Nutrition Policies

PETER DAVIS, NICHOLAS NISBETT, NAZNEEN AKHTAR, AND SIVAN YOSEF

REMARKABLE IMPROVEMENTS IN welfare and human development indicators in Bangladesh—including a notable reduction in the poverty headcount—have accompanied recent economic growth.[1] Some aspects of nutrition have been part of this success story. For example, the percentage of underweight children declined by 1.1 percent per year and stunting rates declined by 1.3 percent per year between 1997 and 2007.[2] And this trend has continued, with rates of child stunting falling to 36 percent in 2014 (Figure 12.1). Other countries may have experienced shorter, quicker reductions, but the Bangladesh story reflects "one of the fastest prolonged reductions in child underweight and stunting prevalence in recorded history."[3]

This chapter tells the story of nutrition change in Bangladesh, drawing on primary research into nutrition-relevant policies and programs and 293 life history interviews, carried out in 2007, that reflect community-level changes in the country (see Box 12.1).[4] Five rounds of Bangladesh's Demographic and Health Survey, covering the period 1997–2011, provide supporting evidence about the broad drivers of nutritional change, particularly those related to the reductions in stunting.[5]

Bangladesh's Nutrition Achievements

Bangladesh has pursued nutrition-specific interventions, but according to stakeholders involved, these have been hampered by problems of governance and implementation since the outset, which have limited their contribution to nutrition improvements. The first large-scale nutrition policy intervention in the country, the National Plan of Action for Nutrition adopted in 1995, focused on behavior change communication, supplementation, and deworming, using the country's strong network of nongovernmental organizations (NGOs).[6] Although the program reached 16 percent of the rural population, the World Bank and other international development partners considered progress inadequate to meet the Millennium Development Goal (MDG) nutrition target.[7] The initial program was revamped in 2002, and the new program reached about 30 percent of the population through volunteer community nutrition promoters working out of community nutrition centers. However, weaknesses in program design, including a lack of capacity within these health centers and interruptions in service delivery, reportedly prompted the Government of Bangladesh, with persuasion from donors such as the World Bank, to end this initiative by 2011.[8]

In 2011, the National Nutrition Services announced as its new objective implementation of a "mainstreamed, comprehensive package of nutrition services to reduce maternal and child malnutrition ... and strengthen coordination mechanisms with key relevant sectors."[9] While it is too early to draw conclusions about the current policy, an interim assessment points to a number of challenges in delivering adequate nutrition interventions, particularly at the community level, including the poor training of frontline health assistants and family welfare volunteers.[10] Taken together, both past and recent experiences highlight challenges in delivering nutrition-specific interventions. What then contributed to Bangladesh's successes? The following sections explore the factors that likely were the main drivers of change.

Pro-Poor Economic Growth Leading to Poverty Reduction

Pro-poor economic growth is associated with a significant part of the improvement of nutrition indicators in Bangladesh. Over the past two decades the proportions of the population in both extreme and moderate poverty have declined substantially.[11] Extreme poverty is commonly accompanied by malnutrition and high morbidity, and increases in household wealth are strongly linked with nutrition improvements. Poverty reduction also likely contributed to the decline in stunting in Bangladesh. In times of household crisis, extremely poor people often cut back on meals—eating two meals per

FIGURE 12.1 Trends in nutritional status of children under 5 years of age in Bangladesh, 1996–1997 to 2014 (%)

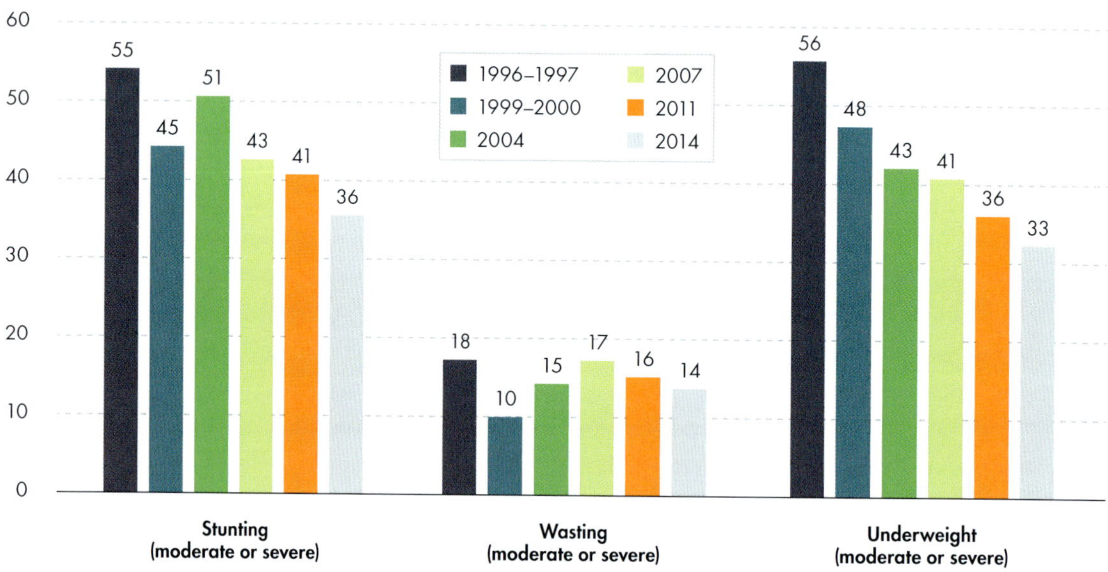

Source: Authors' compilation. 1996–1997 data are from National Institute of Population Research and Training (NIPORT), Mitra and Associates, and Macro International, *Bangladesh Demographic and Health Survey 1996–1997* (Dhaka, Bangladesh, and Calverton, MD, US: 1997); 1999–2000 data are from NIPORT, Mitra and Associates, and ORC Macro, *Bangladesh Demographic and Health Survey 1999–2000* (Dhaka, Bangladesh, and Calverton, MD, USA: 2001); 2004, 2007, 2011, and 2014 data are from NIPORT, Mitra and Associates, and ICF International, *Bangladesh Demographic and Health Survey 2014: Key Indicators* (Dhaka, Bangladesh, and Rockville, MD, USA: 2015).

day instead of three—and on expensive food items, such as meat, fish, milk, fruit, and vegetables, in favor of cheap rice, lentils, vegetables, and small fish.[12] Women and girls often suffer disproportionately.[13] With the decline in poverty, however, acute food shortages have also declined. Fewer households have been forced to cut food expenditures even in the famine-prone areas in the northwest of Bangladesh and in the pre-harvest season when food is scarcest.[14]

Wider analysis complicates this picture. Dietary diversity of Bangladeshis did not improve between 2005 and 2013, despite an increase in per capita consumption expenditure.[15] However, several of the life histories noted that hunger did not reach the extent and intensity experienced in the 1970s and 1980s, and for most people, with the exception of the declining number of extremely poor, hunger was no longer a problem.

Livestock are common household assets in rural Bangladesh, serving as a productive investment and contributing directly to improved nutrition through increased availability of meat, dairy, and eggs. Among the life history interviews, more than a quarter of interviewees considered livestock among the main causes of improvement in people's lives.[16] Livestock investments were usually accompanied by other improvements associated with gradually increasing wealth: investments in education for children, better use of qualified health providers, better water and sanitation, electrification, and a better quality diet. All these changes—including increased wealth in households and community-level improvements, such as improved infrastructure and electrification—are likely mutually reinforcing and support better health and nutrition.

Increased availability of nonfarm and manufacturing work has also been part of the story of economic development in Bangladesh in recent years.[17] These new opportunities have been particularly important for women working in manufacturing,

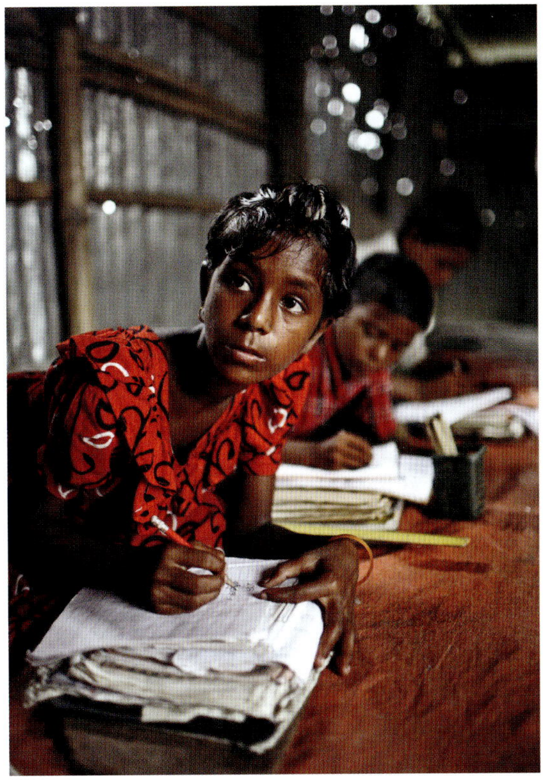

Panos/G.M.B. Akash

Bangladesh used stipends to encourage families to send their children to school, and increases in enrollment likely contributed to improvements in nutrition.

especially in the ready-made garments sector. In addition, Bangladesh's wide range of social protection policies likely helped by providing an income and food security floor for the poorest families, although the relationship of these policies to nutrition outcomes has not yet been demonstrated directly. However, a recent preliminary study in Bangladesh suggests that safety-net cash transfers that included nutrition behavior-change communication had a large and positive impact on child stunting reduction.[18]

Agriculture

Increased agricultural production linked to the Green Revolution contributed to Bangladesh's economic development from the late 1960s into the

BOX 12.1 Well-being in Bangladesh: An individual story of gradual change

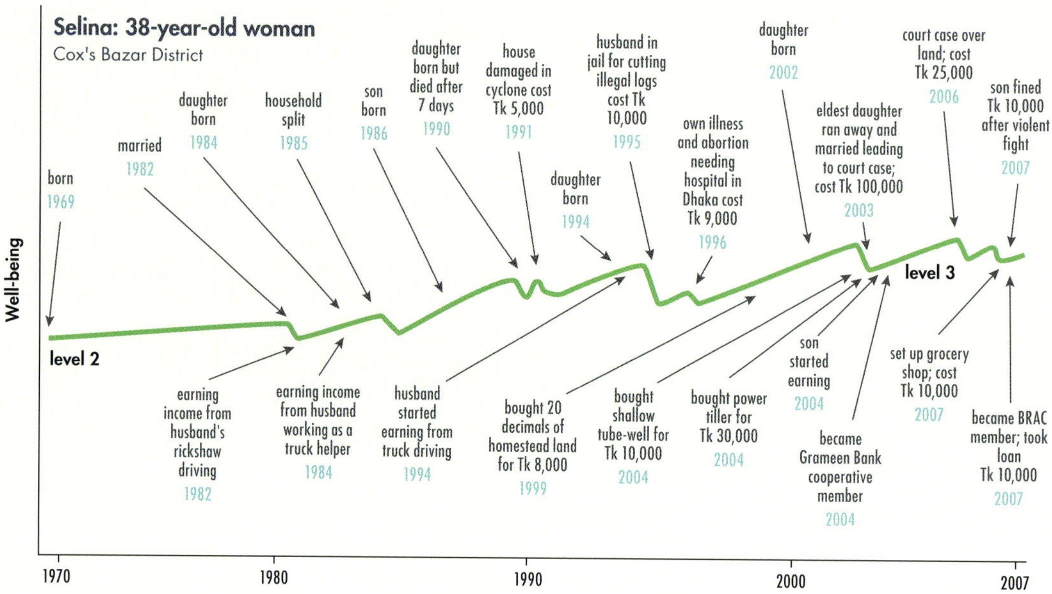

Note: 1 decimal of land = approximately 40.5 square meters. Tk = Bangladeshi taka.

The timeline above summarizes one of the 293 life histories recorded in Bangladesh in 2007. Like many of these histories, Selina's story illustrates the gradual improvement in well-being that can be linked to economic and agricultural development, provision of health and family planning services, and accumulation of household assets. As shown by the timeline, she moved from moderate poverty (level 2—below the poverty line but with some assets) to just above the poverty line (level 3). The poverty level used is multidimensional and includes an assessment of how well the respondent was able to eat.

Selina was 38 years old in 2007 when she was interviewed. She was living in a hilly area of Cox's Bazar District with her husband, Babul (43), their two daughters (13 and 5), and one son (21). Babul worked as a truck driver. Their eldest daughter (23) was married and lived separately.

Selina's life trajectory shows gradual progress from a moderately poor childhood and early married life to a less vulnerable position. In 1982, when she was newly married, her family frequently was forced to miss meals. Their economic situation improved largely because of her husband's income from truck driving starting in 1994, and more recently, her son's income from sharecropping, working with a power tiller, and running a grocery shop. Selina herself was also active in various income-generating ventures supported by loans from NGOs. This gradual improvement in life circumstances was not without setbacks, including problems with Selina's health, the death of a baby, and a number of costly court cases related to the marriage of her eldest daughter, land disputes, and a fight over irrigation water. This pattern of gradual increase in economic well-being, interspersed with setbacks and accompanied by improvements in nutrition, is typical of many stories from the life history interviews.

Source: Life history interview conducted by Peter Davis, Dilara Hasin, and Anowara Begum, Cox's Bazar District, 2007. For a description of the methods used, see P. Davis, "Patterns of Socio-economic Mobility in Rural Bangladesh: Lessons from Life History Interviews," in Methodological Challenges and New Approaches to Research in International Development, edited by L. Camfield (Basingstoke, UK: Palgrave Macmillan, 2014).

Note: All names have been changed to protect the identity of research participants.

1980s. High-yielding varieties of rice and wheat, widespread irrigation, greater use of fertilizers and pesticides, introduction of completely new crops to some areas, such as potatoes and maize, and more intensive farming of vegetables have all boosted production.[19] Since independence, Bangladesh has more than doubled its production of cereal grains.[20] Although the population also more than doubled over the same period, the country is now self-sufficient in rice production. Much of this increase is attributable to the introduction and expansion of *boro* (dry season) rice varieties, grown over the winter season with the aid of irrigation from tubewells.[21] These increases in agricultural production and supply have likely played a significant part in generating nutritional improvements in Bangladesh, although data limitations preclude calculation of that contribution.[22] However, it is not clear if the same progress has been achieved in improving dietary diversity.[23]

Although seasonal food shortages have become less common, minimum dietary availability and dietary diversity have been slow to improve in recent years for all households. The majority of the population remains dependent on cereals for much of their calorie intake.[24] This stagnation has been linked to a research and policy bias toward rice as well as broader drivers of food prices coinciding roughly with the period covered by this review.[25] The prices of lentils and meat have increased steadily in comparison with rice over this period, making it more difficult for the poorest households to adequately diversify their diets.[26] In 2013/2014, Bangladesh experienced price spikes in the cost of its food basket owing to supply disruptions related to election protests and a fuel price hike, even during a time of relatively low and stable global food prices.[27]

Family Planning and Demographic Trends

Bangladesh's demographic and family planning successes, particularly in reducing fertility and child mortality, may be one of the strongest drivers in its nutrition success, along with the closely related improvements in women's empowerment and education. At the time of independence in 1971, fertility in Bangladesh was high and contraceptive use low. Less than 10 percent of couples were using contraception in 1969, and the total fertility rate was around seven.[28] Following the war for independence, a number of programs have been successful in expanding family planning support, including female family-welfare assistants promoting family planning directly in communities. Key stakeholder interviews cited these government programs, along with NGO-based programs, as contributing to increased use of contraception. Such programs have been linked to strong performance on some health indicators in the wider literature.[29] The total fertility rate declined slowly at first, but progress became more rapid after 1979, with a decline from 6.8 to 4.6 by 1988. More recently, the total fertility rate for 2008–2010 was 2.3 and was expected to be about 2.0 in 2016.[30]

Reduced fertility is associated with some improvements in nutrition outcomes.[31] Changes in attitude have accompanied the large demographic shift, with implications for improved nutrition. Field interviews found widespread understanding among interviewees of the importance of having small, healthy families, which reflects the national trend toward declining family size. Interaction with family planning, visiting primary health professionals, and NGO staff have likely contributed to these attitudinal changes.[32]

Health Services

The association between improved health services and improved nutrition in Bangladesh is strong in some respects but mixed in others. Health sector success stories include impressive vaccination coverage, availability of relatively cheap medicines, spread of private health clinics, and more

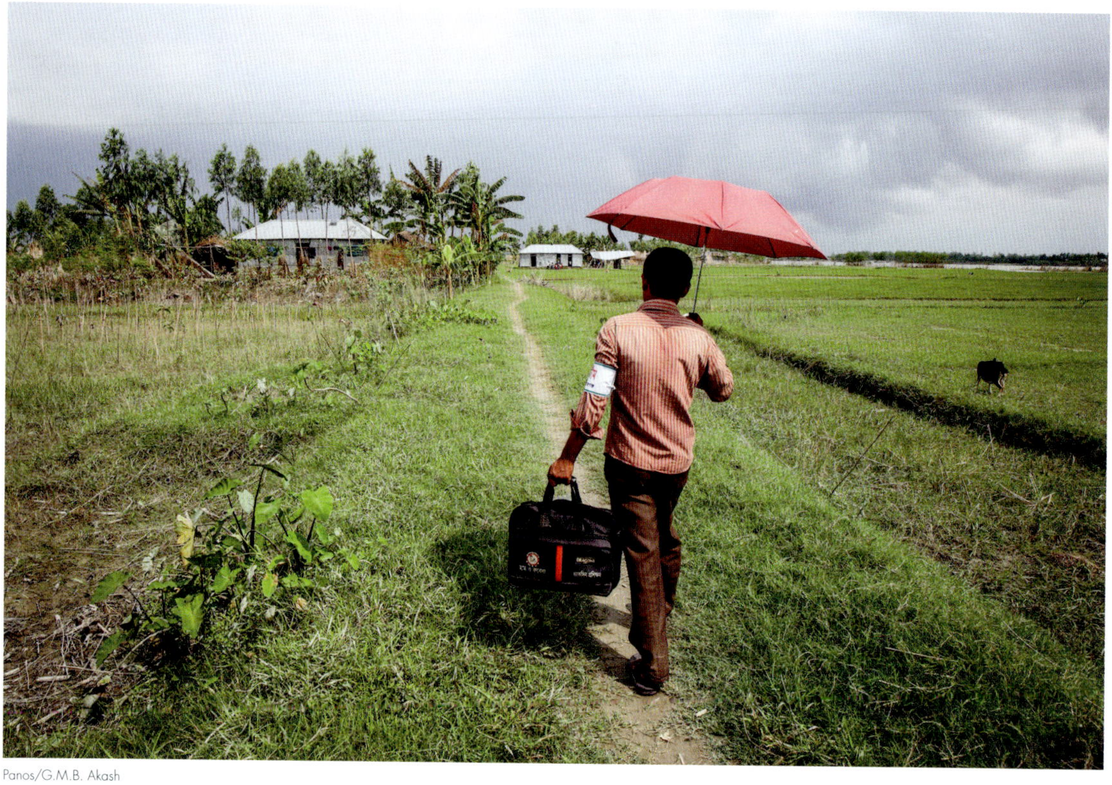

Panos/G.M.B. Akash

A community health care provider makes his rounds, reaching people on this island in Bangladesh's Brahmaputra River.

recently, the establishment of community clinics providing improved coverage for a range of primary health, family planning, and, increasingly, nutrition services.[33]

There have been marked achievements in neonatal, postnatal, and children's health. Maternal and infant mortality have declined, as have stunting rates. Antenatal coverage for births increased from 58 percent in 2004 to 79 percent in 2014, and 64 percent of women in 2014 benefited from services by a trained antenatal care provider.[34] Birth attendance by a skilled provider nearly tripled over a decade, from 15.6 percent in 2004 to 42.1 percent in 2014.[35] Statistical analysis underlines the significance of improved maternal health as a potential driver of stunting reductions—accessing facility birth and antenatal care was significantly associated with childhood stunting declines.[36]

Paradoxically, these successes have occurred despite a relatively weak health system. While indicators such as mortality and birthrates have plummeted, general levels of morbidity remain high. Nutrition indicators for women and children stand out as particularly poor in comparison with the rapid rates of improvement in other health areas.[37] Child stunting levels remain high, despite the rapid decline, as do a number of other indicators. For example, only 36 percent of mothers and children in 2013 received postnatal care within two days of delivery, and in 2013, 17 percent of women aged 19–49 were undernourished.[38]

Education

School attendance in Bangladesh has increased rapidly in recent years, with stipend programs at primary- and secondary-school levels contributing to improved enrolment rates.[39] Bangladesh has a long history of incentive programs for sending children to school. Beginning in 1993, the Food for Education (FFE) program provided wheat (and sometimes rice) to parents of children attending school. In 2002, FFE was replaced by the cash-based Primary Education Stipend. Although the amounts provided, in actual terms, are small and therefore have limited impact on poverty reduction, and coverage was rolled out slowly, the stipends have encouraged school attendance and provided relief for very poor families.[40] As reported in the life histories, parents usually used the money for school-related expenses, such as stationery and food. A Female Stipend Program for girls at the secondary-school level, which was introduced in 1994, increased enrollment rates, reversed the gender gap in grade attainment, and coincided with an increase in the marriage age of women.[41] The program has also likely contributed to improved nutrition. Although this is difficult to demonstrate conclusively, one study shows that parents' level of education was positively related to nutrition outcomes.[42] Children whose parents had both completed high school were expected to be taller than children of parents who had never attended school.

Sanitation and Improved Access to Clean Drinking Water

Bangladesh has made significant strides in providing access to improved drinking water sources and sanitation. The percentage of population with access to improved water sources increased from 68 percent to 87 percent from 1990 to 2015—enough to meet the MDG of halving the number of people without access to safe drinking water. Rural provision has increased faster and disparities between urban and rural areas have disappeared.[43] While access to clean drinking water has direct health benefits, it also has indirect nutrition benefits, particularly in reducing childhood illnesses, which in turn can exacerbate poor nutrition.[44]

The picture on sanitation is also positive; Bangladesh is one of 16 countries that reduced open defecation by over 25 percentage points in the MDG period.[45] Reductions in open defecation figure strongly as a likely driver of stunting reduction.[46] Change in rural communities appears to have been particularly significant, with the practice of open defecation falling dramatically from 34 percent to 3 percent of the population from 1990 to 2012. Unusual for South Asia, the gains have been broad-based, with progress among the poorest in rural communities being much faster than in any other country and largely driving the reduction in open defecation. Even with open defecation now negligible, access to improved sanitation facilities is still low, at 61 percent.[47] Large variations in access persist, particularly between wealth quintiles in the growing urban population.[48]

Women's Empowerment

Looking at the link between nutrition outcomes and women's empowerment, a recent analysis could not detect a significant relationship between nutrition and indicators of women's empowerment. These indicators included the ability to travel alone to a health clinic, an indicator that may not capture wider dimensions of women's empowerment well, and various dimensions of women's decision making in households. These results contradict, to some extent, another observation in the same analysis: although both parents' education levels were significantly associated with changes in stunting, more of the change in child stunting was "explained" by mothers' education than fathers' education.[49]

Another recent study in Bangladesh found that increases in a measure of women's empowerment in agriculture are positively associated with calorie availability and dietary diversity.[50] However, the same study also found that household wealth, education, and occupation were more strongly associated with adult nutritional status than women's empowerment.

The life history interviews elicited similar observations. Although women's empowerment is difficult to measure, the life histories support the view that women have become more empowered over recent decades and that this change is likely to have contributed to improved nutrition. Dimensions of empowerment include markedly increased levels of educational achievement and gender parity in secondary enrollment rates, widespread participation of women in NGO-supported income-generation and other activities, and increased employment of women along with control of their income.[51]

Both community- and stakeholder-level interviews highlighted how employment opportunities for young women are helping to delay the age of marriage and first pregnancies by empowering and valorizing the contribution of girls. Assistance for girls through the secondary education stipend program is having the same effect. The community interviews revealed fairly widespread acceptance of a national narrative that emphasizes the positive role of women in the country's development and the importance of having small families of well-educated, healthy children.

Lessons Learned

Much of the improvement in nutrition in Bangladesh in recent years is likely explained by what can be seen as nutrition-sensitive drivers within a wider enabling environment of pro-poor economic growth. Pro-poor economic growth is linked in turn to improved agricultural production and diversification, a vibrant NGO sector supporting income generation, expansion of nonfarm business and manufacturing sectors creating employment opportunities, remittances from labor migration, and improving infrastructure and electrification. In addition, significant contributions have been made by improved access to education (especially for girls); health and family planning service use and availability; demographic change, such as smaller family sizes, increased birth intervals, and lower age at first pregnancy; and more widespread use of safe water sources and better sanitation. These likely drivers of nutritional improvement have multiple impacts and are mutually reinforcing. These drivers are also predominantly indirect—that is, they are largely the result of economic and social development, not of programs and interventions specifically intended to improve nutrition.

Yet many millions of children in Bangladesh still grow up stunted because of poor nutrition.[52] So while we still need to recognize the major contribution of indirect drivers, and their importance in sustaining gains, the challenge is to make further improvements. Interventions directly aimed at improving nutritional status have been expanding in scope and coverage, but their impact has been limited compared with broader drivers of nutrition-sensitive development. Looking to the future, however, the heavy lifting done by these drivers—including significant gains in income, health, lowered fertility, and sanitation—may not continue at the same rate. Nutrition-specific interventions will need to take on a greater role in Bangladesh.

CHAPTER 13

Reaching New Heights

20 Years of Nutrition Progress in Nepal

KENDA CUNNINGHAM, AKRITI SINGH, DEREK HEADEY, POOJA PANDEY RANA, AND CHANDNI KARMACHARYA

DESPITE SIGNIFICANT ECONOMIC growth, South Asia remains notorious for its alarmingly high rates of undernutrition. This "Asian enigma" has long puzzled both researchers and policy makers. However, Nepal's recent experience presents yet another enigma: a rapid reduction in maternal and child undernutrition during a period of civil war and prolonged political and economic instability. From 1996 to 2011, the prevalence of stunting among children under two years of age fell from 48 to 27 percent, and the prevalence of maternal underweight decreased from 28 to 20 percent.[1]

How did such remarkable improvements take place and how can Nepal sustain this impressive progress? Answering these questions is challenging because many factors influence nutritional well-being and these various determinants interact in complex ways.[2] Globally, multistakeholder, multisectoral platforms are being recommended to address nutritional challenges, precisely because the underlying determinants relate to a wide range of social and economic sectors.[3] Nepal's success in reducing undernutrition may shed light on which sectors require prioritization and coordination and on how to address undernutrition in remote and poor rural settings.

Trends in Nutrition Outcomes, Feeding Practices, and Underlying Determinants

Nepal's progress in reducing child stunting[4] and maternal undernutrition[5] is remarkable. Indeed, the rate of reduction of child stunting in Nepal from 1996 to 2011 has been one of the fastest in the world (Table 13.1). However, despite rapid progress, millions of Nepalese remain undernourished: more than one out of four children under two years of age are stunted and one out of five mothers are underweight.

Understanding Nepal's progress in reducing maternal and child undernutrition requires close examination of both nutrition-specific factors (such as infant and young child feeding practices) and nutrition-sensitive factors (including wealth and education; access to healthcare; and water,

TABLE 13.1 Maternal and child undernutrition in Nepal, 1996–2011 (%)

Year	Maternal underweight[a]	Child stunting[b] (ages 0–60 months)	Child wasting[c] (ages 0–24 months)
1996	27.6	47.8	15.5
2001	26.0	41.1	11.7
2006	25.9	34.0	12.9
2011	20.3	27.0	11.3
Annual % change	−1.8	−2.9	−1.8

Source: Authors' estimates from the 1996 and 2011 rounds of the *Nepal Demographic and Health Survey* (DHS).

Notes: [a] Maternal underweight is defined as a body mass index (BMI) < 18.5; [b] Stunting is defined as a height-for-age Z-score (HAZ) < −2.0 SD from the median of the reference population, based on the 2006 World Health Organization growth standards; [c] Wasting is defined as a weight-for-height Z-score (WHZ) < −2.0 SD from the median of the reference population, based on the 2006 World Health Organization growth standards.

sanitation, and hygiene facilities), as well as the broader political-economic context.

Infant and young child feeding (IYCF) practices are very poor in Nepal and have remained largely unchanged over time. Between 2001 and 2011, Nepal saw no improvement in rates of exclusive breastfeeding—about 80 percent—among children 0 to 6 months of age. Complementary feeding should occur from about age 6 months to 24 months, as children transition from breastfeeding to family foods, but in Nepal only about 60 percent of children 6 to 8 months of age eat solid or semisolid foods. Less than 20 percent of children 6 to 24 months of age consume foods from at least four of seven globally recommended food groups. The only IYCF indicator to improve was minimum meal frequency, defined as the appropriate number of feedings given the child's age and whether he or she is breastfeeding.[6] Progress in minimum meal frequency likely reflects increased household socioeconomic status and food security.

For nutrition-sensitive determinants, a range of indicators are relevant (Table 13.2), but health care, demographic factors, household asset ownership, parental education, and water, sanitation, and hygiene (WASH) may be particularly important for nutrition. Between 1996 and 2011, the Nepalese experienced large improvements in access to and use of health and sanitation services. For example, hospital deliveries increased from 9 to 41 percent, and toilet use increased from 18 to 52 percent. There were also sizable reductions in fertility rates (as proxied by average birth order) and increases in birth spacing, which could be a result of family planning programs, increased wealth and education, or increased overseas emigration—usually of male members of the household—which generates remittances and tends to increase households' access to cash. Asset ownership and parental education, particularly among women, also rose rapidly (Table 13.2). These two factors could influence nutrition through multiple channels, such as by raising food and nonfood expenditures relevant to nutrition and empowering women, which can improve the nutritional well-being of both mothers and their children.

A Statistical Exploration of the Drivers of Nutritional Change over Time

Many factors that underlie good nutrition have improved in Nepal in recent decades, but it is not immediately clear which ones actually made significant contributions to improving the country's maternal and child nutrition indicators. To help shed light on this question, we analyzed statistics

TABLE 13.2 Trends in underlying drivers of nutritional change in Nepal, 1996–2011

Driver	1996	2011	Annual change (%)
Toilet use (%)	18.2	51.6	12.2
Four or more antenatal care visits (%)	6.3	29.6	24.7
Maternal empowerment (%)	9.6	19.9	7.2
Maternal education (years)	1.2	3.9	15.0
Iron supplements during pregnancy (%)	11.6	82.3	40.6
Paternal education (years)	4.0	5.7	2.8
Household asset ownership (1–10)	1.5	4.9	15.1
Child born in health institution (%)	8.6	41.1	25.2
Child fully vaccinated (%)	25.9	51.2	6.5
Water source: piped (%)	30.0	37.1	1.6
Water source: tubewell (%)	32.7	43.7	2.2
Maternal height (centimeters)	150.5	151.1	0.0
Birth order of child	3.3	2.5	-1.6
Birth interval (years)	3.9	4.6	1.2

Source: Authors' estimates from the 1996 and 2011 rounds of the *Nepal Demographic and Health Survey* (DHS).

Note: Asset ownership: 10-component index including electricity access and ownership of radios, TVs, and bicycles; maternal education: years of formal schooling; paternal education: years of formal schooling; antenatal care visits: dummy if mother had four or more check-ups during pregnancy; iron supplements: dummy if mother received iron supplements during pregnancy; health institution: hospital, medical clinic, or health post; birth order: ranking of child's birth order, with a first-born child equal to one; birth interval: time between birth of present child and last-born child; tubewell water: dummy if household drinking water sourced from tubewell; piped water: dummy if household drinking water from a piped source; maternal empowerment: equal weighted index of mother's involvement in three decisions (on her own health, on major household purchases, and on visiting relatives).

from the *Nepal Demographic and Health Survey* (DHS) datasets to see which changes in underlying factors were associated with which improvements in nutritional indicators (Figure 13.1). An underlying factor could possibly explain nutritional change if it has significant and large associations with nutrition outcomes and if it has changed rapidly over time (Table 13.2).[7] The results in Figure 13.1 should not be interpreted in a strictly causal sense, however; rather, they are estimated contributions based on how well different factors statistically correspond with changes in nutrition over time.

The most important factor associated with improvements in child growth was increased access to health services (antenatal and neonatal care), but household asset accumulation and parental education—mostly maternal education—were also important correlates of child growth. Unsurprisingly, maternal height—a slow-moving intergenerational driver—seems to have played only a modest role in improving child height-for-age Z-score (HAZ). Interestingly, though, a large share of the improvement in HAZ between 1996 to 2011 was not explained by the statistical model, possibly because the model did not include certain factors, such as climate shocks, agricultural production, and food security, and access to nutrition-specific programs.

For improvements in child and maternal weight gain, better sanitation appears to have been the most important factor, suggesting that increased toilet access may have led to large declines in maternal and child infections. Increased access to health services (antenatal and neonatal care) was also significantly associated with the improvements in maternal BMI and child weight-for-height Z-score

(WHZ), and household asset accumulation and education played roles as well. In contrast, increased access to piped water seems to have played only a small role. It is important to note that the WHZ model overpredicts nutritional change (that is, estimated changes in WHZ were larger than actual changes between 1996 and 2011), though the model of maternal BMI explains total BMI change quite accurately.

Community Perspectives on Changes in Nutrition and Underlying Determinants over Time

Qualitative interviews of 20 mothers complemented the quantitative findings, giving mothers' perspectives on both nutrition-specific and nutrition-sensitive changes in their communities during roughly the same time period. The women interviewed were selected from two *terai* districts—Rupandehi and Chitwan—and were known to have given birth in one of five five-year periods: 1990–1995, 1995–2000, 2000–2005, 2005–2010, and 2010–2015.[8]

All mothers reported that they had breastfed their babies; their perceptions of their own milk supply determined how long they engaged in both exclusive and predominant breastfeeding. Most mothers reported that they had not introduced most complementary foods to their children at age six months, indicating a general late introduction. Many mothers reported having received antenatal care checkups at a health facility, though this was much more common among mothers who had given birth recently. Similarly, mothers who had given birth more recently reported taking iron supplements during pregnancy and delivering at a health facility. Even some mothers who

FIGURE 13.1 Underlying factors' estimated contributions to improvements in child growth, child weight gain, and maternal weight gain in Nepal

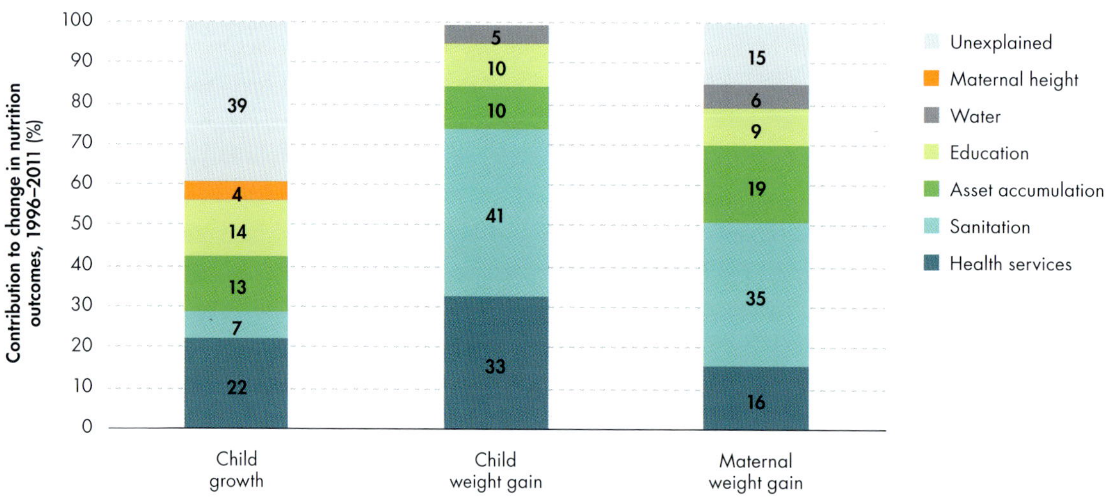

Source: Authors' estimates from the 1996 and 2011 rounds of the *Nepal Demographic and Health Survey* (DHS).

Note: Child growth is based on height-for-age Z-scores (HAZ) for children 0 to 2 years; child weight gain is based on weight-for-height Z-scores (WHZ) for children 0 to 2 years; maternal weight gain is based on body mass index (BMI). The statistics in the figure report the share of total nutritional change estimated by the decomposition model for 1996–2011. The decomposition model is a simple decomposition at means, where the change in each nutrition outcome due to an explanatory variable is the change in means of that variable over the period 1996–2011, multiplied by its regression model coefficient for a pooled model covering all four *Nepal Demographic and Health Survey* (DHS) rounds over 1996–2011.

had previously delivered at home gave birth to their youngest child at a health facility.

In terms of wider community development changes in areas known to have potential contributions to nutrition, mothers noted improvements in housing, income, education, and availability of improved water sources, toilets, and contraception. Mothers noted that houses now tend to be larger and constructed with more permanent roof and wall materials. Most mothers stated that their husbands or sons had left Nepal to work in India, Malaysia, and the Middle East and reported migration-related household income growth, though the positive economic benefits of migration were not universal. Younger mothers were more educated than older ones, and all mothers spoke about sending their children, including daughters, to school. Many mothers stated that they now had a toilet at home and mentioned improvements in access to clean drinking water. Mothers who gave birth recently had one or two children, whereas those who gave birth before 2010 had up to five children. Some mothers talked about the increasing availability and use of permanent contraception over time.

The qualitative interviews thus tended to confirm quantitative findings and shed light on mothers' perspectives, including how and why there had been progress, or a lack thereof, in certain areas. For example, mothers noted limited improvement in infant and young child feeding practices despite many other positive changes, including improvements in access to and use of health services and overall community development.

The Role of Policies, Programs, and Socioeconomic Changes

Nutritional improvements have been driven by economic and social changes, and many of these changes are likely associated with increased public investments, better provision of public services, and an increasing role for NGOs in public service delivery.

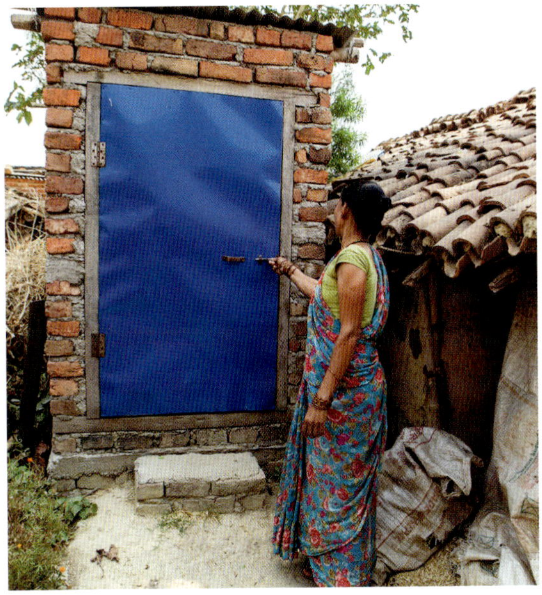

K. Das Shrestha

Better sanitation, including access to latrines like this one, may have led to large declines in infections in mothers and children in Nepal.

Greater access to and use of health services, including antenatal care and hospital delivery, are leading factors associated with reductions in undernutrition, and consistent with the results of other child nutrition studies in Nepal.[9] This progress stems from several factors. First, public spending on health, as a percentage of total public spending in Nepal, rose from about 4 percent in 1988–1992 to 7 percent in 2001–2006.[10] Second, Nepal increasingly decentralized its health services and made a sustained effort to improve people's access to basic health services across the country. Instrumental in this effort was Nepal's expansion of healthcare institutions, including primary healthcare centers and female community health volunteers (FCHVs) working at the sub-village, or ward, level. Since the 1990s, Nepal has increased the number of FCHVs working in rural villages and extended the range of goods and services they provide. These volunteers not only distribute vitamin A but also treat child illness, offer family planning, care for pregnant women and newborns, and serve as the first point of referral to health facilities in cases of severe health complications.[11] In 2005 Nepal introduced the Safe Delivery Incentive Program, which provides cash to women giving birth in a health clinic and provides incentives to health workers to attend deliveries.[12] An evaluation showed that this program increased delivery with a skilled attendant by 17 percent if mothers were aware of the program before childbirth.[13] These health initiatives were specifically designed to overcome the widespread problem of physical isolation in Nepal, as well as the cultural barriers that women face in gaining access to health services, especially during pregnancy.

Micronutrient deficiencies in the Nepalese population have long been a major concern. Although the Ministry of Health and Population has included iron and folic acid supplementation for pregnant and lactating women as part of antenatal care since 1998, coverage has been limited. In 2003 the Intensification of the Maternal and Neonatal Micronutrient Program improved coverage by using health workers and FCHVs to distribute iron and folic acid in communities.[14] As a result, coverage of iron and folic acid supplementation rose from 12 percent in 1996 to 82 percent in 2011. This maternal iron supplementation has been found to be important for child nutrition: in Nepal, iron and folic acid supplements and antenatal care contribute to preventing low birth weight.[15]

Although Nepal has made only limited improvements in supplying households with improveed

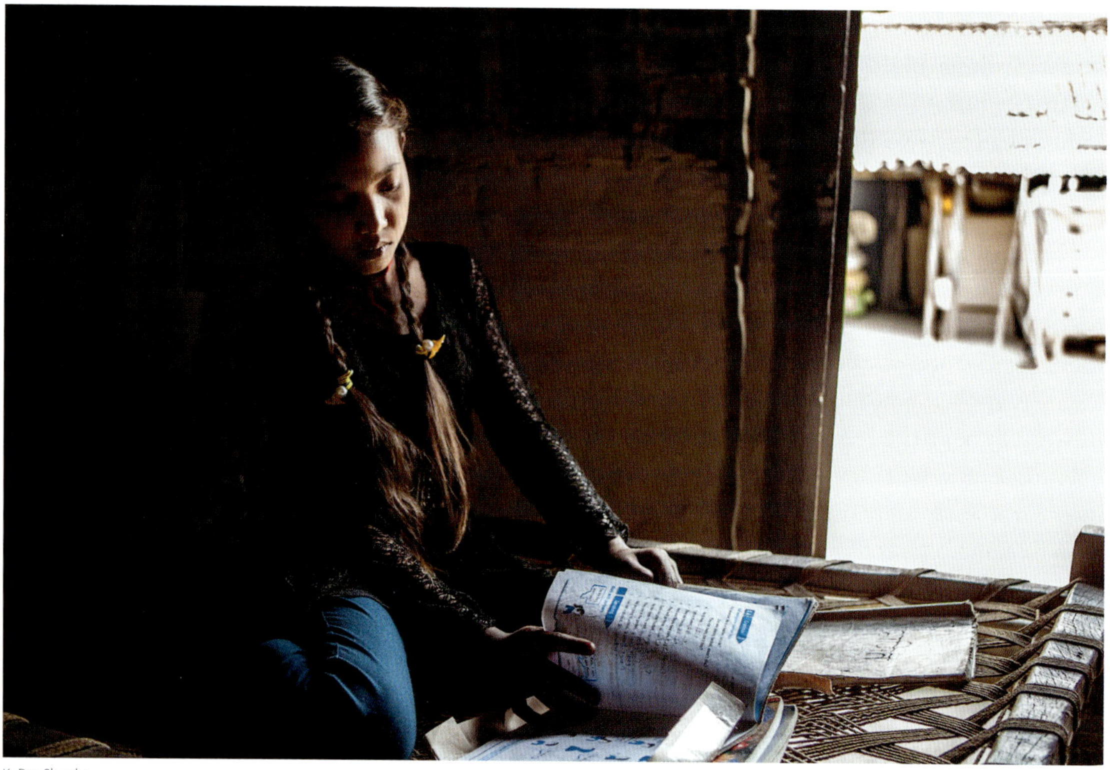

K. Das Shrestha

Nepal has significantly raised its investment in girls' education, which is correlated with the growth of girls' future children.

sources of clean water, which is an important issue for densely populated areas,[16] it has made significant advances in toilet coverage, which have been strongly associated with reductions in undernutrition for both mothers and children. Nepal has had water and sanitation policies in place for decades, but toilet construction and use had made slow progress. In the 2000s, however, there were renewed public and NGO efforts to expand toilet use, and hygienic behaviors (which are difficult to observe) more generally. In 2003, inspired in part by Bangladesh's success, Nepal piloted community-led total sanitation (CLTS) as a sustainable way to use mass sensitization activities to trigger communities to construct and use basic toilets, as opposed to the traditional approach of providing costly hardware support.[17] A wide range of NGO and development partners then rapidly scaled up CLTS. The recognition that an analogous approach was needed for schools, particularly to improve attendance by girls, led to adoption of the school-led total sanitation (SLTS) approach in 2006, which mobilized school-based clubs. By the end of 2015, 27 of Nepal's 75 districts had been declared free of open defecation.[18]

Other important factors associated with reductions in maternal and child undernutrition include improved socioeconomic status and parental education, especially maternal. In Nepal, between 1995 and 2010, the share of people living below the \$1.25-a-day poverty line fell from 42 to 25 percent.[19] While this may not be closely linked to any particular policy, overseas emigration and resulting remittance flows are widely thought to be a major driver of income growth and poverty reduction in Nepal.[20] In particular, the 2000s saw a shift in emigration destinations, with growing numbers of men and some women emigrating to more lucrative employment positions in the Persian Gulf countries rather than to neighboring India. Growth in agriculture—the largest domestic employer—has struggled to keep pace with population growth. Nepal has been in a food deficit since 2006, meaning it is a net food importer; at the same time, public investments in agriculture have been declining.[21] However, the current Agriculture Development Strategy 2015–2035 aims to boost this sector.[22] Tourism—another important sector—was hit hard by the civil war starting in the mid-1990s but recovered strongly after the war ended in 2006.[23]

In education, the government has played a more direct role, committing increasing financial resources to this sector. In 1990 education only received about 10 percent of the overall budget, but by 2011 it received nearly 20 percent.[24] Following the World Conference on Education for All in 1990, Nepal adopted a National Plan of Action, which included gender parity as one of six goals.[25] Since then, improvements in women's educational attainment have been rapid and sustained.

Finally, the government of Nepal has—in more recent times—made a concerted effort to adopt a more explicit multisectoral approach to addressing malnutrition. In 2009, the World Bank and other development partners commissioned a Nutrition Assessment Gap Analysis (NAGA), and in 2011, following its evidence-based recommendations, Nepal adopted the Multi-Sectoral Nutrition Plan (MSNP).[26] The MSNP serves as a national roadmap for addressing undernutrition by engaging various ministries, including health, education, urban development, agriculture, and local development. This roadmap is used to mobilize resources and align projects and programs for nutrition.

Lessons Learned and Future Challenges

Nepal has made huge strides in reducing maternal and child undernutrition in the past 20 years, despite a period of civil conflict and political instability, and without the stellar economic growth of China, India, or Vietnam. In this investigation into Nepal's success in reducing maternal and child undernutrition, four main factors stand out: (1) improvements in access to and use of health services, (2) increased toilet coverage, (3) wealth accumulation, and (4) parental education, especially maternal. Underlying these advances were important policy and programmatic changes, particularly in health, education, and WASH. Across these policies and programs, better delivery of services was vital, given that many households are extremely isolated geographically and socially, and many women and girls as well as individuals belonging to specific castes are marginalized. Also striking is the involvement of multiple actors, including different levels of government, multilateral and bilateral development agencies, a wide range of NGOs, and communities themselves, often through volunteer organizations.

Despite these remarkable improvements, the present situation remains unsatisfactory; there still exist many challenges to achieving further reductions in undernutrition. Nepal will need to scale up nutrition-related policies and programs and perhaps find new creative ways to operationalize plans and policies to help those who have thus far remained beyond their reach. As of 2011, only about 30 percent of births were preceded by adequate antenatal care, just over 40 percent took place in a medical facility, and just over 50 percent of children were fully vaccinated.[27] Despite rapid expansion of WASH facillities, as of 2011 at least half of Nepali households still practiced open defecation and almost two-thirds continued to be without access to piped water.[28] During interviews, mothers also noted the continued lack of adequate road networks, health facilities, education, and job opportunities in rural areas, as well as the long road ahead to creating equal opportunities for all people, regardless of gender or caste. Poverty and food insecurity are also still widespread, especially in the wake of the earthquakes, floods, and the fuel crisis of 2015.

In Nepal, some traditional beliefs and practices are harmful for nutrition and may curb further reductions in undernutrition unless they are addressed. Our quantitative results showed that infant and young child feeding practices have not improved over time, and interviews with mothers revealed that knowledge gaps and cultural beliefs contribute to poor household diets and child feeding practices. Mothers said they had given meat, fish, and eggs to their children only after 12 months of age because they believed that a baby could not digest these foods earlier. Several mothers reported missing antenatal visits because services were not available, but many also noted being bashful about pregnancy or remaining unconvinced that healthcare visits were really necessary.

Cultural norms and practices are often embedded in longstanding gender norms that influence household-level nutrition in many ways. In Nepal, women's empowerment is particularly low even in comparison with other South Asian countries and has only improved modestly in the past 25 years.[29] Results from the 2011 Demographic and Health Survey suggest that mothers play only a small role in household decision making, with 42 percent of mothers reporting that other people made their healthcare decisions. But women's lack of autonomy and decision-making power also affects food allocation and utilization in the household, access to and control of income, freedom of movement, and division of time on a daily basis between work and household chores including cooking, feeding, and caring for young children. All of these can influence women's own nutritional well-being and that of their children.[30] Patriarchal structures present deep-rooted challenges but also open opportunities for policies and programs across a range of development domains—such as agriculture, health, microfinance, education, and WASH—to catalyze women's empowerment.

In addition to the need to tackle deeply ingrained cultural norms, policymakers face significant institutional challenges. The MSNP is a national roadmap for coordinating—or at a minimum, aligning—the many diverse programs and activities across sectors, agencies, and actors, operational at different administrative units, that can contribute to eradicating undernutrition. Working across sectors, however, will require carefully coordinating and managing many ministries and development partners in order to plan, implement, and monitor large-scale packages of interventions operating at the district and subdistrict levels. Nepal also faces many gaps in human resources and institutional capacity, including staff shortages, frequent turnover of frontline workers, and technical and managerial gaps at all levels. An additional challenge—and opportunity—has recently emerged: to align the multisectoral coordination of nutrition efforts with Nepal's newly adopted federalist constitution and its emerging decentralized governance structures. The new subnational government structures will be tasked with public service delivery and broader economic development, which are essential for solving the persistent problem of undernutrition.

Finally, other important nutrition-related topics have yet to be addressed in Nepal. For example, anemia among women and children is an even more pervasive problem nationally than stunting or underweight. Also, the prevalence of overweight among children and women of reproductive age is rising and will likely continue to do so as urbanization and incomes rise; many programs that currently target undernutrition could also be leveraged to prevent overnutrition and noncommunicable diseases. Feeding and care of children during illness remains poor despite its crucial importance for reducing child mortality and morbidity. Food hygiene and safety are also neglected, as is the role of migration in the health and nutritional well-being of both the migrants and the family members left behind.

Despite these challenges, Nepal has an excellent opportunity to sustain and even accelerate its nutritional improvements. In the MSNP the country has not only a roadmap for pursuing a more comprehensive and coordinated multisectoral nutrition strategy, but also substantial political momentum for sustaining its progress and continuing the important process of decentralizing public service delivery. In addition to solidifying its political and financial commitments, the challenge for Nepal will be to effectively operationalize the MSNP and other plans and policies supporting the nutrition agenda and improve their implementation, with specific attention to targeting and scale-up to further address the persistent public health and development burden of maternal and child undernutrition.

CHAPTER 14

Commitments and Accountability

Peru's Unique Nutrition Journey

SIVAN YOSEF AND JAY GOULDEN

PERUVIANS HAVE MUCH to celebrate in regard to the rapid progress the country has made in reducing malnutrition. In 2013, only 3.5 percent of children under five years of age in Peru were underweight.[1] Even smaller proportions—0.5 percent and 0.1 percent—were moderately or severely wasted.[2] But the statistic that many nutritionists point to when lauding the country as a nutrition success is Peru's rate of childhood stunting (Figure 14.1). In 2014, 14.6 percent of children under five years of age were stunted.[3] While this rate is not as low as the country's other nutrition indicators, it reflects a remarkable improvement. Less than a decade earlier, the prevalence was twice as high (29.5 percent).[4] How was this rapid progress achieved—not only at a national level, but across all of Peru's diverse regions, even poor rural ones including the Andean Highlands, and even amongst the poorest 20 percent of the population?

A first glance suggests that strong economic growth may have been the main driver of this dramatic change in nutrition. From 2002 to 2010, Peru enjoyed a 6.4 percent average annual economic growth rate.[5] In about the same period, the public budget doubled.[6] However, an analysis of economic performance and fiscal spending alongside changes in malnutrition rates by region shows little correlation. Nor is there a direct correlation between malnutrition reductions and other factors such as urbanization or mining revenues.[7] While clearly important, economic growth cannot fully account for the nutrition transformation.

Closer examination reveals three main factors that likely underlie Peru's successful fight against child malnutrition over the past decade.[8] The first is multisectoral cooperation, with central roles played by civil society and national and regional levels of government, and the use of "sheltered conveners," that is, actors who can coordinate others without being hampered by institutional conflicts. The second is political will, underlined by a pledge to invest in and prioritize nutrition that has sustained momentum for the fight against malnutrition through multiple political administrations. And third is a prevailing commitment to accountability that extends from national-level politics to more mundane, day-to-day budgetary processes. This chapter looks at the role of these factors and the ways they interconnect across Peru's recent journey in nutrition, to help us understand how countries can achieve and sustain national- and regional-level improvements in nutrition.

Setting the Stage: 1970–2005

Peru's early years of nutrition policy focused on food distribution. In the 1970s and 1980s, the country's efforts on hunger and malnutrition were largely limited to food aid, coordinated primarily by nongovernmental organizations (NGOs) and two large food assistance programs, Programa de Asistencia Directa (PAD or Direct Assistance Program), an employment-based program targeted to marginalized urban and rural areas, and Vaso de Leche (Glass of Milk) targeted to children under six years of age. In the 1990s, the National Program for Food Assistance managed most of the country's food assistance programs, including a network of nearly 20,000 direct feeding sites or soup kitchens (Comedores Populares). PAD was eventually merged into the National Program for Food Assistance along with other food-related programs, with the exception of Vaso de Leche.[9]

By the early- to mid-2000s, Peru was at a crossroads. In 2000, Vaso de Leche and Comedores Populares comprised nearly 60 percent of Peru's food assistance budget but were having no discernible impact on malnutrition, such as child height.[10] Rates of childhood malnutrition, especially in the form of stunting, had been stagnant since 1996—the slow national rate of decline of 0.3 percent per year persisted and rural rates of malnutrition

FIGURE 14.1 Child stunting in Peru, 2004–2006 to 2014

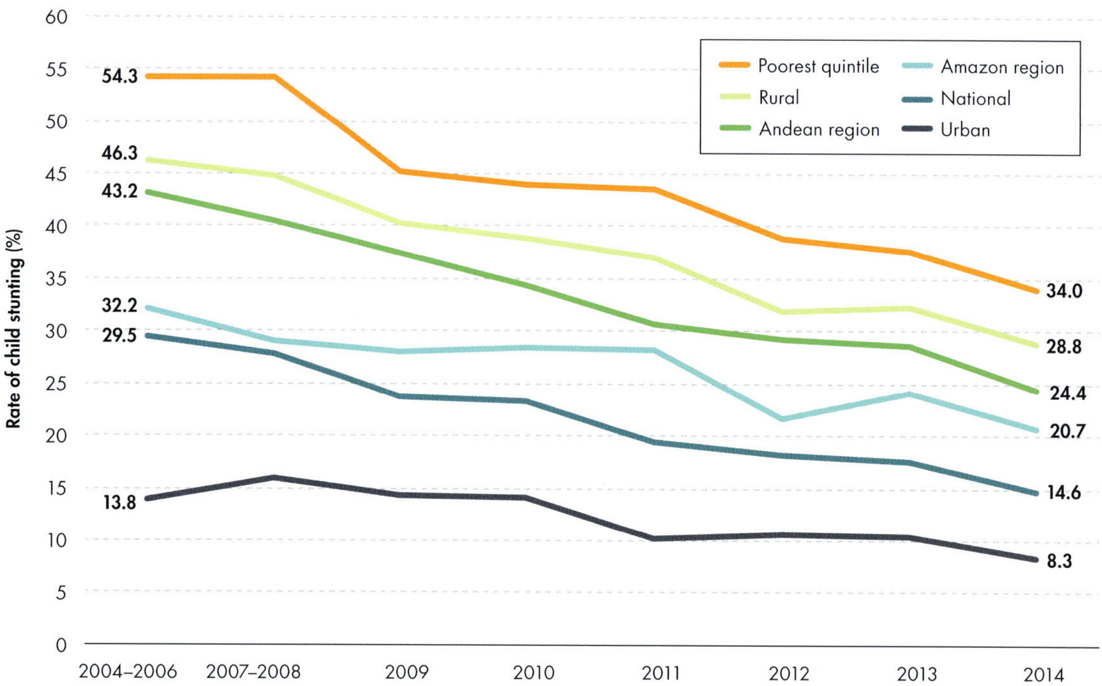

Source: Authors, based on Demographic and Health Survey data.

remained unchanged at 40 percent between 1995 and 2005.[11] The prevalence of stunting was among the highest in Latin America and the Caribbean, 7 percentage points above the regional average—surprisingly high considering Peru's status as a middle-income country that was enjoying the second-highest rate of economic growth in the region.[12] Furthermore, only 28 percent of individuals eligible for services from food assistance programs were able to access them.[13]

In 2001, newly elected President Alejandro Toledo launched a broad reform of social policy that included guaranteed access to healthcare and greater government accountability, promoted the Millennium Development Goals, and created institutional infrastructure for social protection as a poverty-reduction strategy. The National Strategy for Food Security approved in 2004 was never implemented but nevertheless established the organizational processes that supported a later poverty and nutrition program (CRECER).[14] In 2005, President Toledo also set up Juntos, a conditional cash transfer program designed to reduce poverty as well as malnutrition and mortality among children and infants. The prime minister's office was responsible for running this program, which included mechanisms to promote intersectoral coordination.

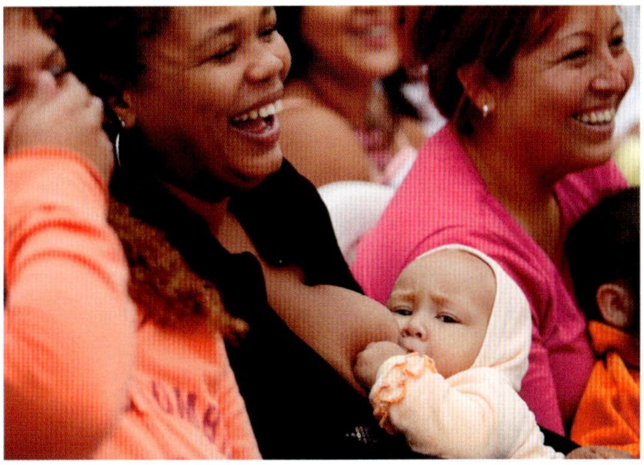

Reuters/E. Castro-Mendivil

Peru's CRECER program aimed to improve nutrition during the first 1,000 days of a child's life.

Under Juntos, households received a monthly transfer of 100 *soles* (US$30) on condition that they keep their children in school, complete health visits including prenatal and postnatal visits, and use the National Nutrition Assistance Program package for children under three years of age.[15] Uniquely for a social protection initiative, Juntos also provided reparations to communities affected by violent conflict. Unfortunately, the program did not include an impact evaluation framework at its outset, which would have facilitated evaluation.[16] The program expanded rapidly, from serving 110 districts and 37,000 households in 2005 to 1,140 districts and 810,000 households in 2012.[17]

Momentum Builds: 2006–2011

In 2006, momentum increased significantly for improving nutrition in Peru. The Child Nutrition Initiative (CNI), an advocacy coalition of civil society, UN agencies, and donors working on health and nutrition, with CARE-Peru in a coordination role, was formed. CNI took on a central role in the nutrition movement—advocating for making nutrition a key part of all poverty-reduction initiatives, promoting greater coordination of external donor funding, and publicly monitoring political commitments to nutrition. Rooted in this monitoring work, CNI launched a nutrition campaign during the 2006 presidential election season that enlisted 10 presidential candidates to pledge to "5 by 5 by 5" if elected: to reduce chronic child malnutrition by 5 percent in children under 5 years of age within 5 years. The pledge also included a commitment to closing the urban-rural gap in malnutrition rates. To our knowledge, this type of high-level advocacy on nutrition had never been undertaken before anywhere in the world.

When President Garcia was elected, he went a step beyond the "5 by 5 by 5" pledge and, with support from CNI, increased the national goal

BOX 14.1 **Results-based budgeting**

The annual budget for the CRECER strategy more than doubled between 2007 and 2011, from US$216 million to US$495 million.[18] Much of this funding was administered through results-based or performance-based budgeting. Beginning in 2008, the Ministry of Economy instituted this approach for five programs, including the Joint Nutrition Program, a new nutrition funding mechanism, and the Newborn and Maternal Health program. These programs were funded according to activity lines that reflected international evidence on effectiveness, and were monitored regularly based on annual evaluations. Findings from the evaluations were incorporated into subsequent program reforms. This process was a significant one, considering its uniqueness and the scale of funds. Progress was measured according to the program's success in achieving planned outcomes and in achieving efficiency and equity (spending per household affected). Consensus-based monitoring was undertaken both at the national and regional levels and involved the participation of civil society, including women and farmer groups. These processes now need to be improved at the municipal level, although there is disagreement as to whether municipal governments have the same technical capabilities as regional governments to absorb and use funds accountably.[19]

for stunting reduction to 9 percentage points over 5 years. He also set up a temporary strategy team (ST-CIAS) to coordinate across ministries and to report progress on nutrition directly to the prime minister, reflecting the priority given to nutrition.

The new government also created a multisectoral strategy, CRECER ("to grow" in Spanish), by executive decree in 2007, managed directly from the prime minister's office. CRECER took the government's existing portfolio of more than 82 social programs and winnowed it down to 26 programs focused on poverty and child malnutrition. These programs heeded the call of CNI and the Pan American Health Organization to go beyond food distribution and moved to promote initiatives in other sectors considered critical to achieving nutrition gains, such as complementary foods (foods other than breast milk or formula fed to an infant); water, sanitation, and health; and conditional cash transfers. CRECER also focused attention on the first 1,000 days of a child's life, from conception to 2 years of age, considered to be the window of opportunity for making lifelong nutrition impacts. Results-based budgeting was introduced by the Ministry of Finance and supported by the World Bank, with a nutrition program as one of the first priorities (see Box 14.1).

Under a program of decentralization, responsibility for these nutrition-related initiatives was devolved to several ministries and to regional and municipal governments, in partnership with civil society and NGOs, with significant funding support from the national government and external donors. Decentralization was strengthened when regional presidents—convened by the government with the support of CNI—signed the Lima Declaration on Child Nutrition in 2006, which aimed to reduce chronic child malnutrition by 5 percent by 2011. Facilitated by legislation that devolved the CRECER agenda to municipal and regional governments, CRECER was implemented in more than 1,100 districts, targeting the two lowest poverty quintiles of the population.[20] Regions and provincial and district municipalities were encouraged to develop explicit targets for nutrition, with mixed results.[21] Indeed, regional disparities remain large, with some regions suffering from stunting prevalence rates as high as 35 percent (Huancavelica), while others boast rates as low as 3.7 percent (Tacna).[22] Nevertheless, between 2007 and 2012, CRECER-targeted districts experienced a 21.4 percentage point reduction in the prevalence of stunting in children under five years of age (54.7 to 33.3 percent), compared to a 10.4 percentage point reduction nationally (28.5 to 18.1 percent).[23]

Many of CRECER's interventions focused on health, with a significant amount of funding also going to Juntos. In 2007, Juntos was redesigned to include nutrition-related conditionalities, such as growth monitoring and promotion.[24] An evaluation of Juntos in 2012 found that the program reduced moderate and extreme poverty gaps among beneficiaries by 14 percent and 7 percent, respectively. The household transfer of 100 soles represented 15 percent of total monthly household consumption, considered moderate compared to other conditional cash transfer programs in Latin America.[25] Beneficiary households consumed 15 percent more food items.[26] A more recent study found that the prevalence of severe stunting was reduced among Juntos participants, with a sizeable increase of 0.13 in height-for-age Z-scores (HAZ or linear growth).[27] Another found that participation in Juntos was associated with a 0.43–0.52 increase in HAZ among boys aged 7–8, and a 0.60 decrease in body mass index-for-age Z-score and 2.7 percentage point decrease in overweight among girls aged 7–8.[28]

Multisectoral coordination also characterized this period in Peru's nutrition journey. CRECER was placed within the prime minister's office, under the interministerial Commission for Social Affairs, to ensure that CRECER had sufficient political and institutional leverage to carry out its mandate, in terms of both implementation and evaluation. The commission was able to coordinate the nutrition activities of CRECER with ministries such as Agriculture, Education, Finance, Health, Woman and Development, and Work and Job Creation.[29] CNI continued to release annual progress reports, and helped develop national and regional guidelines and strategies for presentation to the president, prime minister, and ministries. It also launched national and local media campaigns around its reports and during national and subnational elections. In 2010, the country joined the international Scaling Up Nutrition (SUN) movement.

Nutrition data formed the cornerstone of Peru's renewed commitment to accountability. Annual Demographic and Health Surveys provided vital information on nutrition trends, and possible links between nutrition results and various initiatives. The availability of such data on a yearly basis was impressive, and the sample sizes were large enough to allow for changes to be tracked at the departmental level and for large geographic groupings, such as urban and rural areas, the Andean highlands, and the Peruvian Amazon region. The Ministry of Finance also provided line-item data on budgeting and expenditures, which were used for sophisticated monitoring of equity and efficiency in the consensus-based monitoring mechanism.

Testing the Commitment: 2011–2016

A new election cycle in 2011 raised the question, would Peru's commitment to nutrition weather a new political administration? Nutrition proponents within CNI decided to not wait to find out: a pre-election campaign was launched once again to garner commitments from national and regional candidates.

With the election of President Ollanta Humala, political will was indeed renewed. Humala set new targets of reducing stunting from 23 to 10 percent and reducing childhood anemia from 50 to 20 percent, both by 2016. He reorganized the administration of nutrition within the government, creating a Ministry of Development and Social Inclusion (MIDIS) and immediately tasking it with coordinating a revised nutrition strategy as part of the government's overall social inclusion strategy—Incluir para Crecer (Include for Growth). Incluir

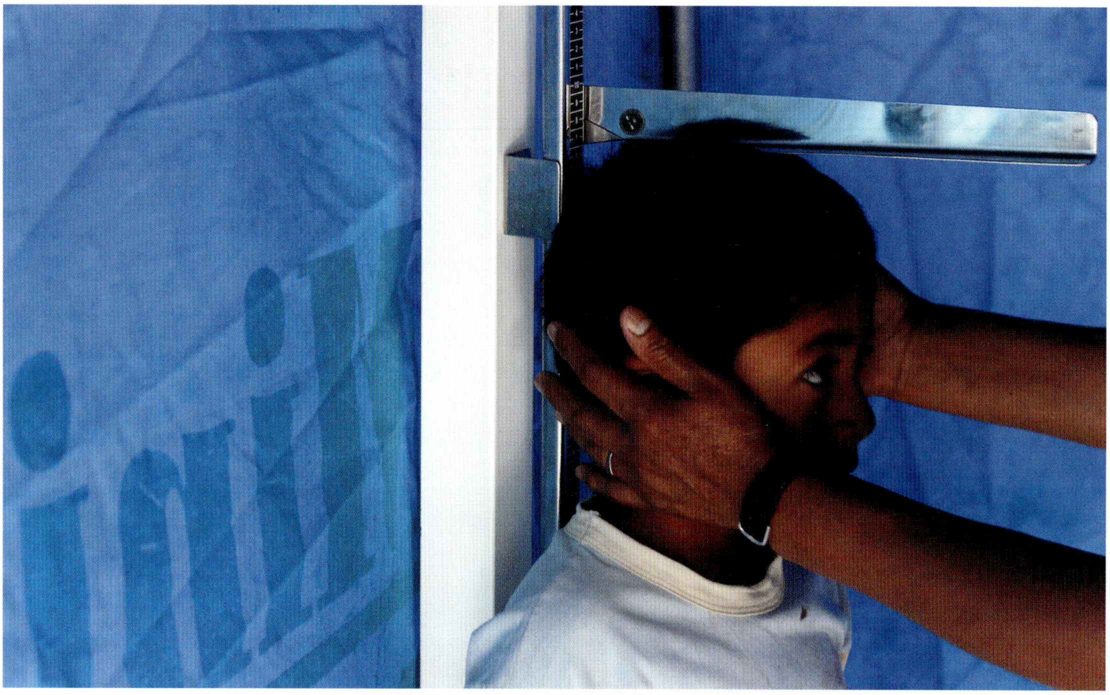

Reuters/M. del Triunfo

A boy gets a height check during a health campaign; Peru cut its rate of child stunting in half in less than a decade.

para Crecer provides interventions throughout the life cycle of at-risk individuals, from early childhood through adolescence, adulthood, and old age. It also seeks to reduce gaps in access to basic social services for the vulnerable, and improve the performance of public management for social programs and services. The new ministry was also responsible for five social programs.

The new administration showed an understanding of the key role decentralization was playing in Peru's nutrition fight. With financial assistance from the European Community and the World Bank, local governments were provided incentives in the form of funding increases of up to 50 percent for successfully aligning their health and nutrition policies with those of the national government, under a conditional transfer program known as the Municipal Incentives Plan. While experience with this scheme has reportedly been positive, a recent assessment suggested that regional governments were often more motivated by a desire to maintain good relations with the Ministry of Economy and Finance than by financial incentives, and that poorer areas and less densely populated ones performed worse than more affluent, urbanized areas.[30] Regions were also given incentives to meet region-specific targets. The majority of the indicators under the Incentives Plan relate to project management, but a few are focused on nutrition and health: immunization coverage; growth monitoring; iron supplementation for children; and iron/folate supplementation for pregnant women. As of 2013, targeted regions have received approximately 75 percent of the total incentive funds they would get for perfect performance.[31]

Lessons Learned

Peru's nutrition journey continues today. The country faces disparities in nutritional status among its regions and between urban and rural areas, particularly small, remote communities. And iron-deficiency anemia remains a serious problem.[32] However, Peru's success in reducing childhood stunting deserves recognition and provides some lessons. The use of sheltered conveners emerges as a critical determinant of the country's success. During the 2006–2011 administration, for example, Peru delegated responsibility for moving nutrition forward to a single player—the prime minister's office—that had the leveraging power, sanctioned by the president, to convene multiple sectors, mostly free of institutional conflicts.[33] Strong support for a multisectoral approach that allows for coordinated policy interventions and approaches is essential for improving nutrition. Interestingly, the radical changes in Peru's approach to nutrition took place in a context of widespread mistrust of government and other public institutions. As of 2008, Peru had much lower levels of public confidence in its Congress and political parties than neighboring countries (12 percent of Peruvians trusted Congress and 11 percent trusted political parties compared with the Latin American averages of 32 percent and 21 percent, respectively).[34] Also of note was that members of Congress and of political parties had very limited knowledge of nutrition policy. On the one hand, this shielded the process from political influence and partisanship; on the other hand, nutrition initiatives can benefit from congressional support, including nutrition legislation, monitoring of the executive branch, and direct accountability to voters.[35]

Strong buy-in to the idea that nutrition matters among diverse stakeholders and at high levels, including buy-in from presidential candidates and government ministries, also likely contributed to Peru's success. The clear and shared narrative on nutrition created by the members of CNI, including a clear framework of the direct and underlying causes of malnutrition, also fostered a strong commitment on nutrition.[36] This seemingly simple narrative was not only useful for seizing opportunities, such as national elections, but also ensured that nongovernmental actors—civil society, donors, academic institutions, and UN agencies—were coordinated and aligned in their engagement with the government. Indeed, joint projects carried out by UN agencies and some of the primary civil society organizations supported implementation of the CRECER and Incluir para Crecer strategies. Such coordination seems to be relatively rare. In many other countries participating in the SUN movement, there are separate SUN networks for civil society, donors, UN agencies, and other sectors (such as academia or business), and a clear, shared position or approach is not developed.

The Peru case also underlines the importance of collecting national and subnational data, allowing for timely monitoring of vital nutrition indicators. The availability of annual data on results, coverage, and financing was critical for enabling a collaborative approach to monitoring and to adjusting programs as required. High-quality data can flag potential problems with program design. An early evaluation of Juntos, for example, suggested that impacts on diet quality were mixed. Beneficiaries were consuming greater quantities of nutritious foods such as vegetables (2.86 *soles* monthly per capita expenditure versus 2.52 in control) and fruit (2.06 versus 1.40), but also more breads and cereals (10.15 versus 8.15) and sugar (3.17 versus 2.65).[37] These numbers suggest that nutritional implications need to be more carefully assessed in any future redesign of Juntos, especially considering that obesity in Peru doubled between 1996 and 2011.[38]

One challenge that lies ahead for Peru is the need to build capacity for implementation and monitoring and evaluation at the regional and municipal levels.[39] The government's commitment to decentralization and the alignment of donor, NGO, and local strategies with the national strategy were key factors in its success. However, decentralization combined with results-based budgeting meant that districts with better results, usually those with more NGOs present, received more technical assistance. This may have left poor performers lagging further behind. These lagging regions and municipalities need greater capacity to receive and process nutrition funds, as well as to implement programs and comply with targets. Capacity building will be critical so that Peru can sustain its successes in nutrition and increase its focus on the geographical and population groups where the highest rates of malnutrition are now concentrated.

CHAPTER 15

On the Fast Track

Driving Down Stunting in Vietnam

MEAGAN KEEFE

VIETNAM HAS MADE dramatic progress in improving nutrition over the past three decades. Following the introduction of Vietnam's Doi Moi ("renovation") economic policies in 1986, the country's economic performance began to improve rapidly. By the 1990s, Vietnam was among the fastest growing economies in the world. From one of the five poorest countries in the world in 1984, Vietnam rose to a rank of 167 out of 206 by 1999.[1] As the country transitioned to a market-oriented economy, rapid economic growth was accompanied by a similarly dramatic decline in the poverty rate, which fell from nearly 75 percent of the population in 1984, to 58 percent in 1993, and down to 37 percent by 1998.[2] Economic growth enabled the country to provide improved health services, which contributed directly to reductions in child malnutrition.[3]

Major progress was made in reducing stunting rates among Vietnamese children under five, particularly in the mid-1990s, when stunting prevalence decreased from 50 percent to 34 percent (1993–1998).[4] Significant changes were made in the health sector as part of the country's economic reforms in this period, including legalization of private medical practice, liberalization of the pharmaceutical industry, and deregulation of retail sales of drugs and medicines, all of which contributed to improvements in health services.[5] A range of nutrition and health policy initiatives introduced by the National Institute for Nutrition in the 1990s likely had an impact on child malnutrition too. Programs to improve the energy and protein content of diets, breastfeeding promotion efforts, salt iodization, increased child immunization efforts, increased availability of oral rehydration therapy, reduced costs of drugs and medical care, and increased health insurance coverage of school children all likely played a role.[6]

Vietnam's rapid economic growth continued throughout the 2000s, and by 2014, it ranked as the world's 55th richest nation. Great strides were made in poverty reduction as well, with the poverty rate reduced to just 2 percent by 2012.[7] However, despite these achievements, the substantial reductions in stunting prevalence achieved in the 1990s were not sustained in the new decade. The decline

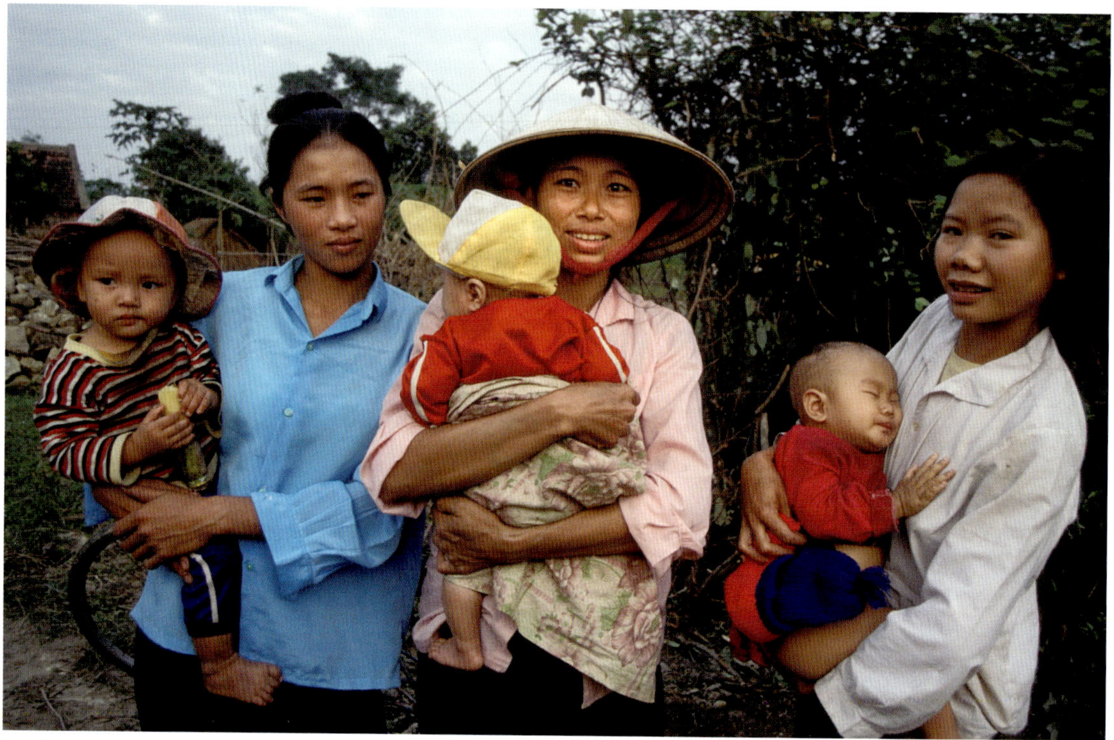

Panos/S. Sprague

To help raise its relatively low rate of exclusive breastfeeding, Vietnam adopted several measures designed to make breastfeeding easier.

in malnutrition was much less than expected, given increased household incomes, food price declines, and increased agricultural production throughout the country.[8] In terms of nutrition outcomes, the prevalence of underweight in children under five was reduced significantly, from 32 percent to 18 percent between 2000 and 2010, but stunting prevalence was only marginally reduced, from 35 percent to 30 percent, during that period.[9] Despite improvements in many health indicators over this time, child malnutrition rates lagged behind, indicating the need to focus particular attention on reducing stunting.[10]

After this slowdown, progress on reducing stunting prevalence resumed at a rapid pace in 2010. Stunting prevalence dropped from 29 percent to 19 percent between 2010 and 2013.[11] Although little research has looked at what is driving these rapid changes, this chapter examines key factors that have likely contributed to this accelerated progress.

Successes in Nutrition-Relevant Policy and Programming

At least three achievements have likely contributed to the reduction in child stunting: prioritization of nutrition by the national government, policies designed to improve infant and child feeding practices, and efforts to reduce micronutrient deficiencies.

Prioritizing Nutrition at a National Level

Vietnam's commitment to reducing malnutrition was strengthened by a series of events between 2006 and 2012. Internally, the first-ever review of the National Nutrition Strategy was conducted in 2007 to evaluate progress and inform future strategy. A Plan of Action to Accelerate the Reduction of Child Stunting in Vietnam was drafted in a coordinated effort to target the country's child stunting problems. At the same time, the country hosted several high profile international events, including the launch of the *Lancet* Series on Maternal and Child Undernutrition and the United Nation's Standing Committee for Nutrition (SCN) Annual Conference.[12]

These events set the stage for an increased focus on nutrition for Vietnam both within the country and internationally. The development of the new National Nutrition Strategy in 2011–2012 put the spotlight on reducing stunting and on development of specific targets for reductions in stunting and underweight by 2030. Vietnam also was one of the few countries to incorporate the World Health Organization's new indicators into its National Nutrition Surveillance System. These indicators emphasize infant and young child feeding and support better monitoring of key nutrition outcomes. While highlighting Vietnam's commitment globally, these events also served to bring the country's National Assembly into the nutrition discussion and to promote the critical importance of nutrition issues within the Ministry of Health.[13]

Implementing Policies to Improve Infant and Young Child Feeding

Beyond the new nutrition strategy, Vietnam also reinforced its emphasis on nutrition with a series of nutrition-sensitive policies. Despite a relatively robust public health system and high usage of health services, little specific action had been taken to improve infant and child feeding practices through education and support to mothers. Beginning in 2010, Vietnam began to promote breastfeeding and to enact policies aimed at increasing knowledge about the importance of breastfeeding and feeding practices for infants and young children.[14] The 2011–2020 National Nutrition Strategy incorporates infant and young child feeding as a critical area for improving nutrition and pays specific attention to reducing stunting and underweight alongside reducing obesity. Vietnam also developed a National Infant and Young Child Feeding Action Plan to put the strategy into practice.

Because many mothers were turning to breast-milk substitutes as a result of their work schedules, in 2012 Vietnam's National Assembly voted to extend paid maternity leave from 4 to 6 months in an effort to reduce this important barrier to breastfeeding. The National Assembly also expanded the country's ban on advertising of breast-milk substitutes, which was a critical step in reducing misinformation about the benefits of infant formula. Although Vietnam remains one of the countries with the lowest prevalence of exclusive breastfeeding in the region, the rate of exclusive breastfeeding for infants under 6 months increased significantly between 2011 and 2014, from 17 percent (where it had been stalled since 2006) to 24 percent.[15] Other recent reforms reflecting the government's focus on improving infant and young child feeding practices include the introduction of new hospital certification criteria (2013), a new national breastfeeding code (2014), and a decree on providing lactation spaces in workplaces to make them more breastfeeding-friendly (2015).

Reducing Anemia

Vietnam has also made strides in reducing the prevalence of anemia in both women and children over the last decade.[16] The government prioritized the control and prevention of micronutrient deficiencies in both its 2001–2010 National Nutrition Strategy as well as the current strategy and targeted the prevention of iron deficiency in particular, which has likely contributed to the progress in combatting anemia. With a focus on reducing child malnutrition, the National Plan of Action for Nutrition targeted the prevention of iron, vitamin A, and iodine deficiencies through a range of activities, including supplementation, diet diversification, and food fortification. Although national data on vitamin and mineral deficiencies are limited, Vietnam is currently on course to meet the World Health Assembly's 2025 anemia target and may even exceed its target of 6.7 percent prevalence by 2025.[17]

Despite the progress shown in reducing anemia, micronutrient deficiencies are still a problem in the country, with much of the population at risk for zinc, vitamin A, folate, and vitamin B12 deficiencies, and the 6–17 month age group particularly at risk.[18] The low micronutrient and protein content of complementary foods typically fed to this age group, including rice flour and rice porridge, point to the importance of improving child feeding practices.[19] To develop interventions that target existing deficiencies, better national data on vitamin and mineral deficiencies are needed.

In addition to specific interventions to improve food diversity and quality, food fortification of everyday products—such as rice, soy sauce, and fish sauce—is also being explored in Vietnam to address some of these critical micronutrient deficiencies. A 2003 Ministry of Health decree set voluntary fortification standards for a number of staple foods and condiments, which prompted various initiatives to assess the feasibility of fortification in Vietnam.[20] Currently, the government is working to mandate fortification of salt and wheat flour to better address some key micronutrient deficiencies.[21]

Remaining Challenges

Vietnam still faces nutrition challenges related to inequities between groups and rising rates of obesity and overweight.

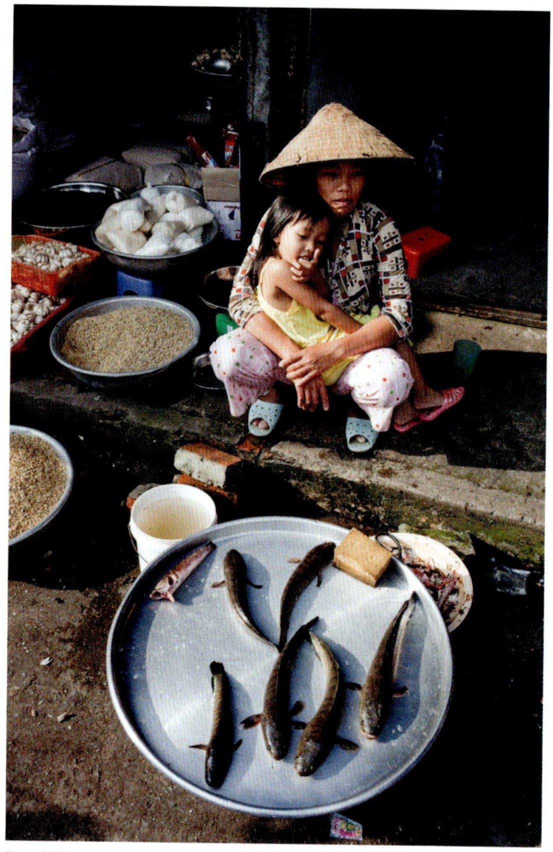

Panos/J. Visser

Vietnam is exploring the idea of fortifying everyday foods like fish to help address micronutrient deficiencies.

Inequities

Inequities persist between key vulnerable groups (rural, poor, and minority populations) and the nonpoor, in terms of both poverty and nutrition.[22] Ethnic minorities make up only 15 percent of the population in Vietnam but account for nearly half the remaining poor in the country.[23] Similarly, children of rural households, poor households, and ethnic minority backgrounds are significantly more likely to be malnourished. Across the 63 provinces, the prevalence of stunting ranges from 7 percent to 40 percent, suggesting that the improvements taking place in the country are still failing to reach the rural poor and minorities.[24] Improving nutrition policy implementation at the local level and addressing these inequities is critical to reducing malnutrition in these vulnerable groups.[25]

As the central government has begun to decentralize, turning more authority over to the provinces to fund and carry out district- and commune-level activity, Vietnam has experienced difficulties in translating national policy into service provision and action at the local level.[26] While planning at local levels should theoretically allow for tailoring of targeted plans and specific nutrition actions to local contexts, the current top-down approach does not allow for provincial-level decision making on goals, priorities, or funding decisions.[27] Some evidence suggests that the relatively unsuccessful decentralization process is actually increasing inequities between provinces, through inadequate targeting of interventions and insufficient budgets.[28] Decisions are still made within the largely centralized ministerial structure in Hanoi. To achieve further success in reducing malnutrition in Vietnam, it will be critical to build capacity for subnational planning and implementation of nutrition policy—through data-driven processes that can be tailored to local contexts.[29] A strategic multiyear approach to nutrition policy could potentially strengthen the subnational planning process and address the difficulty of translating national policy into action at the local level.[30]

Rising Obesity and Overweight

With Vietnam's rapid economic development and urbanization, overweight and obesity problems have begun to emerge alongside the country's undernutrition challenges. This dual burden of malnutrition can be seen in children, adolescents, and adults, with higher prevalence of overweight in urban areas.[31] At the national level, prevalence of overweight and obesity among adolescents was 6 percent and 1 percent, respectively, in 2013. In Ho Chi Minh City, however, prevalence has been found to be much higher, and was already at 18 percent and 3 percent, respectively, by 2010.[32] As Vietnam continues its battle against undernutrition, it will need to acknowledge the emerging public health challenge of overweight and obesity and ensure that its nutrition policies address the dual burden of malnutrition.

Conclusion

Vietnam has firmly established malnutrition on the national agenda. Nutrition successes have been achieved in a rapidly changing environment, providing an example of the progress that can be made with a harmonized approach, key nutrition-sensitive legislation, and coordinated development-partner initiatives complemented by socioeconomic development. With its National Assembly enacting nutrition-relevant policies and laws and the National Institute for Nutrition putting nutrition-specific initiatives into place, Vietnam has made tackling malnutrition a priority. Rapid acceleration in the reduction of stunting over the last four years shows that Vietnam's approach works. Sustaining this progress now depends on improving subnational nutrition planning and implementing targeted nutrition interventions, while addressing existing inequities and the growing challenge of obesity.

CHAPTER 16

Agriculture, WASH, and Safety Nets

Ethiopia's Multisector Story

ANDREA WARREN

OVER THE PAST 25 years, Ethiopia has made remarkable headway in addressing the country's nutrition situation. Despite ongoing challenges, significant progress has been made toward meeting the United Nations Millennium Development Goals, including halving child mortality, doubling the number of people with access to clean water, and quadrupling primary school enrollment. Ethiopia is also on track to eradicate extreme hunger and poverty.[1] The country was one of the top five performing countries in the 2000s in terms of reducing stunting by reducing its prevalence from 57.4 percent in 2000 to 44.2 percent in 2011, although levels remained high at 40.0 percent in 2014.[2] The same 2014 Demographic and Health Survey found that a further 9 percent of children younger than 5 years old experience wasting, and only 4 percent of children meet the standards for a minimal acceptable diet (a World Health Organization [WHO]/UNICEF indicator for complementary feeding).[3] Significant regional differences persist, with the highest rates of stunting (52 percent) found in Amhara and the lowest found in Gambela (27 percent) and Addis Ababa (22 percent). Overall, stunting is more prevalent in rural (46 percent) than in urban areas (36 percent).[4]

The Government of Ethiopia has been proactive in addressing the myriad determinants of undernutrition. Programs, strategies, and partnerships developed since at least 2005 reflect a consideration of both immediate determinants, addressed through "nutrition-specific" interventions, and underlying determinants, addressed through "nutrition-sensitive" interventions.[5] More-immediate determinants, including health status and nutrient intake, are addressed through the government's National Health Extension Program, which has expanded rapidly since 2003 and works to address knowledge gaps pertaining to nutrition at the household level.[6] The government's Community-Based Nutrition Program is another initiative addressing the more immediate determinants of poor nutrition using community-based child growth monitoring and directly engaging communities through nutrition education.[7] In addition, the government is working to fortify wheat

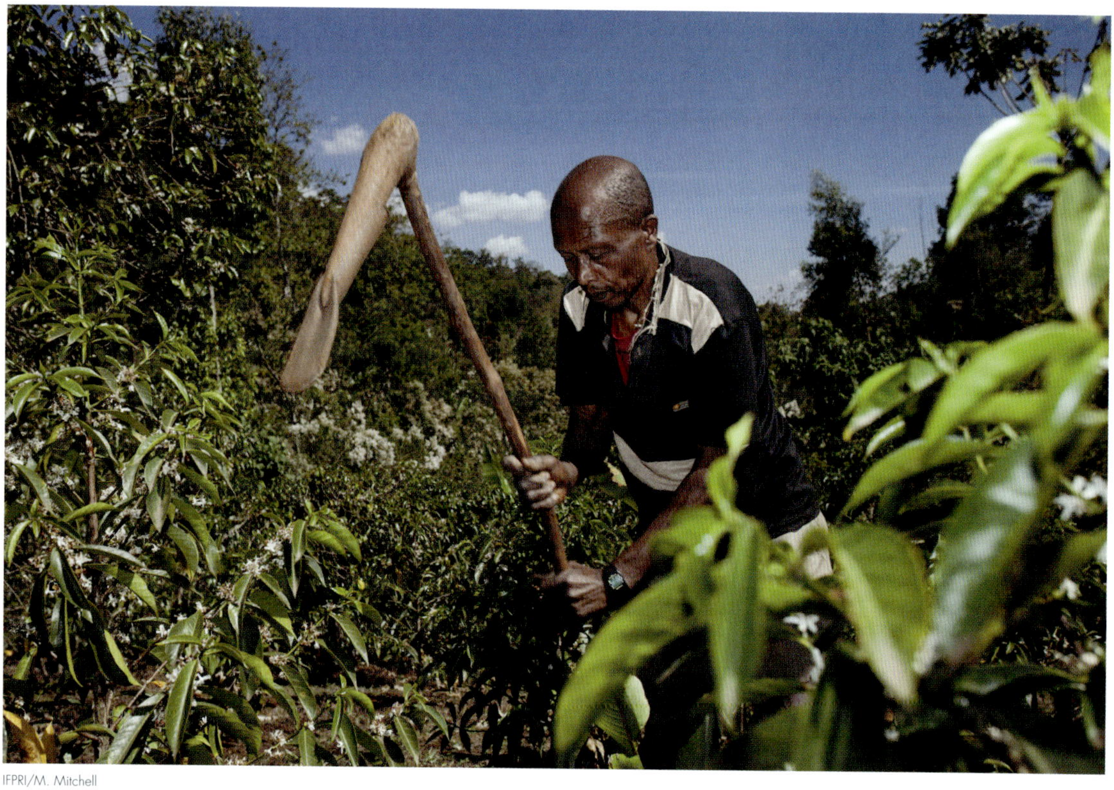

IFPRI/M. Mitchell

Nutrition-sensitive agriculture programs have played a large role in Ethiopia's nutrition improvements.

flour through a Feed the Future–supported public-private partnership known as the African Alliance for Improved Food Processing.[8] The government also works with UNICEF and the Global Alliance for Improved Nutrition (GAIN) on the Universal Salt Iodization Partnership.[9] The government developed the National Nutrition Program (NNP) (2013–2015), which outlined a comprehensive range of both nutrition-specific and nutrition-sensitive approaches to addressing undernutrition. A key feature of the program, now extended to 2020, has been its emphasis on developing explicit multisectoral linkages and initiatives to address inadequate nutrition.[10]

Significant progress has also been made toward addressing the underlying determinants of undernutrition, including education, sanitation, and food security. Government expenditures on education increased from 8.8 percent to 16.7 percent, and social protection program expenditures grew from 7.0 percent to 19.8 percent between 2000 and 2010.[11] Widespread efforts to end open defecation have been implemented through government systems for more than a decade.[12] The government recently introduced explicitly nutrition-sensitive provisions into its Productive Safety Net Program (PSNP).[13] As will be discussed further in the following sections, the PSNP is a large national social protection program administered by the Ministry of Agriculture and dedicated to improving food security among the most vulnerable people in the country. Discussion has recently centered on ways of incorporating nutrition into other flagship agricultural programs. For example, the Agricultural Growth Program, which focuses on increasing crop production in high-production areas, recently undertook a pilot study to assess potential nutrition-sensitive pathways for its 2016–2020 phase.[14]

Working with international partners, the Government of Ethiopia developed a Comprehensive Africa Agriculture Development Programme (CAADP) compact, which is a plan to reduce hunger through agricultural development to which other countries in Africa have committed. The government participates in global forums attendant to the CAADP, including the New Alliance for Food Security and Nutrition.[15] Additionally, Ethiopia was one of the first ("early riser") members of the Scaling Up Nutrition (SUN) Movement when it joined in 2010. Since 2008 several working groups and technical committees concerned with addressing food security and malnutrition have been set up, including the UNICEF/UK Department for International Development (DFID)–convened Nutrition Development Partner Group and the Ethiopian-initiated National Nutrition Task Force and National Nutrition Coordinating Body.[16]

Despite the recent development of both nutrition-specific and nutrition-sensitive programs, policies, and frameworks, it may be argued that the most significant contributions to reductions in stunting nationwide have come from the incidentally nutrition-sensitive effects of growth in the agricultural sector, along with widespread improvements in sanitation.[17] Headey hypothesized, based on the limited data available, that growth in the agricultural sector may correspond to some increase in basic food security, which may be partly responsible for the overall trend toward reduced stunting observed since 2000.[18] Indeed, food production per capita has steadily increased, growing an average of 1.9 percent per year from 2002 to 2007 and 3.3 percent per year from 2007 to 2012, along with total agricultural production per capita, which grew 2.1 percent per year from 2002 to 2007 and 3.1 percent per year from 2007 to 2012.[19] Cereal crop yields have also risen quickly since 2008 relative to the rest of the continent. Sanitation improvements (particularly reductions in open defecation) were associated in recent analyses with reductions in anemia in pregnant women.[20] This improvement in maternal health in turn is associated with increased birth size, making sanitation one of the potential factors driving observed stunting reductions between 2000 and 2010.[21] The push to implement improved sanitation has been a notable policy success story, as will be discussed in the following sections.

This chapter uses household interviews to contribute to a discussion of improvements in agriculture and sanitation and their possible effects on lives and livelihoods at the community level. The discussion of agricultural improvements pays particular attention to nutrition-sensitive recent efforts in the study area (though these efforts were not termed "nutrition sensitive" at their inception). The discussion of sanitation describes in detail the strong commitment to implementing improved sanitation countrywide and identifies areas for ongoing improvements. Looking to the future of nutrition, we discuss the changes being made to the country's PSNP—a flagship government-led social protection program under the Ministry of Agriculture that is concerned primarily with alleviating food insecurity and preventing asset depletion for the most vulnerable households.[22] Recent changes to the program to make it explicitly nutrition sensitive demonstrate positive momentum toward improving nutrition and serve as evidence that nutrition is making its way into the policy mainstream. We conclude by discussing lessons learned from the different programs in place.

Background and Setting

The original data discussed in the following sections derives from research conducted for Stories of Change, a Transform Nutrition project designed to narrate the changes surrounding nutrition programming in several countries with high burdens of undernutrition. The research team conducted 30 in-depth, semistructured qualitative interviews with a sample of households practicing rain-fed subsistence agriculture in the zone of Wolaita, located in the Southern Nations, Nationalities, and Peoples Region (SNNPR) of Ethiopia. All households were chosen from a single village in one *kebele* (the lowest unit of government administration) to better assess shared experiences of changes in the community over time (Figure 16.1).

Agricultural Growth and Nutrition

Improvements in agricultural production nationally have been one of the three major drivers of economic growth in Ethiopia since 2004, along with investment in the public sector and an expansion of the service sector.[23] The agriculture sector averaged 7.6 percent growth per year between 2004 and 2014. Within the agriculture sector, crop production has seen the greatest growth per year—8.8 percent on average—and accounts for one-third of all GDP growth. The widespread distribution of improved seed and fertilizer is claimed to have been one of the most significant drivers of overall increases in crop production.[24] Notably, the government has invested significantly in environmental rehabilitation in degraded areas using physical labor from the public works arm of the PSNP, though this has not necessarily been a major driver of crop production nationally.[25]

The village under study was located on rocky, mountainous terrain that could be termed a less-favored area.[26] While villages less than 20 kilometers away had experienced rapid and significant improvements in agricultural productivity from the use of improved inputs over the past five years and were able to introduce irrigation, this area had undergone a progressive decline in soil fertility and water retention owing to extensive erosion and a lack of watershed management.[27] The issue of land degradation was compounded by dwindling farm sizes, with the majority of the study sample farming 0.5 hectare or less.

A recent initiative for environmental rehabilitation and watershed management halted the decline. Measures such as improved terracing, trenches, and bunds had been introduced, along with a World Bank–funded project to replant forests at the top of the mountain. The government had also been intensively promoting the use of improved seed and fertilizer through the agricultural extension service, and extension agents (known as development agents or DAs) began making regular visits to households despite the remoteness of the area.

Farmers reported that the environmental rehabilitation initiatives and efforts to increase crop yields had intensified since 2010. Much of the pathway between agriculture and nutrition appeared to consist of leveraging agriculture as a source of food, with less consideration being given to the issue of dietary diversity.[28] Nonetheless, farmers were quick to mention the benefits of recent agricultural programs to their crop yields and household food security. Several farmers reported that crop yields had doubled as a result of increased application of fertilizer, improved seed, and improved soil and water conservation techniques, though yields remained low relative to nearby *kebeles* owing to the recent history of land degradation and small farm sizes. Many noted that they were better able to meet their household food requirements, though all respondents had difficulty meeting all of their consumption needs through farm activities alone. Farmers suggested that the emphasis on production was beginning to shift toward an acknowledgment of the importance of consumption patterns. Several households reported that DAs had started advising them to grow and consume a variety of fruits and vegetables where possible.

The events in the study area over the past several years illustrate the thoroughness of the government's approach to agricultural intensification. Although parts of the country could benefit from the direct application of fertilizer and improved seed, Ethiopia is home to a vast array of landscapes and climatic zones, making a one-size-fits-all approach to agriculture impractical. To illustrate, a village representative from an adjacent *kebele* with fewer erosion and soil degradation problems reported that the use of fertilizer and improved seed had allowed households in that area to meet close to 100 percent of their consumption needs through farming.[29] This area's unique needs had to be addressed through environmental rehabilitation efforts before the benefits of modern inputs could be realized. According to farmers, the physical conservation measures had made the effective application of improved seed and fertilizer possible.

Sanitation

Change was stirring nearly 10 years before environmental rehabilitation took place, this time related to sanitation. In 2007, the Water and Sanitation Program[30] described a reportedly successful effort in the region from 2003 onward to promote "small doable practices" to improve sanitation and hygiene, emphasizing latrine-building and hand-washing at critical times. Households in the area reported that it took them several years to fully accept the idea of sanitation and hygiene, but with the strong

FIGURE 16.1 Administrative regions of Ethiopia

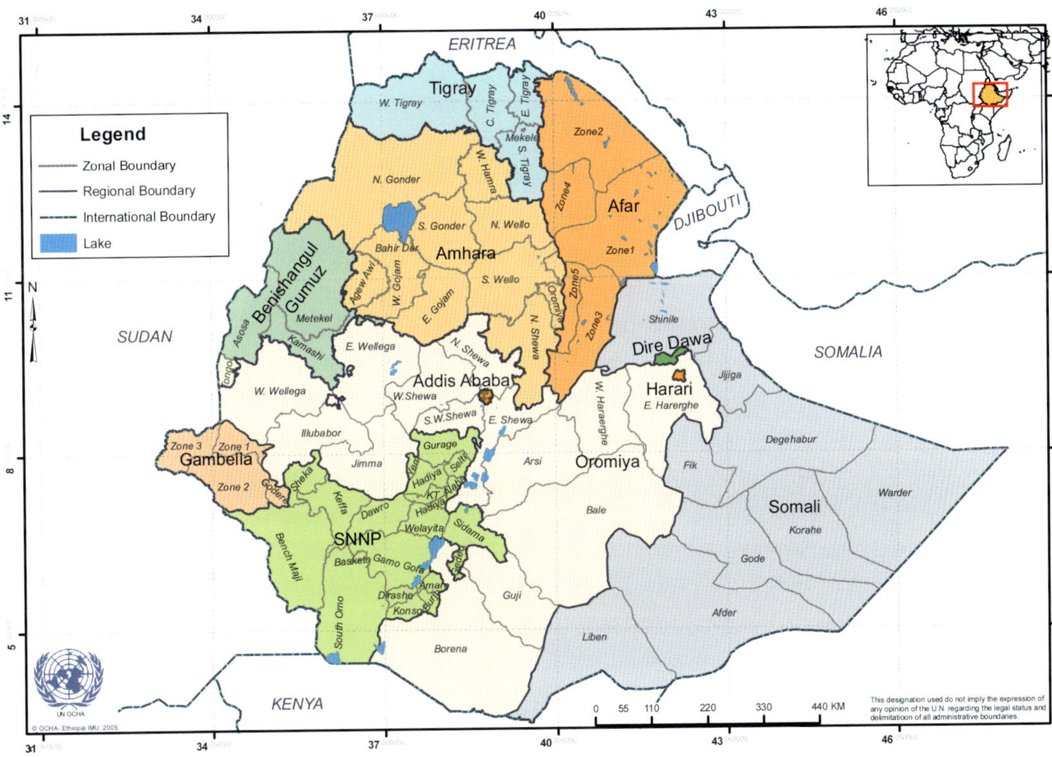

Source: Adapted from Relief Web, Administrative Regions of Ethiopia, http://reliefweb.int/sites/reliefweb.int/files/resources/73A2361742549480852572120070071 0-ocha_REF_eth051031.pdf.

commitment of the government, eventually all households reported that they had built pit latrines and adopted more hygienic practices. The study area was unique for its strong record in promoting improved sanitation and hygiene practices. At the district level, this area had recently received a Certificate of Excellence in water, sanitation, and hygiene from the federal government.

In the early 2000s, the government shifted from a curative to a preventative approach to healthcare. Sanitation, seen as one of the key low-input, high-impact interventions, was embraced as a cost-effective fit for the government's tight budgetary constraints.[31] In the SNNPR, a high-impact approach advocated by John Snow International and USAID, combined with elements from the successful Community-Led Total Sanitation (CLTS) program, was piloted in 20 districts before being scaled up to the entire region. Notably, the "small doable practices" approach promoted by CLTS was consonant with discussions with households: that is, incremental, practical changes should be made first. Project implementers highlighted the SNNPR as one of the more successful regions in which this approach was implemented.[32] Households reported anecdotally that they had noticed a decrease in diarrheal diseases in their children, a change potentially supported by national Demographic and Health Survey data suggesting that sanitation has an important effect on child growth outcomes.[33]

The push to implement improved sanitation had strong government support, and commitment was apparent at all levels of government, including dedicated budgetary support. National implementation was facilitated by clear hierarchical structures in place from the federal to the ground level, which ensured knowledge dissemination and accountability.[34] To implement health programming and disseminate knowledge thoroughly at the community level, the government's National Health Extension Program relied on what are known as 1:5 and 1:30 networks, in which one household acts as lead knowledge disseminator for five others, which are then organized into groupings of six or more, to form the larger 1:30 networks, also overseen by one leading household.[35] Latrine-building and hygiene initiatives were implemented and scaled up through the government's existing National Health Extension Program with support from international nongovernmental organizations and donors, including John Snow International and the Water and Sanitation Program.[36]

At the community level, ownership of latrines is now widespread, albeit not all are up to a satisfactory standard. Based on their positive experiences in their own homes, some respondents suggested that as a next step, constructing public latrines would benefit the community. While official project reports suggest generally positive outcomes in the SNNPR, an independent study of water and sanitation in the Shebedino district of the SNNPR concluded that implementation of project activities was overly supply-driven, and the limited community participation in planning and decision making led to unsatisfactory outcomes.[37] For example, only 37 percent of study respondents had a ventilated improved pit latrine, and only 27 percent considered their latrine complete, with walls, floor, and roof. Furthermore, follow-up and continued health education have reportedly been absent in the study area. This omission is echoed by concerns regarding sustainability and ownership discussed in Baye[38] and in a brief by the Water and Sanitation Program,[39] and is part of the issue of lack of monitoring around sanitation and hygiene programs identified by Plan International[40] and in a more recent report by the Water and Sanitation Program.[41] Given the potential importance of sanitation for improving nutrition outcomes, ongoing attention should be given to these issues.

Future Directions: The Productive Safety Net Program

Ethiopia's PSNP began in 2005 as a way to focus and coordinate repeated appeals for humanitarian aid to alleviate drought-related crises. When the program was introduced, it represented a marked shift in perspectives on poverty and vulnerability, seeking to build resilience among the most vulnerable households and to reduce poverty over time. Donors coalesced around these ideas, and the program, which was government led and implemented largely through government structures, began operating as a cash or food transfer program in the country's historically vulnerable districts. It is now one of the largest social protection programs in Africa south of the Sahara.[42] Since 2005, the PSNP has played an important role in improving food security for its beneficiaries as well as serving as a platform for disseminating improved agricultural technology and developing rural infrastructure.[43]

In its previous three phases, the program reached nearly 8 million of the most vulnerable individuals.[44] The program is designed to help beneficiaries get through the lean season without depleting household assets. Beneficiaries participate in public works activities in exchange for food or cash transfers for part of the year. If physically unable to work, beneficiaries may receive direct support. To achieve a more holistic approach to reducing poverty and increasing resilience, targeted livelihood packages were added on through the Household Asset Building Program.[45] Nutrition-sensitive provisions were added to the third phase of the program. For example, descriptions of possible linkages between the PSNP and the National Health Extension Program were provided, and the

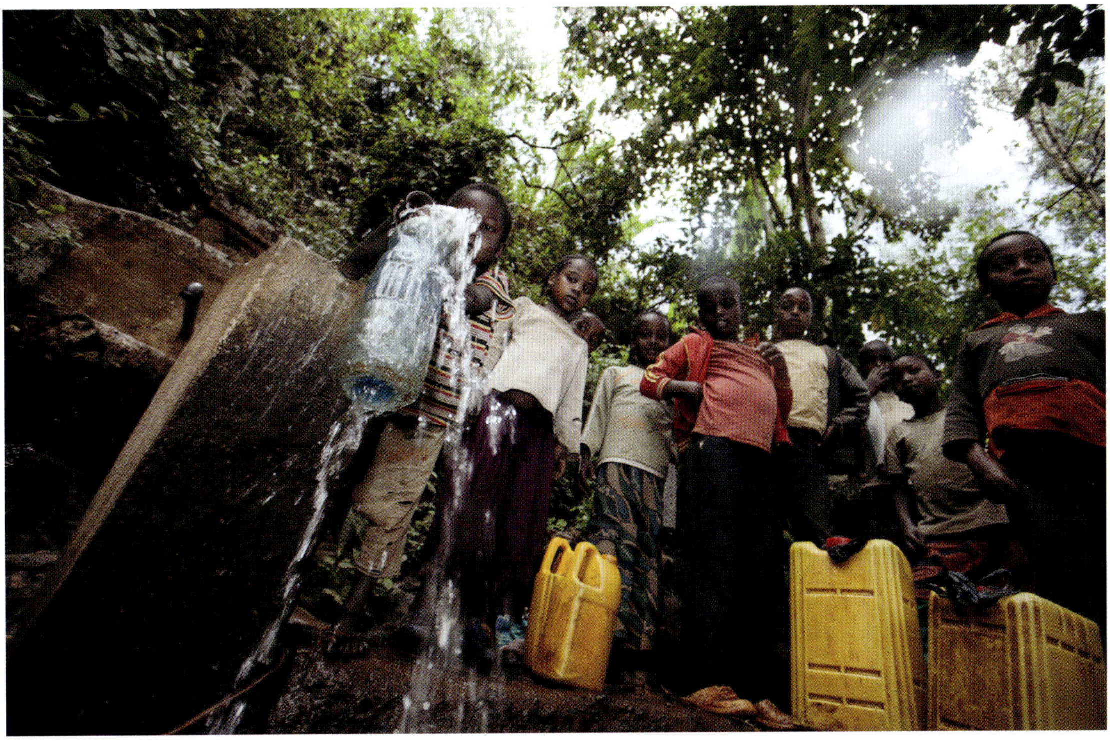

IFPRI/M. Mitchell

Better sanitation and hygiene in Ethiopia appear to have boosted children's growth.

list of eligible public works was expanded to include attending classes for nutrition education. However, capacity constraints and a lack of guidance and monitoring are claimed to have prevented most of the provisions from being fully realized.[46]

The changes to the PSNP, which went into effect in June 2015, will attempt to explicitly tie agriculture and health efforts together with a unified vision for improving nutrition outcomes nationwide through nutrition-sensitive programming. A social protection program at its core, the PSNP also serves as a space for experimentation and innovation in improving food security, economic status, and overall well-being. Over the course of its fourth phase (PSNP4, 2016–2020), the program aims to roll out nutrition-sensitive interventions and services as part of its normal operations and to put in place appropriate indicators and monitoring mechanisms to facilitate implementation.[47]

Among other measures, PSNP4 will renew the focus on multisectoral coordination to effectively implement nutrition-sensitive measures and increase monitoring capacity to ensure accountability. These changes will include stronger linkages with the Ministry of Health to connect clients with health services. In partnership with the health sector, behavior-change communication materials focusing on nutrition will be developed, and clients will be given the option to replace a portion of their public works obligations with behavior-change communication.[48] Pregnant women will immediately be transferred to direct support, which they will receive for up to one year after they give birth. Targeting criteria will be increasingly sensitized to "nutritionally vulnerable" households, such as those with pregnant or lactating women. Public works will be made more sensitive to gender and feature reduced physical requirements for women. Households with temporary nutrition emergencies will be considered for temporary inclusion. PSNP4 will also renew its focus on livelihood development and support but with a nutrition-sensitive spin.[49]

As a new frontier for promoting nutrition and an important space for innovation and experimentation, the results of PSNP4 will provide lessons and examples of how agriculture and nutrition can be linked through social protection programming.

Conclusions and Lessons Learned

In this chapter, we highlighted and discussed agricultural growth, sanitation, and the PSNP as examples of "stories of change" around nutrition in Ethiopia. The first two topics represent a cascade of interventions that demonstrate commitment and coherence from the federal to the ground level, although limited community participation in decision making on sanitation investments detracted from achieving full benefits. They also illustrate the importance of nutrition-sensitive interventions for improving livelihoods and living conditions as well as setting the stage for further improvements in health, food security, and economic growth. The changes to the PSNP are an important step toward advancing nutrition in development agendas more broadly and suggest the future directions and potential staying power of nutrition in nontraditional or multisectoral contexts.

Until recently, agricultural programs focused largely on the sectoral mandate of increasing food production, while giving less attention to the consumption aspect. Farmers reported that this emphasis, too, was changing, with the recent advice from DAs to grow and consume a variety of fruits and vegetables. Increases in crop production do not inevitably translate into better nutritional outcomes in the immediate term but can lay the foundation for more diversified pathways between agriculture and improved nutrition to come. Further research is needed to fully describe these potential sequences and linkages, particularly in marginal or less favored areas.

Lessons from the record of implementing sanitation improvements in Ethiopia are twofold. While improved sanitation appears, based on preliminary results, to have had a significant impact on improving child growth outcomes, research and evaluation reports indicate that greater community participation, more dedicated follow-up, and monitoring and evaluating such programs are necessary to achieve even greater impact and to sustain recent progress.

The changes to the PSNP are significant and have the potential to serve as a model for other countries interested in sensitizing social protection programs to nutrition. The program, however, reaches only 11 percent of the population and targets those most vulnerable to food insecurity.[50] For the rest of the population, a continued emphasis on the quality and reach of agriculture and health service provision will be important to drive further improvements in overall well-being.

Currently, inhabitants of the study area are not asking for more health or agricultural information as the road to health and well-being; instead, they are asking for tangible roads to be built in their area. Investment in rural infrastructure and transportation networks has consistently been one of the major drivers of economic growth in high-potential agricultural areas. Moreover, research on investments in rural infrastructure in India demonstrated that road building in low-potential, rain-fed areas alleviated poverty much more significantly than did similar investments in higher-potential areas.[51] Recent research in Ethiopia indicating that access to markets is a key determinant of children's diets also highlights the importance of seeing nutrition through multiple lenses.[52] This perspective points to the need to consider new pathways to engage support and interest in improving nutrition from a wide range of stakeholders as well as to broaden the horizon for what "counts" as nutrition sensitive.

An important takeaway of the research for Stories of Change is that the success of a single nutrition-specific initiative (such as dietary supplementation or the promotion of proper infant and young child feeding practices) is conditioned on meeting ongoing, deeper-rooted challenges to livelihoods, food security, and health. Nutrition-sensitive interventions have the potential to go much further to address the underlying determinants of undernutrition. Not only are both types of intervention needed to generate significant and sustained impacts, but they are likely to be mutually reinforcing.

CHAPTER 17

25 Years of Scaling Up

Nutrition and Health Interventions in Odisha, India

PURNIMA MENON, NEHA KOHLI, MARA VAN DEN BOLD, ELISABETH BECKER, NICHOLAS NISBETT, LAWRENCE HADDAD, AND RASMI AVULA

ODISHA, A STATE of 42 million people in eastern India, is one of the poorest in the country. It has faced many development challenges over the years, including insurgent movements, large pockets of extreme deprivation among scheduled tribe communities,[1] social disparities, and natural disasters, as well as a relatively late fiscal turnaround (in 2004–2005) in comparison with other states. Yet Odisha has made significant progress in reducing child undernutrition—less than India as a whole, but more than many other richer states. How has it achieved this progress?

Data from three rounds of India's National Family Health Survey (NFHS) and the Rapid Survey on Children (RSOC)[2] show that, in Odisha, the proportion of stunted children younger than 3 years of age fell from 49 percent to 44 percent between 1998–1999 and 2005–2006 (compared with an all-India decline from 51 percent to 45 percent during the same period). Between 2006 and 2014, stunting among children younger than 5 years in Odisha fell from 45 percent to 38 percent (compared with an all-India decline of 48 percent to 39 percent). The rate of stunting decline in Odisha has accelerated from 1.8 percent a year to 2.1 percent a year in the past 10 years, but it remains slower than the all-India rate of decline. This lag is unsurprising, given the challenging conditions in Odisha. Nevertheless, Odisha's rate of decline in childhood stunting is at least three times the rate of decline in other similarly poor states, such as Bihar.[3] Not all nutrition indicators showed such advances: anemia rates among children and pregnant women increased or remained stagnant in Odisha between the early 1990s and the mid-2000s, hovering between 60 and 70 percent.

In 2005–2006, Odisha's undernutrition levels were close to those of the state of Gujarat, which is richer and better endowed. That same year, Odisha's performance on delivering health services and Integrated Child Development Services (ICDS) interventions was among the best in India, ranking below only one other state.[4] More recently, data from 2014–2015 showed that Odisha had outpaced richer states, such as Gujarat, Madhya Pradesh, and Uttar Pradesh, in

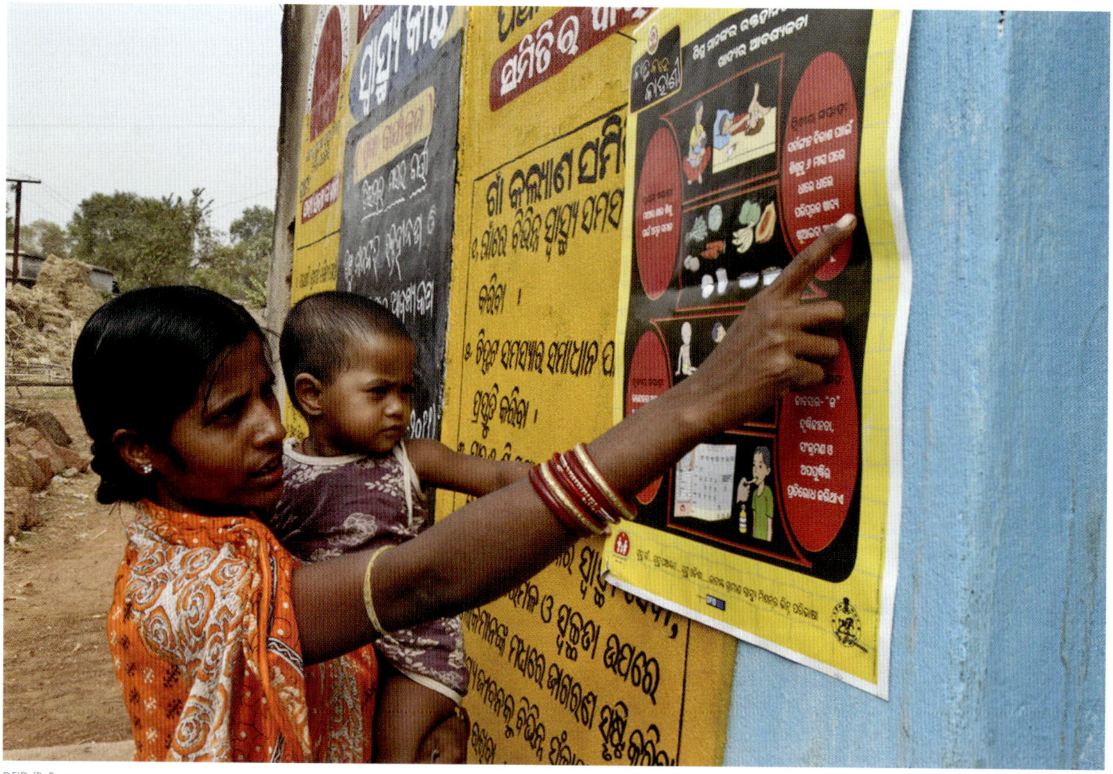

DFID/P. Ranger

A mother reads the latest advice on how to feed children from the health information wall in her village.

several areas. Odisha had better nutrition outcomes, such as stunting levels. It performed better in terms of immediate determinants, such as infants 6–8 months old receiving solid, semisolid, or soft foods and minimum dietary diversity during complementary feeding. And it had greater coverage of nutrition-specific interventions, such as mothers of children younger than 3 years old who received three or more antenatal care checkups and children 12–23 months old who were fully immunized.[5] A recent analysis of nutrition progress across states in India explicitly recognized Odisha as a leading state for nutrition-relevant social sector programs, including those targeting health, nutrition, and food security. The authors of that paper called Odisha a "positive deviant in nutrition policymaking" in areas related to nutrition.[6] Given the unusual emphasis on nutrition policy making for a poor state such as Odisha, we sought to conduct a Stories of Change study there to understand the drivers of success in establishing supportive social policies and scaling up effective programs for health and nutrition.

This chapter seeks to explain how changes in the delivery of nutrition-specific programs (specifically the ICDS) and the National Rural Health Mission (NRHM) came about over time in Odisha. We also aim to identify the policy and programmatic factors that enabled the changes in these important programs over time, drawing on diverse sources of data, including interviews with present and former officials and stakeholders involved in designing and implementing nutrition and child health policies and interventions.[7] While we argue in this chapter that the continuity of key actors in Odisha—rather unique in India—is an asset, we recognize that relying on such sources for assessing performance potentially entails a conflict of interest. Thus, we used a recent framework for scaling up the impact on nutrition to ground our analysis of these factors.[8] Because child-level data on the nutritional status of children in 2014–2015 are still not available for analysis for Odisha—or indeed, for any other state in India—we restricted our use of quantitative data to reporting statistics rather than performing an empirical econometric analysis.

Nutrition-Specific Interventions, Programs, and Policies in Odisha That Target Children's First 1,000 Days

Nutrition and health services in Odisha have been delivered primarily through the nationwide ICDS program and the health system. Our review of available data shows that, during the 25-year period from 1991 to 2015, coverage of antenatal care, institutional deliveries and assisted births, immunization, vitamin A supplementation, and the use of key ICDS services all went up in Odisha (Table 17.1). For some of these services, improvements in coverage were substantial. Despite variability across the state in these improvements and the continuing challenges of providing services in tribal areas, evidence also suggests that intervention coverage became more equitable.[9]

Trends in the Focus and Shape of Health and Nutrition Policies and Programs over Time

HEALTH INTERVENTIONS (1990–2015)

Odisha started health sector reforms in the early 1990s, with support from key development partners. As early as 1995, India launched National Immunization Days to address polio in particular; Odisha also carried out "Pulse Polio" days—specific campaign days only for polio vaccination. These efforts expanded into a national initiative called the Reproductive and Child Health Programme in 1997, which aimed to deliver an integrated package of health and nutrition services for pregnant and lactating women, children, and adolescents. In 2001, the state launched the Infant Mortality Rate (IMR) Mission, ramping up efforts to reduce the IMR.[10] As part of this effort, Odisha emphasized implementation of antenatal care and newborn care.[11] In addition to strengthening the implementation of existing interventions, the mission introduced interventions to prevent malaria among pregnant women and incentives to promote institutional deliveries.[12] The state government also developed a vision document for health in the early 2000s.

Over the past decade, especially between 2004 and 2015, the state health delivery system experienced major enhancements with the launch of the State Health Mission in 2005 under the NRHM. Under the NRHM, the budgetary outlays for public health increased, a new cadre of health workers including accredited social health activists was appointed, a conditional cash transfer scheme (Janani Suraksha Yojana) to incentivize institutional deliveries was introduced, and nutrition rehabilitation centers for facility-based treatment of severely acutely malnourished children were launched in 2005–2006.[13] The goal of the mission was to reduce the IMR, the maternal mortality rate (MMR), and the total fertility rate by strengthening reproductive and child health services.

Odisha also strengthened the delivery of its immunization program, rolled out a vitamin A supplementation campaign during 2005–2010[14] and adapted the national guidelines for Village Health and Nutrition Days, renaming it the Mamata Diwas—a single platform for delivering multiple maternal and child nutrition interventions. In addition, guidelines were released for screening and identifying severely malnourished children under age 5 for treatment at rehabilitation centers

TABLE 17.1 Changes in nutrition and health outcomes, immediate determinants, and interventions in Odisha state and India, various periods, 1990 to 2015

Outcome indicator	Study timeline								
	1990–1995		1995–2000		2000–2005	2005–2010		2010–2015	
	Survey data periods								
	1992–1993[a]		1998–1999[b]			2005–2006[c]		2013–2014[d]	
	India	Odisha	India	Odisha		India	Odisha	India	Odisha
Stunting (%)[e]	NA	51	51	49	NA	45 (48)	44 (45)	(39)	(38)
Wasting (%)[e]	NA	28	20	30	NA	23 (20)	24 (20)	(15)	(18)
Infant mortality rate	79[f]	112[f]	68[f]	81[f]	NA	57[f]	65[f]	NA	56[g]
Maternal mortality rate	437[h]	NA	540	NA	NA	NA	NA	178[i]	230[g]
Women with body mass index < 18.5 kg/m2	NA	NA	36	48	NA	36	41	NA	30[j]
Women aged 15–49 yrs. with anemia (%)	NA	NA	52	63	NA	56	63	NA	77[j]
Children (aged 6–35 mos.) with any anemia (%)	NA	NA	74	72	NA	79	74	NA	NA
Children (< 3 yrs.) breastfed within 1 hr. of birth (%)k	10	18	16	25	NA	24	54	45[k]	73[k]
Children (< 6 mos.) exclusively breast-fed (%)	NA	NA	NA	NA	NA	46	50	65	69
Children receiving solid/semi-solid food and breast milk (%)	31	30	34	30	NA	56	68	51[l]	56[l]
Children (0–59 mos.) with diarrhea in the past 2 weeks (%)	10[m]	21[m]	NA	NA	NA	9	12	7	9
Children (< 5 yrs.) with diarrhea in the past 2 weeks who received ORS (%)	18[n]	17[n]	27[n]	35[n]	NA	26[n]	41[n]	54	71
Women received/bought iron–folic acid supplements during pregnancy (%)	51	50	58[o]	68[o]	NA	65	83	31[p]	45[p]
Mothers who had $\geq$ 3 antenatal care visits for previous birth (%)	44	35	44	48	NA	52	62	63	75
Receipt and use of ICDS supplementary nutrition during pregnancy (%)	NA	NA	NA	NA	NA	21	45	41	61
Births in a health facility (based on past 2 births in the 3 yrs. prior to survey) (%)	26	14	34	23	NA	41	39	79	81
Receipt and use of ICDS supplementary nutrition during lactation (6 mos. after birth) (%)	NA	NA	NA	NA	NA	17	40	42	77
Children (12–23 mos.) fully immunized (%)	36	36	42	44	NA	44	52	65	62

(Table 17.1 continued)

Outcome indicator	Study timeline: 1990–1995		1995–2000		2000–2005	2005–2010		2010–2015	
	Survey data periods: 1992–1993[a]		1998–1999[b]			2005–2006[c]		2013–2014[d]	
	India	Odisha	India	Odisha		India	Odisha	India	Odisha
Children (12–35 mos.) who received vitamin A dose in the past 6 mos. (%)	NA	NA	17	26	NA	25	30	46[q]	57[q]
Receipt and use of ICDS supplementary nutrition for children (%)	NA	NA	NA	NA	NA	26[r]	53[r]	49[s] 44[t]	89[s] 67[t]

Sources: National Family Health Survey (I, II, III), India, reports and fact sheets (http://rchiips.org/nfhs/); Rapid Survey on Children 2013–14 (http://wcd.nic.iNActs/rapid-survey-children-rsoc-2013-14); Annual Health Survey 2012–13 Fact Sheet (http://www.censusindia.gov.in/vital_statistics/AHSBulletins/AHS_Factsheets_2012-13/FACTSHEET-Odisha.pdf); and Special Bulletin on Maternal Mortality in India 2010–12 (http://www.censusindia.gov.in/vital_statistics/SRS_Bulletins/MMR_Bulletin-2010-12.pdf).

Notes: Percentages have been rounded to whole numbers; NA = not available; ORS = oral rehydration salts; ICDS = Integrated Child Development Services; [a] National Family Health Survey – I (1992–1993); length/height data were not collected for five states; hence, India average data are not available; [b] National Family Health Survey – II (1998–1999); [c] National Family Health Survey – III (2005–2006); [d] Rapid Survey on Children (2013–2014); [e] Indicator calculated for children < 3 years old; figures in parentheses are for children < 5 years old; [f] Per 1,000 live births for the 5 years preceding the survey; [g] Annual Health Survey 2012–13 Fact Sheet; [h] Per 1,000,000 live births for the 2 years preceding the survey; [i] Special Bulletin on Maternal Mortality in India 2010–12; [j] Clinical, Anthropometry and Biometry Census Survey (2014); [k] Indicator calculated for children aged 0–23 months; [l] Indicator calculated for children aged 6–8 months; [m] Indicator calculated for children aged < 4 year; [n] Indicator calculated for children aged < 3 years; [o] Includes tablets and syrup; [p] Indicator specifies 100 or more tablets; [q] Indicator calculated for children aged 6–59 months; [r] Indicators calculated for children aged < 6 years; [s] Indicator calculated for children aged < 3 years; [t] Indicator calculated for children aged > 3 years.

on a designated day in a month (Pustikar Diwas). Between 2011 and 2013, the state launched three nationally driven initiatives that included free transportation for institutional delivery (the Janani Express);[15] medical care and other facilities for pregnant women and sick newborns (Janani Shishu Suraksha Kayakaram); and early detection and treatment of physical problems in children younger than 18 years.[16]

Taken together, all these state-level initiatives over the years have built on national health initiatives. They have summed up to create an overall set of services to support better maternal and child health, mostly with a focus on reducing mortality.

ICDS INTERVENTIONS (1990–2015)

The ICDS program, which began in October 1975, was designed to deliver services to pregnant and lactating women, children younger than 6 years old, and adolescent girls through the *anganwadi* centers (AWCs). The services include supplementary nutrition, health education, immunization, health checkups, and referrals, all delivered by *anganwadi* workers; most of these services are delivered in coordination with the health program (see Chapter 2).

In Odisha, the ICDS program was started in 85 AWCs in the Subdega block of the Sundargarh district.[17] Over the past two decades, it has evolved and expanded, largely following national guidelines but also experimenting and enlarging its set of services. Odisha laid a strong foundation for the ICDS program in the early 1990s by building the capacity of the program staff and facilitating coordination with the health department. The ICDS projects and the AWCs continued to grow from the early 1990s until 2014, with major expansions occurring in 2004, then in 2009, and again between 2010 and 2014. These expansions were largely the result of the state government's adherence to the Supreme Court of India's order to increase the number of

AWCs, as part of the national public interest litigation case on the Right to Food.[18]

In the late 1990s and early 2000s, the ICDS focused on identifying and providing solutions for moderately and severely malnourished children (*Ami bhi paribu*—"We too can," a positive deviance initiative) and investing in medical referral for chronic cases. To comply with the Supreme Court of India's 2006 judgment, the Department of Women and Child Development (DWCD) implemented decentralization, in which the existing self-help groups under "Mission Shakti" took charge of procuring and preparing food supplements.[19] Mothers' committees were set up in 2006 and rejuvenated in 2012 to monitor the ICDS services. The Government of Odisha, along with its development partners, made significant efforts to identify key barriers to ICDS service provision and use and in the late 2000s established a Nutrition Operational Plan.[20]

Factors Contributing to Policy and Program Changes in Odisha

An analysis of state-level stakeholder interviews and documents points to a confluence of factors that facilitated changes in the health and ICDS programs. We examine these factors next using the recent framework for scaling up impact on nutrition.[21]

A Vision for Impact

Odisha's work on scaling up key health and nutrition interventions was stimulated by its poor ranking within India on IMR and high levels of infant and maternal mortality, so changing both of these was a driving goal. The state's goals were to accelerate reductions in the IMR, MMR, and total fertility rate by strengthening reproductive and child health services. As evidence, mostly global, emerged on the links between poor nutrition and mortality outcomes, during the past two decades Odisha broadened its agenda to include nutrition as well.

Delivering Interventions through Multiple Operational Platforms

Over time the government implemented interventions through both the health and ICDS programs in order to capitalize on both platforms, and it supported cross-platform convergence on the common goal of mortality reduction in several ways,[22] which likely had positive implications for scaling up interventions. Over the years, the types of interventions delivered through the ICDS steadily evolved and expanded. The mortality-reduction goal led to the use of the ICDS platform to identify and rehabilitate severely malnourished children who were at the greatest risk of dying. When the NRHM came into being in 2004, Odisha, after a somewhat slow start, began rolling out key mortality-reduction interventions, such as antenatal care and immunizations, whose rapid scale-up was likely facilitated by the existing state government goal of reducing mortality. Early government orders and a culture of working together across two operational platforms—the health department and the ICDS—continued to support the use of both platforms to deliver interventions that worked toward the overarching mortality-reduction goal. Finally, Odisha's investment in establishing the *Mission Shakti* women's self-help group within the same department that ran the ICDS program enabled the state to respond rapidly to guidelines that stipulated decentralized production of food supplements by the self-help groups.

Catalysts, Champions, and Ownership

Catalysts for action against malnutrition in Odisha included the state's poor national ranking on infant mortality (which spurred internal reflection and action planning) and intense human rights commission monitoring of starvation and other deaths in tribal districts in the state. The choice of Odisha for sector support from the UK's Department for International Development (DFID) technical assistance program likely also contributed to an infusion of resources and support to strengthen the area's systems.

Several individuals across the two government departments were named, along with the chief minister, as key leaders for health and nutrition in the state. The Odisha political leadership had consistently appointed well-qualified and motivated bureaucrats to manage social sector programs; these individuals took ownership of the vision for improving mortality rates and realizing the programs' potential.

Several observers mentioned the notion of "political/policy intent," which conveyed the goals' focus, as well as the existence of "bureaucratic space" that enabled operations, innovation, and learning. Individual commitment and leadership influenced both policy support and implementation of programmatic changes. For example, at the state level, the chief minister's interest in women's empowerment, and the potential political gains from supporting women, led to initiatives such as the Mission Shakti self-help groups in 2001. These later provided an operational framework for scaling up the decentralized production of supplementary food. The chief minister was also credited with providing "enabling leadership"—that is, clearly stating policy intent but staying removed from operational details.

Several dynamic and committed secretaries and directors of the health department and the DWCD were acknowledged to have provided leadership in moving the agenda forward in the state and to have taken ownership for state goals. Longer tenures by leaders than in other states were also thought to have led to a combination of problem and solution ownership, as well as accountability for results. There was said to have been a sense of responsibility and collegiality among the bureaucrats of the health department and the DWCD and a desire to effectively implement the programs that facilitated coordinated action: "Odisha is a special case in that coordination is ensured from the highest level. Joint letters were sent to the district collectors to ensure that the ICDS and health departments work together from the district level below. This is rarely done," remarked one bureaucrat who worked at the state level during the mid-2000s, when nutrition was beginning to take center stage.

Diverse Pathways for Scaling Up

Our analysis and interviews showed that scaling up took different pathways in Odisha. Expansion of child care centers and frontline workers in the ICDS, the frontline workforce in the NRHM, and the number of women's self-help groups all led to delivery platforms' becoming available for interventions as well as innovative operations. Once these basic structures and functions were replicated statewide, the scaling up of interventions followed a more functional pathway, and new interventions or operational strategies to achieve coverage could be added to available platforms. For example, eggs were added to the ICDS and midday meal scheme across the state, special child nutrition days (Pushtikar Diwas) were added to improve coverage of weighing and screening for severe malnutrition,[23] and self-help groups were used to produce foods for the ICDS.[24] However, limited evidence exists on the impacts of these specific innovations.

Gradually Building Up Strategic and Operational Capacities

Scaling up these interventions was enabled by strengthening both strategic and operational capacities. Over time, a diverse set of capabilities had been built statewide. It is unclear how many of these were intended from the start, but it is apparent that the combination of investments clearly paid off for the state.

From a strategic capacity perspective, the chief minister appointed high-caliber bureaucrats to the social sector departments, including health and ICDS. This move clearly signaled the strategic importance of the social sector across a bureaucracy that typically deprioritizes it by not appointing high-caliber individuals to these positions. Several of Odisha's bureaucrats were well trained for their sector: two senior bureaucrats had midcareer degrees from top public health universities in the United States, and the lead of the NRHM state unit was a doctor with significant public health experience.

From an operational capacity perspective, several years of supporting and strengthening the system readied it to respond. Strengthening measures included establishing training arrangements, transparently recruiting frontline workers and supervisors, and reducing the capture of frontline positions by local elites. It is possible that the state policy ensuring that all ICDS frontline and supervisory staff were women led to greater motivation within a sector that focused on women and children. District collectors, relatively junior in the bureaucratic hierarchy, were noted to have good communication with secretaries, who were more senior, and to have invested in ensuring robust program implementation. Because of high-level support of social sector programs, district collectors routinely included social sector programs in their monthly district reviews. And at the grassroots level, administrative changes were made in how frontline

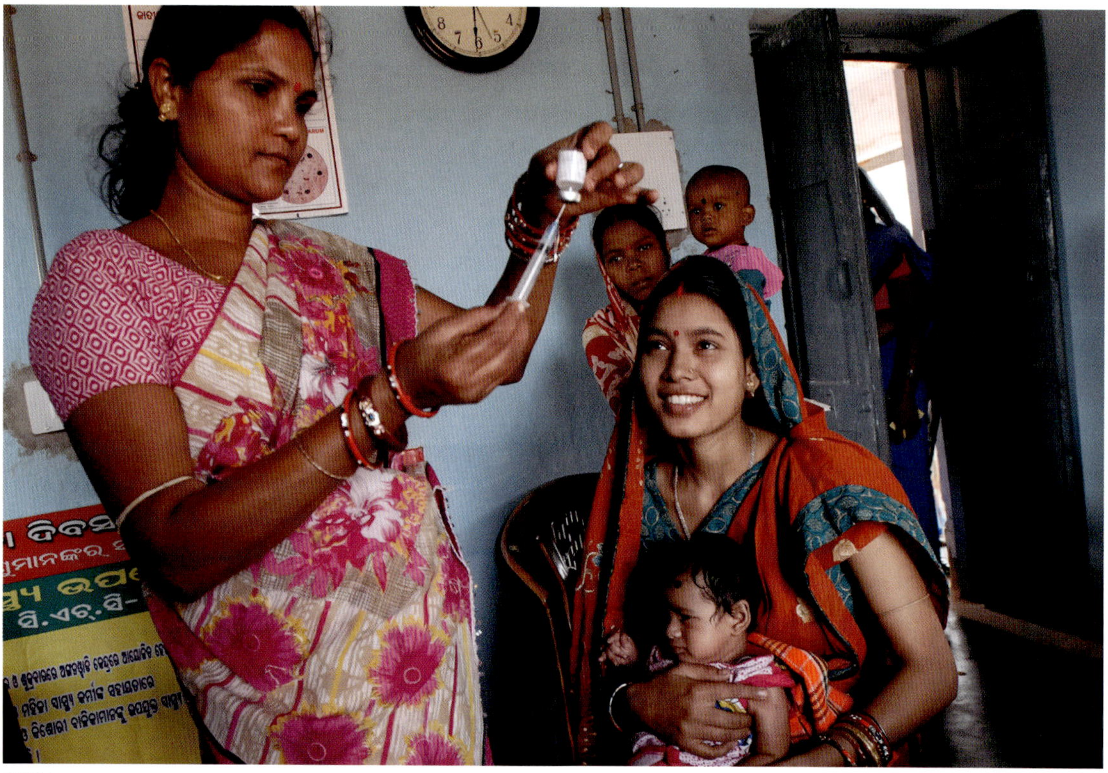

DFID/P. Ranger

From 1991 to 2015, coverage of antenatal care, institutional deliveries, immunizations, and other interventions all went up in Odisha.

workers were selected. "[Frontline workers] continue to be at the heart of [our] success in health and nutrition," remarked one senior bureaucrat in our stakeholder interviews.

Finally, several development partners (UNICEF, DFID, the United Nations Office of Project Services [UNOPS], the World Food Programme, CARE, and the World Bank) were said in interviews to have played significant roles in supporting the operations of the health and ICDS programs. Over the years, UNICEF, DFID, and UNOPS helped implement health programs by giving technical and financial assistance and by working in alignment with Odisha's state goals. The World Bank supported the expansion of ICDS projects in the 1990s, and CARE invested in strengthening delivery systems through its Integrated Nutrition and Health Program (1996–2001 and 2001–2005), which was implemented in collaboration with the ICDS and health programs. And from the mid-2000s, the DFID-supported technical support team invested in systems for strengthening data gathering and documentation. UNICEF was a fairly constant development partner for nutrition throughout the two decades.

Adequate, Stable, and Flexible Financing

For several years, creating the fiscal space for social sector programs in Odisha was a challenge. In 2004–2005, however, space opened up owing to increased national financing for social sector programs, state-level financial restructuring, and significant technical support and direct state budget support to Odisha from DFID. Financial restructuring under the government of Chief Minister Naveen Patnaik was credited with turning around a nearly bankrupt state to reach financial stability, which allowed for investments in social programs and state infrastructure development. Financial restructuring included (1) undertaking fiscal consolidation; (2) reforming tax policy and administration (for example, introducing a value-added tax); (3) restructuring expenditures (such as reducing public-sector employment); and (4) restructuring debt (swapping high-cost debts for low-cost ones).[25] These measures brought together diverse sources of funding to implement national programs, deploy state-level initiatives and innovations, and bring more technical support to the health and nutrition program landscape in Odisha.

Creating an Enabling Policy Environment

Three major elements appear to have contributed to an enabling policy environment for scaling up health and nutrition interventions in Odisha: high-level policy and political backing of social support programs, political and bureaucratic stability, and the emergence of a supportive policy and fiscal framework at the national level. First, Chief Minister Patnaik provided leadership on development issues in the state by sending clear signals of interest in the social sector programs, which were featured in all state reviews and to which he appointed strong bureaucrats. He is said to have established a clear policy intent to deliver on social sector programs and then to have given bureaucrats autonomy to function without political interference. He also signaled a low tolerance for corruption in social sector programs, which limited graft in the systems. Second, an unusual degree of electoral stability for the political party in power enabled several reforms in health and nutrition programs to continue uninterrupted. Coupled with political stability, bureaucrats were assured adequate tenure in their positions to allow them to amass knowledge on health, nutrition, and social programs and to experiment with, learn from, and take credit for innovations in program implementation. Third, overarching policy support—coming from new socially focused policies, programs, and associated financing at the national level—allowed Odisha to expand and experiment in health and nutrition programs. Indeed, this expansion was especially important both for the scale-up and roll-out of the NRHM and for the expansion of the ICDS. In the case of the ICDS, expansion was mandated by the Supreme Court's ruling on the Right to Food.

Measurement, Learning, and Accountability

Data were used to support decisions in different ways as the programs evolved. In the early years, this data-for-action approach focused on "weighing efficiency"—that is, ensuring that all children were weighed monthly to identify the most malnourished. In later years, investments in concurrent monitoring surveys by the DFID-supported technical support unit, and the use and discussion of these data with officials, facilitated the use of third-party data. Odisha also hosted important research studies that informed state-level programming; for example, Odisha is home to Ekjut, a nongovernmental organization involved in major experiments on the use of women's groups for achieving health and mortality outcomes. Overall, a culture of constructive use of data appears to be in place, though it is not without its challenges. For example, multiple sources of state-level data have created some confusion, data are not always available below the district level, the monitoring systems do not capture all necessary indicators, and the state still depends on monitoring systems established by national programs.

Conclusions and Challenges Ahead

Our study reveals Odisha as a state that, over time, steadily managed to chip away at several system-level challenges to scale up, strengthen, and deliver a set of effective health and nutrition interventions. Rather than identifying a single forward-looking strategic master plan, our analysis highlights the convergence of several actors, along with several operational and financial resource pools, which in turn enabled the state to respond positively to major national policy changes and to use national fiscal commitments to health and nutrition to provide better services inside its borders. The key success factors in Odisha included high-level political support for health and nutrition programs, fiscal and policy space to operate, and useful collaborations with committed development partners. In addition, notwithstanding continuing challenges of diversity in levels of undernutrition and progress in program delivery and outcomes across the state, a cadre of committed and technically capable bureaucrats enabled programmatic action despite the challenges of a state that is predominantly poor, rural, and tribal. The common goal of reducing IMRs in the mid-1990s and 2000s contributed significantly to several key actions (antenatal care, immunizations, a focus on severe malnutrition, and others) that were scaled up to successfully reduce mortality.

Several lessons from Odisha's experience may be transferable to other states of India—and possibly even to contexts outside of India. These lessons include the importance of (1) setting goals; (2) ensuring bureaucratic stability, capacity, and motivation to deliver on the goals; and (3) creating an enabling environment with little to no political interference, adequate financing from diverse sources (to ensure flexibility and agility), and adequate technical support. Several states in India now have financial stability, the availability of technical support, and additional resources, as well as highly capable bureaucrats who are keen to make a difference. However, long-term political stability, political commitment to development goals for all, and lack of political interference in social sector programs are not always easy to come by. Could this set of drivers of change in Odisha be replicated, in a more rapid and focused way, in other states? And can Odisha itself succeed in capitalizing on its enabling environment to continue to innovate, expand, and deliver results in areas within the state that are still lagging?

As Odisha looks ahead to improving nutrition further, it becomes crucially important to create similar targets in this area, build on existing technical and system capacities, and capitalize on existing high-level support for such initiatives. The state still faces geographic disparities, which largely reflect challenges in delivering services to the state's tribal populations and in addressing their broader development needs. Therefore, actions will need to engage other government departments, such as the education sector, water, sanitation, and hygiene, and the Rural Development Department, to ensure that some of the known social determinants are tackled on an urgent basis.

Reducing undernutrition in Odisha is an imperative for the state's further development. Can Odisha become a shining beacon of hope, not just for scaling up nutrition and health interventions and reducing mortality but also for bringing together cross-sectoral interventions to more rapidly improve nutrition in one of India's poorest states? Perhaps the time is ripe for Odisha to take the next big leap for nutrition.

Part IV: Leading the Way Forward

CHAPTER 18

Championing Nutrition

Effective Leadership for Action

NICHOLAS NISBETT, ELISE WACH, LAWRENCE HADDAD, SHAMS EL ARIFEEN, SAMANTHA REDDIN, KARINE GATELLIER, NAMUKOLO COVIC, SCOTT DRIMIE, JODY HARRIS, AND SIVAN YOSEF

THE CALLS FOR strong leadership in the fight against global and national malnutrition have multiplied during the past decade.[1] The role of nutrition champions in advocating for nutrition, formulating policies, and coordinating and implementing action in nutrition have increasingly been recognized in such countries as Peru, Brazil, Thailand, and the Indian states of Tamil Nadu and Maharashtra.[2] Global initiatives such as the Scaling Up Nutrition (SUN) Movement, the African Nutrition Leadership Programme, and the European Nutrition Leadership Platform have invested in building up capacity for leadership among national governments, civil society, and the private sector. The World Public Health Nutrition Association's guide on competencies needed to build up the workforce in global public health nutrition identified leadership as key.[3] More widely, leadership within the field of public health has been highlighted as key to moving child and maternal health higher up on the global agenda[4] and tackling critical issues such as HIV and AIDS at the national and community levels.[5]

While evidence within the nutrition and public health arenas points time and again to the role of leadership in successfully crafting nutrition policies and movements, little is actually known about the characteristics of leaders in nutrition: who they are, how they function, with whom they work, and what makes them effective. This chapter—whose main body is extracted from the article "What Drives and Constrains Effective Leadership in Tackling Child Undernutrition? Findings from Bangladesh, Ethiopia, India, and Kenya," published in *Food Policy* in 2015—aims to answer some of these questions.[6] It first reviews the literature on leadership within both nutrition and other disciplines. It then draws on interviews conducted with 89 influential decision makers in four countries with high burdens of undernutrition: Bangladesh, Ethiopia, India, and Kenya.[7] The chapter also highlights a case study on leadership from Zambia (see Box 18.1) and 10 nutrition champions (see Box 18.2) identified as part of a global selection process run by Transform Nutrition in 2015, in order to convey

BOX 18.1 The role of leadership in nutrition change in Zambia

Zambia is a complex landscape of stubbornly high poverty and hunger rates on one hand and an impending problem of overweight and obesity on the other.[8] Child stunting rose from 1992 to 2001 and then fell by 5 percent from 2001 to 2013, but remains unacceptably high at 40 percent.[9] Nonetheless, the country has shown some positive trends in maternal and child survival and child undernutrition indicators, and there have been several targeted efforts to bolster leadership for nutrition in the country.

Zambia has long had a formal institutional structure to provide leadership for nutrition: the National Food and Nutrition Commission (NFNC), formed in 1967 under the Ministry of Health to advise the government on nutrition matters. Although the NFNC is recognized as best positioned to lead and coordinate nutrition action for Zambia, it had been neither well supported nor highly active in the decades since its founding, and there was skepticism about its inherent leadership capacity. In recent years, however, nutrition has seen a revival in Zambia. The country adopted a new nutrition policy in 2006, held national nutrition symposia in 2009 and 2011, joined the SUN Movement in 2010 as an "early riser" country,[10] and drafted the National Food and Nutrition Strategic Plan for 2011–2015. In 2011, recognizing a strategic leadership deficit, it contracted with the African Nutrition Leadership Programme to provide leadership development support for the NFNC. Beyond the NFNC as the technical nutrition arm of government, efforts are under way to improve political leadership on nutrition, and a nutrition group has been created in Parliament as a Special Committee of Permanent Secretaries on Nutrition, with members drawn from key line ministries and chaired by the cabinet secretary.

Nongovernmental organizations (NGOs) have also played important leadership roles on nutrition issues in Zambia. With the renewed focus on nutrition since 2009, formerly sporadic action by civil society coalesced under the coordination of the newly formed Scaling Up Nutrition Civil Society Organization Alliance (CSO-SUN). In 2014, William Chilufya, head of CSO-SUN in Zambia (see Box 18.2), led the way in raising the profile of nutrition in Zambia, partly through the strategic use of media and partly by leading Zambia to become one of the first countries to analyze its budget spending on nutrition.[11] The CSO-SUN Alliance is treading a fine line between working with the government and holding it to account.

Since the early 1990s, the Nutrition Association of Zambia (NAZ) has provided leadership from within the nutrition profession through advocacy, guidance to the profession, and networking. With a less public face and less international backing than the NFNC or CSO-SUN, NAZ has been working largely behind the scenes. This triad of national leadership from government (NFNC), civil society (CSO-SUN), and nutrition professionals (NAZ), backed by forward-thinking donor leadership under SUN, has been key to Zambia's ability to seize nutrition opportunities as they have arisen.

Efforts to boost nutrition leadership have also been made at the local levels. In Mumbwa District, the District Nutrition Coordination Committee (DNCC), catalyzed by the international NGO Concern Worldwide and co-led by nutrition champion Christopher Dube (see Box 18.2), builds local leaders' capacity to put nutrition higher on the agenda and coordinates several ministries and NGOs involved in providing nutrition-related services. Ultimately, DNCC members and their national counterparts envision that stronger strategic capacity at the local level will result in the design and implementation of innovative solutions to help address stunting. And there is evidence that this is starting to happen, as the national nutrition program reaches down to the local level in Mumbwa.[12]

The case of Zambia has shown that support of leadership development can take many forms, just as leadership itself can manifest in different ways—from championing a cause to planning policy and undertaking action. Both strategic and technical leadership are needed not only at the national level, but also at the local levels, where the real action happens. This chapter documents ways that leadership can be built, and Zambia's experience demonstrates that more responsive and context-driven leadership development schemes are required if we are to properly support the next generation of nutrition leaders.

the depth and breadth of the experience of these remarkable leaders.

While the focus is on leaders who have contributed to national-level policy changes in nutrition, this chapter (and the literature) recognizes the importance of leadership in nutrition practice and at different levels of policy and programming. Through this approach, this chapter aims to deepen our basic understanding of leadership within nutrition and offer up ways in which nutrition champions may be identified and supported to lead the fight against malnutrition both globally and within their own countries and communities.

Evidence on Nutrition and Leadership in Development

Research on leadership in nutrition is still nascent and suffers from wide gaps in country-level data. The landmark 2008 *Lancet* series on child nutrition highlighted leadership as integral to making progress on the international and national nutrition stages. Bryce and colleagues[13] and Morris and colleagues[14] identified a lack of capacity to train and support individuals to take on strategic roles in nutrition as a major barrier to conceptualizing and guiding national and subnational nutrition agendas. Heaver[15] identified three types of actors

BOX 18.2 10 leaders in transforming nutrition

The stories of 10 nutrition leaders, identified through a global selection process led by Transform Nutrition in 2015, are varied. They reveal something of the breadth of experience and contexts in which those championing nutrition find themselves in their work to tackle nutrition at grassroots, regional, and national levels around the world. Their stories resonate with earlier research on nutrition that has emphasized the practical and strategic nature of leadership. Charismatic leadership is something that a few may be born into, but most types of leadership can be built up and supported. More information on these and other champions can be found on the Transform Nutrition website: www.transform-nutrition.org/nutrition-champions/.

Manaan Mumma

Regional Nutrition and HIV Officer, World Food Programme Regional Bureau for East and Central Africa, Kenya

While working in maternal and infant nutrition and integrated management of acute malnutrition programs, Manaan Mumma witnessed how children suffering from acute malnutrition could recover when simple solutions were provided by community health workers. "The solutions are within reach. We already know what needs to be done. A lot was already happening at the community level. For me, it was how we amplify this from the subnational level to the national level. For me, that was the drive," says Manaan. Building on her experience from a career in the HIV sector, she realized the gains that could be made in nutrition by deploying advocacy efforts and civil society. While working for the Kenya AIDS NGOs Consortium and serving as an executive committee member of the Scaling Up Nutrition Civil Society Alliance (SUN CSA), Mannan has worked to engage stakeholders and nutrition champions throughout the region to bring attention to nutrition issues at all levels. As a result, the First Lady of the Republic of Kenya, the Honorable Margaret Kenyatta, accepted the role of nutrition champion for Kenya. In 2015, Manaan led the effort to convene representatives from Burundi, Ethiopia, Kenya, Rwanda, Tanzania, and Uganda to discuss regional nutrition issues at the East African launch of the *Global Nutrition Report*. Manaan uses the network of members of Parliament (MPs) developed through her work in the HIV sector to raise their awareness of nutrition through one-on-one meetings and "meet your MP" advocacy days, where community members at the grassroots level all over the country have face-to-face meetings with their MPs.

(Box 18.2 continued)

William Chilufya

Country Coordinator, Zambia Civil Society Scaling Up Nutrition Alliance, Zambia

William Chilufya spearheaded the creation of the Zambia Civil Society Organization Scaling Up Nutrition Alliance (CSO-SUN). Under his leadership, CSO-SUN has engaged with a range of stakeholders to inspire key government officials, civil society, and the media to be vocal advocates for nutrition. CSO-SUN developed "10 Critical Steps to Address Child Under-nutrition in Zambia, Permanently" through consultation among civil society, cooperating partners, and the government to identify key areas for action across sectors that are required to effectively address the nutrition situation in Zambia. William and his team have also worked with the government to ensure that both the National Social Protection Strategy and the National Agriculture Policy include nutrition objectives.[16] With William's guidance, CSO-SUN has been effective in creating strong relationships with key MPs. These include the Honorable Highvie Hamududu, chairperson for the Budget Committee of Parliament and a vocal advocate for nutrition in the Zambian parliament. CSO-SUN has also inspired the formation of the All Party Parliamentary caucus on food and nutrition. William recognizes the role the media can play in nutrition and has worked with his team to increase media interest in nutrition through regular articles in the *Zambia Daily Mail,* interviews and quotes on major Zambian radio and TV stations, and a Nutrition Media Awards ceremony to inspire and reward journalists covering issues of nutrition. Mobilizing civil society to speak with one voice is key. Says William, "The whole aim is forming alliances. When you have that critical mass, it enables the government to listen to you quite quickly for certain key issues that might be a little bit controversial."

Debjeet Sarangi

Director, Living Farms, India

As head of Living Farms, an organization working with landless and marginal farmers and consumers in Odisha, India, Debjeet Sarangi has successfully used participatory methods to help communities mobilize to combat underlying factors of undernutrition in their area. Debjeet and his team support communities to hold monthly meetings to diagnose these factors, identify solutions, and collectively implement and monitor activities. Communities have made major changes based on this strategy; one community, for example, banned the marriage of girls under 19 years of age. Under Debjeet's leadership, the Living Farms program also works with communities to ensure they have sufficient diverse and nutritious food, focusing on how best to use village agricultural land, forests, and other commons to grow and collect food and providing nutrition education and nutritious recipe ideas. Collaboration with local officials ensures that health and nutrition services are efficient and reach those in need, and Debjeet works to collect and share data regularly with key stakeholders. From 2011 to 2014, areas where Living Farms operates saw a 35 percent reduction in the infant mortality rate and a 12 percent drop in newborn deaths. Debjeet says, "When there is a reduction in newborn death, and in the infant mortality rate, you get a sense of peace, you can sleep peacefully."

Christopher Dube

Medical doctor and chairman, Mumbwa District Nutrition Coordination Committee, Zambia

Christopher Dube founded the first District Nutrition Coordination Committee (DNCC) in Zambia, which coordinates from the bottom up all nutrition-related activities led by key ministries. Members of the committee include representatives from five ministries at the district level and nongovernmental organizations (NGOs). Under Christopher's leadership, this committee has grown from 6 members to about 25 members. Christopher and his team engage with representatives from the ward nutrition

(Box 18.2 continued)

development committees, created by the DNCC, as well as representatives from the sub-ward level. Lobbying policy makers on the importance of nutrition and coordinating efforts is a key strategy of Christopher and his colleagues. They hold one-on-one meetings with MPs and policy makers, and they share information through the District Development Coordinating Committee (of which the DNCC is a subcommittee) as well as the Ward Nutrition Committee. The DNCC promotes one common and coordinated way of administering and monitoring nutrition issues in the district—a concept others are keen to replicate in different parts of the country. "The multisectoral approach has helped bridge the gap between stakeholders in the district and has highlighted the concept of nutrition as a cross-cutting issue. This has helped … inform the citizens about the difference between having food and being healthy in terms of nutrition," says Christopher.

SanSan Myint

Head, Three Millennium Development Goal Fund (3MDG Fund), Myanmar

SanSan Myint first started advocating for nutrition interventions in the health programs in which she worked with a range of population groups, including urban and rural communities as well as those affected by HIV/AIDS. These experiences, coupled with her observations of the SUN Movement thriving in countries where she had worked, led her to become the coordinator for the Civil Society Alliance for Scaling Up Nutrition (SUN CSA) in Myanmar, which successfully launched in February 2015. The SUN CSA was formed relatively quickly, owing in large part to SanSan's efforts. She revived her network of contacts within the Ministry of Health, which she had built up during 14 years working there at the start of her career. Recognizing the top-down nature of Myanmar society, she first approached community gatekeepers to get local NGOs and other actors on board. The SUN CSA also tapped into the constituencies and networks of its Steering Committee members. SanSan says, "Working and starting up with this broad group of partners was very instrumental in getting people engaged, interested, and on board, because we each had our own constituencies. We also had our own local NGO networks. That was how we were able to mobilize a lot of people in a very short time." SanSan also worked to ensure that the SUN CSA's activities were participatory and inclusive, that the large media community was engaged, and that advocacy efforts were based on strong evidence.

Christine Muyama

Nutrition Programs Officer, Graca Machel Trust, Uganda

Christine Muyama has held a number of roles building nutritional awareness and advocacy in Uganda and the surrounding region. As national coordinator for the Uganda Civil Society Coalition on Scaling Up Nutrition (UCCO-SUN), she and her team successfully advocated to ensure nutrition was addressed as a key issue in Uganda's National Development Plan (NDP) II. They also motivated the King of Tooro (western Uganda) to declare a week for nutritional awareness—an important accomplishment in a region that is considered the food basket of the country yet has the second-highest level of malnutrition. Christine and her colleagues also engaged with and provided nutrition advocacy training to government officials in the DNCCs from the start. Christine currently serves as the Nutrition Programs officer at the Graca Machel Trust, where she supports civil society alliances in Malawi, Mozambique, and Tanzania to lobby leaders to prioritize nutrition at the national, district, and community levels. Through this work, she has organized nutrition advocacy training with MPs in Malawi, who are now leading the movement to ensure that funds allocated to nutrition reach the community level. In addition to providing evidence papers and statistics, Christine has found that one of the best ways to engage with decisionmakers is to provide them with firsthand human stories that illustrate the

(Box 18.2 continued)

evidence. "This real-life evidence clicks into their brains faster and helps bring life to the statistics you are showing them," she says.

Neerja Chowdhury

Political journalist and member of the Citizens' Alliance against Malnutrition, India

Neerja Chowdhury has used her position as a reputable political journalist to raise awareness about malnutrition issues among government officials and the media in India. Following the election of a large number of young MPs in 2004, she coordinated a visit with eight young MPs to the areas most affected by malnutrition, garnering media coverage and shaping the view that nutrition is an issue that cuts across party lines. The group became known as the Citizens' Alliance against Malnutrition and continued to visit states ruled by different political parties. The Citizens' Alliance has since encouraged the Naandi Foundation to carry out the HUNGaMA (Hunger and Malnutrition) Survey to help fill the wide gap in data and knowledge on child malnutrition in India. The group also facilitated a meeting between film star Aamir Khan and then–Prime Minister Manmohan Singh, which led the government to mount a multimedia campaign on malnutrition with the star.[17] Neerja works with the Citizens' Alliance to identify entry points for nutrition action and attention in the government at the senior level, building on the MPs' connections and her own. The Citizens' Alliance may have encouraged the government to move ahead with its 2010 decision to focus on improving child and maternal health in 200 high-burden districts in the country. The Citizens' Alliance is an advocacy initiative with no formal structure, convener, or funding. Says Neerja, "That's the way we wanted it, rather than become a formal organizational structure. The important thing is that there is a committed core group and they have taken ownership. When momentum flags, I give it a push."

Frealem Shibabaw

Director, Ethiopia School Meal Initiative, Ethiopia

Frealem Shibabaw founded a school meal initiative in Ethiopia that partners with small dairy farms to feed 7,000 kindergarten and primary school students every day before class. Through a formal dialogue with cabinet members and state presidents, Frealem designed the school meal program with an emphasis on local ownership and sustainability. In less than three years, she established the initiative with 23 dairy farms in 5 regional states and an average of 10 cows and 6 dairy farm workers per school. Plans are underway to begin feeding pregnant women and younger siblings of enrolled children. The program has helped increase enrollment rates and has built interest among regional governments, which are considering scaling up the school dairy farm model. The federal government is also looking to turn this approach into a national school meal program. Critical to the success of this program has been Frealem's engagement with key actors, including her strategic selection of top political officials to lobby for it and her focus on those interested in her ideas regardless of their sector. The school meal program team shares regular reports with local and regional officials, nonprofit organizations, community groups, and other stakeholders. Communities' involvement in and ownership of the initiative are vital. Frealem says, "Before we prepare our lessons, I think we should sit down with the community and learn from them first.... What is there, and what is not there, and what will work, and what will not work, and why. Unless you know the community very well, it's very hard to design strategies that work."

(Box 18.2 continued)

Basanta Kumar Kar

Senior Advisor, Coalition for Food and Nutrition Security, India

Basanta Kumar Kar has led or been involved in many successful nutrition initiatives in South Asia while working at National Dairy Development Board in India, ActionAid International, CARE, and the Global Alliance for Improved Nutrition (GAIN). For example, Basanta and colleagues at GAIN helped to roll out a pilot program in Bangladesh on vitamin A fortification of refined vegetable oil; the program ultimately reached 45 million people.[18] Under Basanta's leadership, GAIN partnered with the Bangladesh Ministry of Primary and Mass Education and others to pioneer the Community Led Integrated School Nutrition Program, an innovative school feeding model that emphasized both delivery of high-quality nutrition-rich meals and strong community engagement. Basanta's involvement in nutrition issues has been driven by efforts to build institutional partnerships, for example, with the government, while advocating for the poor and marginalized. As a state program representative at CARE, he served as a member secretary to the first-ever State Nutrition Advisory Committee in Chhattisgarh, India, which set the nutrition agenda in a newly formed tribal-dominated state. He also contributed to the development of a 10-year National Strategy on Prevention and Control of Micronutrient Deficiencies as a member of the strategy's Expert Working Group. Demonstrating context-specific evidence and impact through programs has been key to Basanta's influence on policy makers in South Asia. He says, "Every country wants their policy to be unique ... so you have to bring out or contextualize the policy with the country, with the context, with the local political economy."

V. Ramani

Director General, Mother–Child Health and Nutrition Mission, India

V. Ramani brought nutrition to the forefront of public policy concerns and promoted involvement at all levels of government and civil society to address child malnutrition in Maharashtra. The Mother–Child Health and Nutrition Mission led by Ramani scaled up efforts across the state to significantly reduce malnutrition among young children. Between 2006 and 2012, Maharashtra's stunting rate among children under 2 years of age reportedly declined by 15 percentage points—one of the fastest declines in stunting in the world. Two existing channels were used to address child undernutrition in Maharashtra: the *Integrated Child Development Services* (ICDS) and the public health system. "Our efforts were really aimed at making these two wings of the government work together, centralize their working, and ensure there was collaboration between them," says Ramani. He made it a priority to motivate staff in the ICDS and public health services. Under Ramani's leadership, the Mission sensitized different stakeholders to the various issues in child malnutrition and created confidence that the problem could be tackled in a systematic, time-bound manner by improving public service delivery systems and measuring accountability for outcomes. This model has since been replicated in other Indian states including Gujarat, Jharkhand, Karnataka, Madhya Pradesh, and Uttar Pradesh.

within nutrition: *decision makers,* such as heads of ministries, who are most traditionally nutrition champions; *influencers,* such as donors, mid-level bureaucrats, or civil society actors, who can create networks of nutrition champions and supporters; and *clients,* who rarely have input into policy but can elevate accountability in nutrition programming, thus becoming leaders themselves. A summary of country case studies by the Mainstreaming Nutrition Initiative[19] looks at how these different types of leaders operate within the actual policy process, depending on the context. For example, the analysis contrasts Bolivia, Guatemala, and Peru, where political leaders espoused rhetoric

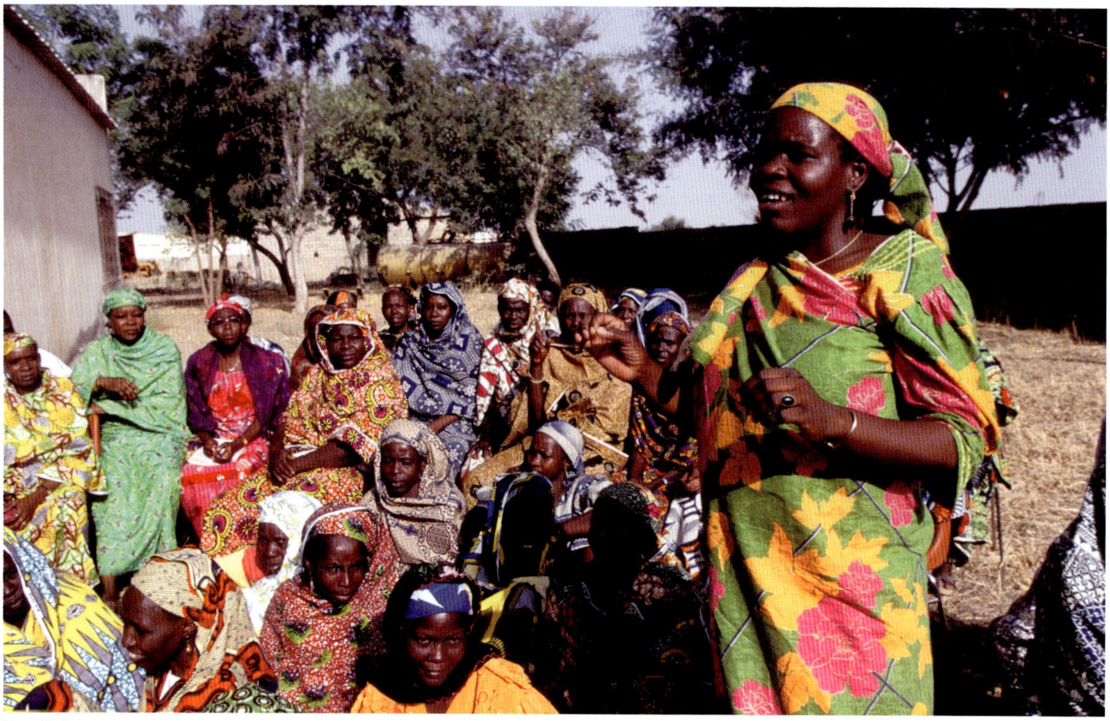

Panos/G. Pirozzi

Local clients of nutrition interventions, like these women in Cameroon, can play a leadership role by strengthening accountability.

during national elections, with other leaders' less politically visible work in Bangladesh and Vietnam.

Also relying on country case studies, the *Analysing Nutrition Governance* series compares nutrition policy process in six countries (Bangladesh, Brazil, Ethiopia, India, Peru, and Zambia).[20] The Zero Hunger campaign in Brazil (see Chapter 11), for example, was tied closely to the administration of President Luiz Inácio Lula da Silva, while the Child Malnutrition Initiative, an advocacy coalition in Peru, converted political leaders to the cause by persuading presidential candidates to sign onto a pro-nutrition pledge (see Chapter 14).[21]

Beyond these studies, many experts in the nutrition literature have called for more and stronger leadership, but these lack a substantial conceptual or empirical base. Reviews of the larger international development field have found a generally poor state of research on leadership and an excessive focus on the personality attributes of leaders in wealthy countries within other fields, such as business studies and organizational and development psychology.[22] The state of the literature makes it difficult to apply these conclusions to political processes related to nutrition in low- and middle-income countries.

Borrowing from the fields of systems science and adult development yields more insights. A systems model presents leadership as an interactive process, rooted in context and history, that changes over time rather than as a top-down managerial concept.[23] Individuals with high levels of adult development—that is, the ability to understand and manage complex situations—can appreciate how to influence and reshape the different perspectives and connections among stakeholders in order to build up a social network that can effect changes in policies or programs.[24]

In summary, wider reviews outside the field of nutrition emphasize the need for a contextually situated—and therefore political—understanding of how leaders operate. In looking at leadership across diverse contexts, our focus on leadership needs to go beyond what leadership is or what it accomplishes to look at how leadership operates.

What Motivates Nutrition Leaders, and What Are Their Capabilities?

The interviews with 89 nutrition leaders yielded interesting insights about their motivations and capabilities (see Table 18.1 for a summary of the findings). Regarding initial motivation, several champions came to their leadership positions by chance, entering nutrition early in their careers and deliberately staying engaged. A few individuals with a clinical practice background had entered nutrition as a result of seeking evidence on the underlying causes of child and maternal health issues. Still others were motivated to make a positive change by the dire situation in their home communities or because of career placements in rural areas. Regardless of their initial intent, nutrition seems to have become an issue about which they care, making the case for exposing potential leaders from other disciplines to both nutrition data and firsthand experience as a way of

TABLE 18.1 Summary of findings from nutrition leader interviews and implications for leadership

Research question	Findings	Implications
What motivates people to become leaders in nutrition? Are there common elements in their backgrounds that lead them to champion nutrition?	• No common origin/catalyst drivers, but several common pathways, including exposure to situations of high malnutrition and desire to understand the root of health problems	• Nutrition is "sticky" for some; need to expose as many potential leaders as possible to the realities of undernutrition
What enables leaders to operate effectively in the nutrition policy sphere? In particular, what are their analytical and political capabilities?	• Most effective leaders are able to deal with complexity, are systemic thinkers, and have reached postconventional levels of adult development • Roles depend on networks: in fragmented networks, they may be boundary spanners; in less fragmented but not cohesive networks, they may be co-creators; individuals may change roles depending on need and capacities	• Find ways to support these capabilities and build them up in others • Encourage development of networks
What are the external challenges and barriers to their effective operation?	• Donor/civil-society politics • Fragmentation and lack of coherent frames • Lack of executive-level political commitment (rhetoric not backed by reality) • Knowledge and data gaps (see below)	• Promote consensus building • Develop accountability mechanisms for top-level commitment • Consult identified leaders on political constraints
What do leaders assess as the knowledge gaps? How do they employ their existing knowledge?	• Gaps: effective multisectorality, timely data, operational research • They employ existing knowledge by using locally sourced and/or translated knowledge to reach policy audiences	• Consult identified leaders on knowledge and data gaps • Support local research supply and demand, local knowledge brokers

Source: Authors' interviews with 89 nutrition leaders.

garnering cross-sector support for nutrition in the future.

The interviews also uncovered a relationship between effective leadership and higher levels of adult development, underlining the need to attract individuals with advanced analytical or "sense-making" capabilities to the field through incentive structures and rewards. Furthermore, the types of leaders and leadership activities that were found to be effective depended on the shape and maturity level of the nutrition social network. Fragmented networks benefited from leaders who could cross boundaries; more mature networks benefited from individuals who could generate an environment of co-creation. This paradigm can also be applied more broadly to the national context: leaders working in countries with high levels of fragmentation could change the shape of the social network rather than try to work within it.

The wide diversity of contexts in which leaders must operate makes the case for helping individuals within the nutrition community increase their levels of adult development. Coaching or participation in programs has been shown, experimentally, to increase adult development levels over long periods of time (nine months or longer).[25] Other options are to increase group-level adult development at the time of engagement with nutrition, such as through participatory stakeholder mapping exercises or support programs that aim to develop broader leadership qualities in nutrition. Examples include the African Nutrition Leadership Programme or summer school run by the UK's Institute of Development Studies and the International Food Policy Research Institute. There is also a need to support existing leaders, financially or institutionally, so that they have the capacity and power to help the nutrition network over which they preside overcome challenges.[26]

What Challenges Do Nutrition Leaders Face?

Leaders' ability to effect change is determined partly by the policy and political environment, which can either promote or hinder nutrition progress.[27] The interviews yielded a view of leadership as a political process[28] during which leaders must navigate such challenges as siloed ministries; inappropriate roles for donors or the private sector; a bias toward food production to the detriment of nutrition; and lack of local knowledge, evidence, and data to inform policy, programming, and advocacy. Even where there was support for nutrition from the prime minister or a cabinet minister, it was often explained as political rhetoric without action to back it up, accompanied by a lack of real commitment and understanding of nutrition at high levels. This finding underlines the importance of creating mechanisms for holding ministers and bureaucrats accountable for meeting their commitments in nutrition. Initiatives such as the Hunger and Nutrition Commitment Index are key in this regard.[29]

Of the four target countries, only respondents from India noted the role of civil society in influencing and driving change, mainly due to the Right to Food campaign and placement of nutrition advocates within the then-ruling Congress Party and its National Advisory Council. In Bangladesh, researchers, pediatricians, and multilateral donors were viewed as being able to shape policy, especially in light of donor pressure to mainstream the National Nutrition Service into existing community health provision. In Kenya, key government officials backed by technical support from donors within government were influential in convening disparate stakeholder groups. Leaders from Ethiopia did not refer to any particular individuals as influential, perhaps reflecting the country's more authoritarian political structure.

A common theme across all the countries (with the exception of India) was disproportionate donor power. Interviewees reported that donors focused solely on their own programs or collected large amounts of data without sharing it. Many interviewees, however, praised particular donors for spurring support for nutrition in their countries. Some interviewees from India did express concerns about donor collusion with the private sector, though there was little reflection overall across the four countries on the role of the private sector.

These reflections do not necessarily paint an accurate picture of the four countries studied. They do, however, reveal a fragmented nutrition landscape that may affect the ability of the nutrition sector to create a cohesive narrative on effective action, both internally within the nutrition community and externally to key decision makers.[30] For example, in Bangladesh and India, the nutrition community reportedly suffers from a rift between breastfeeding advocates and those advocating for a wider range of nutrition-specific interventions, including micronutrients and ready-to-use therapeutic foods for the treatment of severe acute malnutrition. Other splits in the framing of nutrition in Ethiopia and Kenya have occurred between advocates of food-based approaches or food-based emergency nutrition efforts on the one hand and advocates of other nutrition actions such as

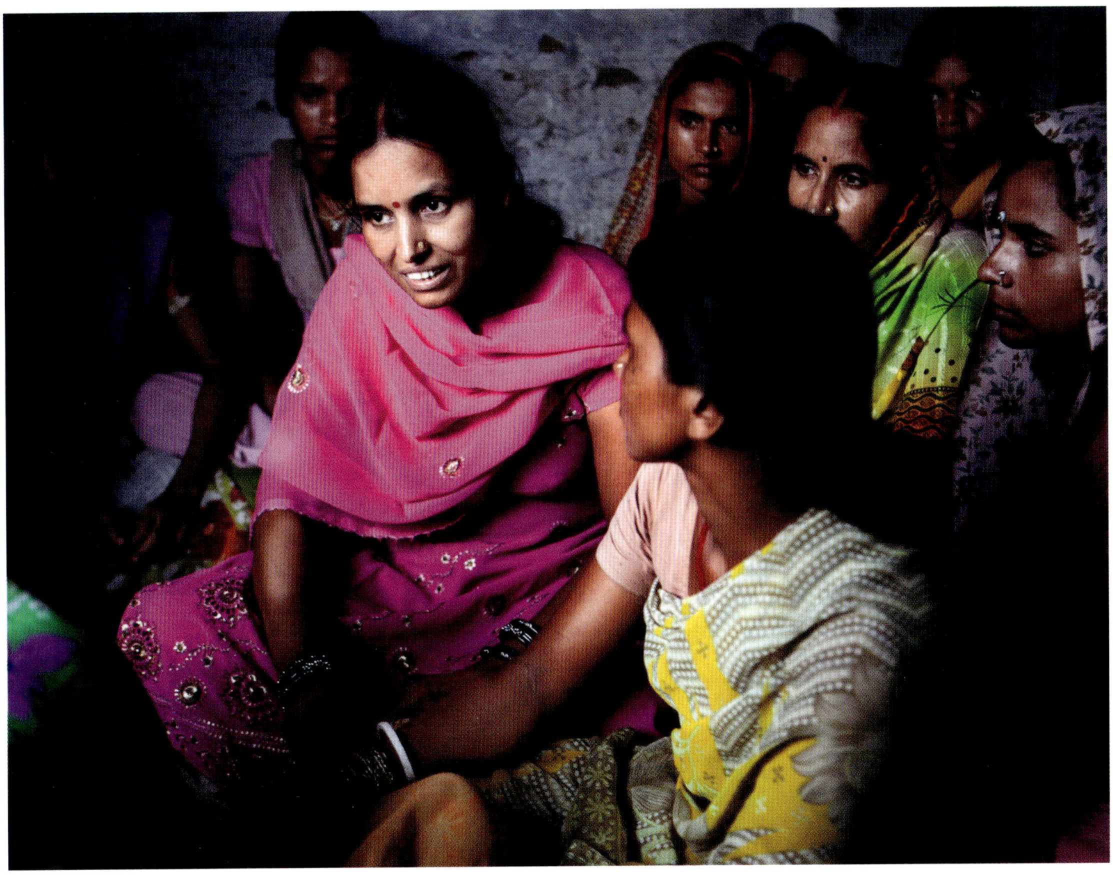

Panos/A. Loke

A woman in the state of Bihar, India, talks about health care at a community meeting.

improvements in water and sanitation or infant and young child feeding on the other hand.

What Do Leaders Assess as the Knowledge Gaps?

Leaders in nutrition seem to have a thorough understanding of the latest evidence on nutrition-specific and nutrition-sensitive determinants and interventions, and the more capable ones translate this knowledge into messages that can be understood by the greater public and that can potentially influence decision or policy makers. The leaders also identified some knowledge gaps, including knowledge about how to coordinate multisectorally and particularly how to commission, collect, and interpret timely and localized research, knowledge, and data.

Generating evidence locally was viewed as critical to getting decision makers to pay attention to research, since many decision makers are perceived as wary of being unduly influenced by foreign donors. Interviewees called on researchers to produce locally applicable frameworks or systems of analysis, to use rapid-fire assessments tailored to specific states and decision makers, and to undertake monitoring and operational studies based on district and regional-level data.

Leaders are the individuals most likely to turn evidence into action, so consulting them before commissioning research can help ensure that the research has a long-term impact. An internally neutral, "unimpeachable" research body that can produce credible research was seen as critical. At the same time, some external arbitration of data and evidence was seen as helpful in forcing difficult decisions.

Conclusion

Leadership is a common factor in successfully promoting action on nutrition globally, regionally, and within countries. At the same time, the nascent and exciting field of leadership in nutrition still suffers from a number of knowledge gaps. We need a deeper understanding of leaders' motivations and how to develop nutrition champions from the wider field of influential decision makers. More case studies are needed describing the impact of individual champions on nutrition success stories, such as those referred to here and in Boxes 18.1 and 18.2.

Equally important, more research is needed to develop the next generation of nutrition leaders and to evaluate existing initiatives in nutrition leadership. These include the REACH partnership (established by the FAO, UNICEF, the World Food Programme, and the WHO), the SUN Movement, and regional initiatives such as the African Nutrition Leadership Programme and Action Against Hunger's support for nutrition champions in West Africa. Quantitative and qualitative work can assess whether investments in leadership pay off in terms of changes to program or policy coverage and impact, quality of services, and program costs. More work is also needed to increase the capacity of leaders to operate within an enabling environment for nutrition policy,[31] connecting these studies to political economy research to fully understand leaders as they operate in complex and adaptive real-world political systems.

CHAPTER 19

New Horizons

Nutrition in the 21st Century

STUART GILLESPIE, JUDITH HODGE, RAJUL PANDYA-LORCH, JESSICA WHITE, AND SIVAN YOSEF

BY WEAVING STORIES together with analysis and description in this book, we have sought to convey the variety of experiences in tackling malnutrition in different contexts throughout the past five decades. This narrative approach is intended to help the reader translate an experience into his or her own context, showing many examples of *what* can be done and *how* success can be achieved. Our aim is not only to inform action, but to inspire.

We focus on change. Success stories emerge in their own time and place, but they do not always endure, especially if the context changes (one well-documented example of this is Tanzania's Iringa project; see Chapter 2). So while it may be difficult to duplicate individual successes, it may be easier to replicate principles and processes—ranging from how malnutrition is conceptualized and measured, to analytical approaches to unraveling its key drivers, to approaches to developing and implementing an appropriate mix of responses. In this short conclusion we highlight some of the key lessons from earlier chapters.

The opening chapter showed how an "either-or" mentality tended to prevail within the nutrition community through the mid- to late 20th century: vigorous debates revolved around whether nutrition was a food issue or a health issue, whether it was within the purview of the Ministry of Agriculture or of Health, and whether it was about macronutrients or micronutrients. This either-or thinking spilled over into discussions of appropriate responses: Which sector should take the lead? Is a top-down or bottom-up approach preferred? What is the appropriate role for the private sector? Major divides split clinical scientists, who had a more medical and curative orientation, from structuralists, who were more holistic and systems-oriented in their analyses and focused more on preventing the problem than on "curing" it. This split was also reflected in the divide between humanitarian nutritionists and developmental nutritionists, who at times appeared to inhabit parallel universes. There were even debates over the rationale for dealing with malnutrition. Utilitarians highlighted the economic benefits of a well-nourished population, citing cost-benefit and cost-effectiveness analyses. Human rights advocates emphasized entitlements, duties, and accountability.

As the new millennium dawned, a more enlightened view of the potential relevance of all of this thinking started to emerge, with the importance of any one response being in large part determined by context. The 1990 UNICEF conceptual framework paved the way for a better understanding among a wide range of stakeholders of their respective roles in multilevel and multisectoral responses to malnutrition. The framework did so by starting not with any one sector, but with the malnourished child, showing how the key drivers of malnutrition emerged and exerted their influence at different levels. Malnutrition began to be understood as a multilevel and multisectoral problem that required engagement by a range of stakeholders.

The three sections of this book mirror the *Lancet* framework shown in Chapter 1 (itself an evolution of the UNICEF framework that includes benefits and interventions), highlighting the three core levels of response to malnutrition. At the level of individuals, malnutrition is caused by inadequate dietary intake, often interacting with disease and poor care. Nutrition-specific interventions—including those aimed at improving infant and young child feeding, addressing micronutrient deficiencies, and managing acute malnutrition (topics addressed in Chapters 3–5)—can make inroads at this level, if well targeted and well implemented. But they cannot solve the problem by themselves, as the roots lie deeper. At the underlying level, corresponding to households and communities, we see the importance of transforming sectoral actions—for example, within agriculture, social protection, and water, sanitation, and hygiene (Chapters 6–8)—to make them more nutrition-sensitive. And at the base of the framework lie country-level enabling environments, in which political commitment, governance, policy, legal frameworks, capacity, and financing are all key (Chapters 10–17).

Many responses to malnutrition depend on community action. Chapter 2, on community nutrition programs, highlights the pivotal importance of a "good process"—driven by active participation, local ownership, and empowerment—in developing and implementing programs. The development of community-based management of acute malnutrition (Chapter 5) enabled local volunteers to detect severe acute malnutrition early. There are many other examples of proactive community action benefiting nutrition, such as community-led total sanitation in Mali (Chapter 8) and community health volunteers' work to expand access to supplementation, family planning, and care for pregnant women and newborns in Nepal (Chapter 13).

In addition, many of the experiences highlighted in this book illustrate the importance of multisectoral approaches and in a sense validate the three-tiered *Lancet* framework. The social protection chapter (Chapter 7), for example, highlights the efforts of Mexico's PROGRESA/ Oportunidades/Prospera program to raise families' incomes, address household food security, create opportunities for maternal and child care and education, and improve child feeding practices. The agriculture chapter (Chapter 6) discusses interventions that combine homestead food production and animal husbandry with behavior-change communication focused on infant and young child feeding, with a strong emphasis on the role of women. But the message of multisectorality may come across most clearly when discussing achievements at the country level. Ethiopia's nutrition story (Chapter 16) is associated with progress on agricultural growth, sanitation, and social protection. In Thailand (Chapter 10), nutrition was explicitly recognized by complementary sectors such as health, agriculture, education, and rural development and woven into micro- and macro-level planning to alleviate poverty. Brazil's nutrition strategy (Chapter 11) similarly hinged on delivering a multisectoral program that focused on income redistribution and pro-poor spending, alongside improving access to education, health, and sanitation. Indeed, pro-poor economic growth was recognized as a factor in several of the country experiences, such as in Thailand and Bangladesh, where improvements in household wealth made a large contribution to various nutrition outcomes (Chapters 10 and 12).

What also becomes clear is that the levels of response to malnutrition are linked vertically, such that nutrition-sensitive sectoral action has the potential to support the scale-up of nutrition-specific interventions, while both need to be underpinned by enabling environments. And these levels of response offer synergies. If attention is paid to all levels simultaneously, the whole—in terms of impact—is greater than the sum of its parts. Many success stories in the book illustrate this synergy: the Alive & Thrive program's achievements in improving breastfeeding and complementary feeding practices in Bangladesh, Ethiopia, and Vietnam, for example, show what can happen at a large scale when a range of actors—such as governments, NGOs, and CSOs—coalesce around common goals (see Chapter 3).

Within the past decade, there has been a coming of age as the global nutrition community has taken on board the political element of change. Political commitment is a fundamental ingredient of any enabling environment, and there are many reasons why malnutrition is political. But generating and sustaining political commitment can be challenging. The overall benefits of improving nutrition often take longer than a politician's time in office to fully manifest themselves and may thus get short shrift. Moreover, undernutrition may be largely "invisible" where it is most prevalent. Stunted children are often so commonplace that everyone from a child's parents to a country's policy makers may see them as the norm (this "normalization" increasingly applies to child overweight and obesity as well). Unlike HIV, for example, undernutrition is not infectious. As ruling elites are thus not threatened by it, and its societal invisibility reduces its prominence as a development issue, it becomes easy to ignore. Nonetheless, huge gains in political commitment have been made in recent years, with the Scaling Up Nutrition (SUN) Movement on the frontline of such political change.

Even if the problem does succeed in capturing the attention of politicians and policymakers, the next challenge is to figure out what to do. As discussed, addressing malnutrition comprehensively and sustainably requires actions by several often unconnected sectors. The role of the private sector can lead to particular challenges. Asymmetries of power and of incentives between governments and multinationals require proactive government regulation of the private sector. Governments have had to take measures to protect breastfeeding, for example, as discussed in Chapter 3, and they have had to cope with junk food manufacturers' attempts to undermine policies designed to tackle obesity, highlighted in Chapter 9.

Commitment is important but actions speak louder than words. Commitment is relevant only when it leads to action that generates impact on the ground. This is the new frontier for nutrition. Commitment and knowledge of what works must lead to large-scale implementation of nutrition-relevant policies and programs. Translating commitment into action requires, among other things, accountability, data, and capacity. With regard to accountability, US$23 billion of funding for nutrition ($4 billion for nutrition-specific programming and $19 billion for nutrition-sensitive programming) was pledged at the 2013 Nutrition for Growth Summit in London. How many of these pledges have been activated and operationalized?

This is one of the key tasks of the pioneering *Global Nutrition Report*: to shine a light on what happened next and whether governments are actually stepping up their investment in nutrition. Global and national accountability is key, but accountability is relevant at all levels and ultimately should be channeled downward to communities where nutritionally vulnerable populations reside. Peru's story (Chapter 14) illustrates this point well: its Child Malnutrition Initiative, a multistakeholder advocacy coalition, is widely credited with enlisting presidential candidates to pledge to improve nutrition and subsequently publicly monitoring these commitments.

Accountability cannot operate in a data vacuum. It is crucial that timely data on trends in different forms of malnutrition and on outcomes of actions and programs become available and accessible in the public domain. More data that are actionable at the subnational level are also needed. More and better evaluations are required—not just assessments of whether a program works but process evaluations that highlight impact pathways—to help understand why, how, and where programs work or don't work.

Finally, the time is ripe for a major long-term investment in strengthening capacity for nutrition. Capacity is needed at different levels—individual, community, organizational, and systemic—and for different purposes. In particular, within the new generation of nutrition professionals, we need individuals with stronger strategic and operational capacities to go along with their technical skillsets. And we need to strengthen the capacity of individuals in other sectors, to empower and motivate them to apply a nutrition lens in their work and to contribute to nutrition-relevant change through their programming and investments.

An example of transformational capacity is leadership. Leaders open doors, turn keys, and inspire others. Leaders in and for nutrition are not necessarily hierarchical; they tend to exhibit lateral leadership—the ability to successfully work across sectors, build collaborations and alliances, and communicate effectively. Nutrition champions and policy entrepreneurs are needed to catalyze social and political change and make development policy in general more nutrition-sensitive. The profiles of current leaders in nutrition (Chapter 18) show how champions may spring from many different quarters. We need to develop the next generation of nutrition leaders and to strengthen existing initiatives, including academies and curricula, that aim to build leadership capacity.

Not all experiences in this book are glowing success stories, and not all successes endured. This is the real world. Changes and challenges are constant. Possibly the greatest challenge is the rising problem of obesity—in fact more people are now overweight or obese than are undernourished. As Chapter 9 underlines, not a single country has shown a decline in overweight in recent years. Systems approaches are needed to change obesogenic environments into enabling environments, and there is a need to ensure that interventions to tackle undernutrition do not inadvertently contribute to obesity. As we have done here with undernutrition (and its longer history), the nutrition world will need to highlight more stories of change in obesity prevention and control in years to come, drawing on promising interventions such as Mexico's tax on sugar-sweetened beverages. As progress is made, new challenges and new frontiers emerge. This is why we called this book *Nourishing Millions*—it is an ongoing process.

APPENDIX

How the Stories of Change in This Book Were Selected

SIVAN YOSEF, JUDITH HODGE, STUART GILLESPIE, AND RAJUL PANDYA-LORCH

THE BOOK EDITORS selected and prepared the case studies included in this book using a five-step process as follows: (1) collect potential case studies using a global call for nominations and review of scholarly and gray literature; (2) develop and apply criteria to create a list of eligible case studies; (3) supplement this list with contributions from Transform Nutrition's Stories of Change project as well as in-depth interviews with experts in the field; (4) select final topic areas and case studies based on discussion with the project's advisory committee; and finally, (5) write the book chapters and conduct peer review.

Step 1: Collect Potential Case Studies

Call for Nominations: June–September 2015

The book editors circulated a call for nominations in June–September 2015. The call for nominations was widely distributed by email, posted on the project's website, and linked to the websites of several organizations.

Literature Review: May–August 2015

A literature search was conducted using a snowballing approach (seeking advice from key experts and then examining references of reviewed or recommended materials) and gray-literature capture, as outlined by Hagen-Zanker and Mallet.[1] The starting point for this process consisted of landmark country case studies, including those of the UN Standing Committee on Nutrition (formerly the ACC/SCN) published in 1991, 2005, and 2013[2]; UNICEF case studies (2009 and 2013)[3]; reviews of nutrition-specific and nutrition-sensitive interventions and the enabling environment in the *Lancet* series on maternal and child nutrition (2008 and 2013);[4] and the *Global Nutrition Report* (2014 and 2015[5]). A search was also conducted for reports from research institute websites such as Eldis, the IFPRI e-brary, and Secure Nutrition; from the World Bank, UNICEF, the Food and Agriculture Organization of the United Nations (FAO), the World Health Organization (WHO), and the Scaling Up Nutrition (SUN) Movement; and from other governmental and nongovernmental organizations and international bodies. Where possible, this review drew on systematic reviews, peer-reviewed journal articles, meta-analyses, and randomized controlled trials. To cast the net wide, we looked at gray literature, including program reports, annual reports, blogs, and websites.

Step 2: Develop and Apply Criteria

The combined process of nominations and literature review yielded 99 potential case studies.

Although criteria had been widely circulated throughout the global call for nominations, the project team reviewed all the case studies carefully to ensure they were indeed eligible. The criteria were the following:

1. Beneficiaries: The program, project, policy, investment, intervention, or innovation operated in at least one low-income or lower-middle-income country and benefited a vulnerable group or groups of people.
2. Date: The intervention was implemented within the past 50 years.
3. Relevance: The intervention engaged nutrition directly or indirectly through related sectors such as education, health, agriculture, water, and sanitation programs.
4. Importance: The intervention addressed an important nutrition security problem or issue.
5. Scale: The intervention operated at a significant scale, defined as national, regional, provincial, or covering a substantial number of beneficiaries. Demonstration or pilot projects were not considered.
6. Nutrition-related outcomes: The intervention had a documented impact on nutrition-related outcome indicators. Examples include changes in anthropometry such as child stunting; individual intake of calories, macronutrients, micronutrients, or specific foods; individual or household dietary diversity; women's status or empowerment linked to nutrition outcomes, production diversity, or dietary diversity; and nutrition-friendly investments in health, education, child feeding and care, water, sanitation, and hygiene, and enabling policy environments.

After applying these criteria and eliminating duplicates, the project team had a final long list of 71 eligible case studies. Using the project's conceptual framework (see Chapter 1), these case studies were then categorized as (1) nutrition-specific programs and interventions; (2) nutrition-sensitive programs and approaches; and (3) interventions that were both nutrition-specific and nutrition-sensitive in approach, worked in multiple sectors, or targeted the enabling environment for nutrition. Within these categories, the case studies were further disaggregated by time period and geographic region.

Step 3: Supplement the List of Case Studies

Contributions from Transform Nutrition

Critical contributions were also provided by Transform Nutrition, a global multipartner research consortium led by the International Food Policy Research Institute (IFPRI). In late 2014, Transform Nutrition launched a research initiative called "Stories of Change," which developed a series of structured case studies focused on national-level successes in six developing countries or regions: Bangladesh, Ethiopia, the state of Odisha in India, Nepal, Senegal, and Zambia. Throughout 2015 and into 2016, country teams undertook in-depth assessments and analyses, using both primary and secondary data, to develop case studies. These case studies will be incorporated into a learning platform linked to existing communities of practice, such as the SUN Movement. Given the synergies between *Nourishing Millions* and Transform Nutrition's Stories of Change projects, the six country case studies were added to the list for consideration. Four were ultimately written up as chapters (Chapters 12, 13, 16, and 17), and one is presented as a box within a chapter (Box 18.1 on nutrition leadership in Zambia).

Key Informant Interviews

To fill in any potential information gaps on nutrition case studies, 10 key informant interviews were conducted with high-level experts. The 40- to 60-minute interviews identified success stories and covered other relevant topics such as historical changes in nutrition. The interviews were recorded, transcribed, and coded for future analysis. Case studies identified by the experts were then added to the list for consideration.

Step 4: Make Final Selections with Input from the Advisory Committee

The project's Advisory Committee (listed on page 218) met on September 30, 2015, to discuss all the case studies in depth. Members provided input on which case studies best met the project's criteria while ensuring a balanced presentation of nutrition-specific, nutrition-sensitive, and country-level stories as well as a coherent storyline. Following the meeting, the project team finalized the list of chapters to include in the book.

Step 5: Write Chapters and Conduct Peer Review

All the chapters were written by the book editors, external authors, or Stories of Change team members. Draft chapters were reviewed by the editors and, in most cases, by additional expert reviewers. They were then revised by the authors before being submitted for peer review. All chapters underwent formal peer review by IFPRI's independent Publications Review Committee (PRC). Upon approval by the PRC, the chapters were edited and finalized.

Notes

Chapter 1

1 World Bank, *Repositioning Nutrition as Central to Development: A Strategy for Large-Scale Action,* Directions in Development (Washington, DC, 2006).

2 The Sustainable Development Goals (SDGs)—all 17 of them—were ratified by the United Nations in September 2015. The second goal is to "end hunger, achieve food security and improved nutrition, and promote sustainable agriculture." The two most nutrition-relevant targets for this goal are 2.1 ("By 2030, end hunger and ensure access by all people, in particular the poor and people in vulnerable situations, including infants, to safe, nutritious, and sufficient food all year round") and 2.2 ("By 2030, end all forms of malnutrition, including achieving, by 2025, the internationally agreed targets on stunting and wasting in children under 5 years of age, and address the nutritional needs of adolescent girls, pregnant and lactating women, and older persons").

3 S. Gillespie, P. Menon, and A. Kennedy, "Scaling Up Impact on Nutrition: What Will It Take?" *Advances in Nutrition* 6 (2015): 440–451.

4 R. E. Luna, "The Storytelling Scientist," *Science* 350, no. 6259 (2105): 391.

5 S. Denning, "Using Stories to Spark Organizational Change," *Systems Thinker* 13 (2002): 2–6, http://www.providersedge.com/docs/km_articles/using_stories_to_spark_organizational_change.pdf, accessed March 14, 2016.

6 In doing this, we draw on several different sources: a review of published literature charting the history of different aspects of nutrition, interviews with key actors who have been involved in international nutrition research and practice through several decades, and a broader review of nutrition literature that reveals how nutrition was seen and programs were enacted at different points in time.

7 These include a history of nutrition in a specific organization (World Bank), histories of emergency nutrition, histories of nutrition policy, histories of infant feeding interventions, and broader histories of international nutrition.

8 World Bank, "Learning from World Bank History: Agriculture and Food-Based Approaches for Addressing Malnutrition," Agriculture and Environmental Services Discussion Paper 10 (Washington, DC, 2014).

9 N. Nisbett, S. Gillespie, L. Haddad, and J. Harris, "Why Worry About the Politics of Childhood Undernutrition?" *World Development* 64 (2014): 420–433.

10 S. R. Gillespie, M. McLachlan, and R. Shrimpton, eds., *Combating Malnutrition: Time to Act* (Washington, DC: World Bank–UNICEF, 2003).

11 U. Jonsson, "Paradigms in Applied Nutrition," paper presented at the 19th International Congress of Nutrition (ICN), Bangkok, Thailand, October 4–9, 2009, http://www.rtfn-watch.org/fileadmin/_migrated/content_uploads/U._Jonsson_-_Paradigms_in_Applied_Nutrition.pdf.

12 E. Kennedy, P. Webb, P. Walker, E. Saltzman, D. Maxwell, M. Nelson, and S. Booth, "The Evolving Food and Nutrition Agenda: Policy and Research Priorities for the Coming Decade," *Food and Nutrition Bulletin* 32, no. 1 (2011): 60–68.

13 E. Kennedy, "Nutrition Policy in the U.S.: 50 Years in Review," *Asia Pacific Journal of Clinical Nutrition* 17, S1 (2008): 340–342.

14 P. Webb, "Malnutrition in Emergencies: The Framing of Nutrition Concerns in the Humanitarian Appeals Process, 1992 to 2009," *Food and Nutrition Bulletin* 30, no. 4 (2009): 379–389.

15 M. H. N. Golden, "The Development of Concepts of Malnutrition," *Journal of Nutrition* 132, Suppl. 7 (2009): 2117S–2122S.

16 S. M. Crowther, L. A. Reynolds, and E. M. Tansey, eds., *The Resurgence of Breastfeeding,* Wellcome Witnesses to Twentieth Century Medicine, vol. 35 (London: Wellcome Trust Centre for the History of Medicine at UCL, 2009).

17 S. J. Knaak, "The Problem with Breastfeeding Discourse," *Revue Canadienne de Santé Publique* 97, no. 5 (2006): 212–214.

18 J. Levinson and M. McLachlan, "How Did We Get Here? A History of International Nutrition," in *Scaling Up, Scaling Down: Overcoming Malnutrition in Developing Countries,* edited by T. Marchione (Amsterdam: Gordon and Breach Publishers, 1999).

19 S. S. Morris, B. Cogill, and R. Uauy, "Effective International Action against Undernutrition: Why Has It Proven So Difficult and What Can Be Done to Accelerate Progress?" *Lancet* 371, no. 9612 (2008): 608–621.

20 L. Potvin, S. Gendron, A. Bilodeau, and P. Chabot, "Integrating Social Theory into Public Health Practice," *American Journal of Public Health* 95, no. 4 (2005): 591–595.

21 A. Berg, "Sliding toward Nutrition Malpractice: Time to Reconsider and Redeploy," *American Journal of Clinical Nutrition* 57 (1992): 3–7; J. Garrett and M. Natalicchio, eds., *Working Multisectorally in Nutrition: Principles and Practice from Senegal and Colombia* (Washington, DC: International Food Policy Research Institute, 2011).

22 P. V. Sukhatme, "Size and Nature of the Protein Gap," *Nutrition Reviews* 28, no. 9 (1970): 223–226.

23 D. McLaren, "The Great Protein Fiasco," *The Lancet* 304, no. 7872 (1974): 93–96.

24 A. Escobar, *Encountering Development: The Making and Unmaking of the Third World* (Princeton, NJ: Princeton University Press, 1995).

25 The conflation of the related but separate problems of undernutrition and hunger, still persists; see D. J. H. te Lintelo and R. W. D. Lakshman, "Equate and Conflate: Political Commitment to Hunger and Undernutrition Reduction in Five High-Burden Countries," *World Development* 76 (2015): 280–292. And some country policies and training programs still erroneously refer to undernutrition as "protein-energy malnutrition."

26 S. Reutlinger and M. Selowsky, *Malnutrition and Poverty: Magnitude and Policy Options* (Baltimore, MD: Johns Hopkins University Press, 1976).

27 A. Sen, *Poverty and Famines: An Essay on Entitlement and Deprivation* (Oxford: Oxford University Press, 1983).

28 H. Geach, "The Baby Food Tragedy," *New Internationalist,* August 23, 1973, http://newint.org/features/1973/08/01/baby-food-action-editorial/, accessed February 26, 2016.

29 UNICEF, *Strategy for Improved Nutrition of Children and Women in Developing Countries* (New York, 1990).

30 For a discussion of the framework's dissemination and use in different contexts, see D. Pelletier, "How Nutrition Policies Change: Lessons from the Promotion and Use of the UNICEF Conceptual Framework," in *Combating Malnutrition: Time to Act,* edited by S. Gillespie, M. McLachlan, and R. Shrimpton (Washington, DC: World Bank–UNICEF, 2003).

31 World Health Organization, *International Code of Marketing of Breast milk Substitutes* (Geneva, 1981).

32 A. Berg, *The Nutrition Factor* (Washington, DC: Brookings Institution, 1973), 1.

33 J. Levinson, "Nutrition Isolationism," in *Combating Malnutrition: Time to Act,* edited by S. Gillespie, M. McLachlan, and R. Shrimpton (Washington, DC: World Bank, 2003).

34 J. O. Field, "Multi-sectoral Nutrition Planning: A Post-mortem," *Food Policy* 12, no. 1 (1987): 15–28. Others, though, saw this time as a learning experience that, far from being abandoned, has evolved into the current focus on multisectoral action (if not "planning" in the sense of the complex models advocated in the 1970s); see H. Alderman, L. Elder, A. Goyal, A. Herforth, Y. T. Hoberg, A. Marini, J. Ruel-Bergeron, J. Saavedra, M. Shekar, S. Tiwari, and H. Zaman, *Improving Nutrition through Multisectoral Approaches* (Washington, DC: World Bank, 2013). The issue of multisectorality continued to dominate country-level studies in the subsequent decades; see J. Harris and S. Drimie, "Toward an Integrated Approach for Addressing Malnutrition in Zambia: A Literature Review and Institutional Analysis," IFPRI Discussion Paper 01200 (Washington, DC: International Food Policy Research Institute, 2012). These are recurrent themes in the next two decades of country studies.

35 Nisbett et al., "Why Worry About the Politics of Childhood Undernutrition?"

36 V. J. Quinn, *Nutrition and National Development: An Evaluation of Nutrition Planning in Malawi from 1936 to 1990* (The Hague, Netherlands: Wageningen Agricultural University Press, 1994).

37 Levinson, "Nutrition Isolationism."

38 J. Grant, "Nutritional Security: An Ethical Imperative of the 1990s," address at the International Conference on Nutrition, Rome, December 5–11, 1992.

39 L. LaViollette and V. Mannar, *Scaling Up and Sustaining Nutrition Interventions: Lessons Learned from Success in the Asia-Pacific Region* (Seattle, WA: National Bureau of Asian Research, 2008).

40 World Health Organization, *Global Nutrition Policy Review: What Does It Take to Scale Up Nutrition Action?* (Geneva, 2013).

41 P. Pinstrup-Andersen, ed., *The Political Economy of Food and Nutrition Policies* (Baltimore, MD: Johns Hopkins University Press, 1993).

42 J. O. Field, "Nutrition Planning to Nutrition Management," in *The Political Economy of Food and Nutrition Policies,* edited by P. Pinstrup-Andersen (Baltimore, MD: Johns Hopkins University Press, 1993).

43 S. R. Gillespie, J. B. Mason, and R. Martorell, *How Nutrition Improves,* ACC/SCN State-of-the-Art Series, Nutrition Policy Discussion Paper No. 15 (Geneva: UN Standing Committee on Nutrition, 1996).

44 E. Clay and B. Schaffer, eds., *Room for Manouevre: An Exploration of Public Policy in Agriculture and Rural Development* (London: Heinemann Education Books, 1984).

45 Gillespie, McLachlan, and Shrimpton, *Combating Malnutrition: Time to Act.*

46 R. Heaver, *Strengthening Country Commitment to Human Development: Lessons from Nutrition* (Washington, DC: World Bank, 2005).

47 World Bank, *Repositioning Nutrition as Central to Development.*

48 Scaling Up Nutrition (SUN) Movement, "About," http://scalingupnutrition.org/about.

49 Nutrition-sensitive interventions are those that "address the underlying determinants of fetal and child nutrition and development—food security; adequate caregiving resources at the maternal, household, and community levels; and access to health services and a safe and hygienic environment—and incorporate specific nutrition goals and actions"; see M. T. Ruel and H. Alderman, "Nutrition-Sensitive Interventions and Programmes: How Can They Help to Accelerate Progress in Improving Maternal and Child Nutrition?" *Lancet* 382, no. 9891 (2013): 536–551.

50 Enabling environments are defined as the "political and policy processes that build and sustain momentum for the effective implementation of actions that reduce undernutrition"; see S. Gillespie, L. Haddad, V. Mannar, P. Menon, and N. Nisbett, "The Politics of Reducing Malnutrition: Building Commitment and Accelerating Progress," *The Lancet* 382, no. 9891 (2013): 552–569.

51 T. Marchione, ed., *Scaling Up, Scaling Down: Overcoming Malnutrition in Developing Countries* (Amsterdam: Gordon and Breach Publishers, 1999).

52 Gillespie, Menon, and Kennedy, "Scaling Up Impact on Nutrition: What Will It Take?"

Chapter 2

1 S. Gillespie and J. B. Mason, *Nutrition-Relevant Actions: Some Experiences from the Eighties and Lessons for the Nineties,* United Nations Administrative Committee on Coordination-Subcommittee on Nutrition (Geneva: ACC/SCN, 1991); J. Jennings et al., *Managing Successful Nutrition Programmes,* ACC/SCN State-of-the-Art Series Nutrition Policy Discussion Paper no. 8 (Geneva: ACC/SCN, 1991); S. Gillespie, J. B. Mason, and R. Martorell. *How Nutrition Improves,* ACC/SCN State-of-the-Art Nutrition Policy Discussion Paper no. 15 (Geneva: ACC/SCN, 1996).

2 UNICEF, *Strategy for Improved Nutrition of Children and Women in Developing Countries* (New York: UNICEF, 1990).

3 O. Abosede and J. McGuire, *Improving Women's and Children's Nutrition in Sub-Saharan Africa: An Issues Paper. Policy, Research and External Affairs,* Working Paper WPS 723 (Washington, DC: Population and Human Resources Department, World Bank, 1991).

4 E. Kennedy, *Successful Nutrition Programs in Africa: What Makes Them Work?* Policy, Research and External Affairs Working Paper WPS 706 (Washington, DC: World Bank, 1991).

5 U. Jonsson, "Success Factors in Community-Based Nutrition-Oriented Programmes and Projects," in *Malnutrition in South Asia: A Regional Profile,* S. Gillespie, ed. (Kathmandu, Nepal: UNICEF, Regional Office for South Asia, 1997).

6 United Nations Administrative Committee on Coordination Sub-committee on Nutrition (ACC/SCN), "Effective Programmes in Africa for Improving Nutrition," *SCN News,* no. 15, www.unscn.org/layout/modules/resources/files/scnnews15.pdf.

7 L. H. Allen and S.R. Gillespie, *What Works? A Review of the Efficacy and Effectiveness of Nutrition Interventions* (Manila: United Nations and the Asian Development Bank, 2001).

8 L. Iannotti and S.R. Gillespie, *Community-Driven Nutrition Programming: Lessons Learned from Sub-Saharan Africa* (Geneva: USAID/LINKAGES and UNICEF, 2002).

9 S. R. Gillespie, M. McLachlan, and R. Shrimpton, eds., *Combating Malnutrition: Time to Act* (Washington, DC: World Bank–UNICEF, 2003).

10 B. Ljungqvist and U. Jonsson, "Nutrition Governance: Iringa Nutrition Program Re-Visited," Statement to the Panel on Nutrition Governance, 3rd Federation of African Nutrition Societies (FANUS) African Nutrition Conference, Arusha City, Tanzania, May 24–29, 2015.

11 UNICEF, *Strategy for Improved Nutrition of Children and Women in Developing Countries.*

12 C. Dolan and J. Levinson, "Country Perspectives: Tanzania," in *Combating Malnutrition: Time to Act,* S. Gillespie, M. McLachlan and R. Shrimpton, eds. (Washington, DC: World Bank–UNICEF, 2003).

13 Government of the United Republic of Tanzania, WHO, and UNICEF, *The Joint WHO/UNICEF Nutrition Support Programme in Iringa, Tanzania. 1983–88 Evaluation Report* (Dare Salaam, Tanzania: Government of the United Republic of Tanzania, 1988); F. Kavishe, "Nutrition Relevant Actions in Tanzania," United Nations Administrative Committee on Coordination/Sub-Committee on Nutrition (ACC/SCN) Country Case Study (Geneva: ACC/SCN, 1993); U. Jonsson, B. Ljungqvist, and O. Yambi, "Mobilization for Nutrition in Tanzania," in *Reaching Health for All,* J. Rohde, M. Chatterjee, and D. Morley, eds. (Delhi, India: Oxford University Press, 1993).

14 Jonsson et al., "Mobilization for Nutrition in Tanzania."

15 Ljungqvist and Jonsson, "Nutrition Governance: Iringa Nutrition Program Re-Visited."

16 Dolan and Levinson, "Country Perspectives: Tanzania."

17 Gillespie et al., *Combating Malnutrition: Time to Act.*

18 M. Gragnolati, C. Bredenkamp, M. Das Gupta, Y.-K. Lee, and M. Shekar, "ICDS and Persistent Undernutrition: Strategies to Enhance the Impact," *Economic and Political Weekly* 41, no. 12 (2006): 1193–1201.

19 Ibid.

20 A. Gupta, "Governing Population: The Integrated Child Development Services Program in India," in *States of Imagination: Ethnographic Explorations of the Postcolonial State (Politics, History, and Culture),* T. H. Blom and F. Stepputat, eds. (Durham, NC: Duke University Press, 2001).

21 M. Gragnolati et al., *India's Undernourished Children: A Call for Reform and Action,* HNP Discussion Paper series (Washington, DC: World Bank, 2005).

22 M. Shekar, *The Tamil Nadu Integrated Nutrition Project: A Review of the Project with Special Emphasis on the Monitoring and Information System,* Cornell Food and Nutrition Policy Program Working Paper no. 14 (Ithaca, NY: Cornell University Press, 1991).

23 S. Gillespie and A. Measham for the World Bank, *Implementation Completion Report for the Second Tamil Nadu Integrated Nutrition Project,* Report no. 17755 (New Delhi: World Bank, 1998).

24 L. Haddad et al., "Maharashtra's Child Stunting Declines: What Is Driving Them? Findings of a Multidisciplinary Analysis" (Brighton, UK: Institute of Development Studies, 2014).

25 UNICEF, *Strategy for Improved Nutrition of Children and Women in Developing Countries.*

26 Jennings et al., *Managing Successful Nutrition Programmes.*

27 D. Headey et al., "The Other Asian Enigma: Explaining the Rapid Reduction of Undernutrition in Bangladesh," *World Development* no. 66 (2015): 749–761.

28 TANGO (Technical Assistance to NGOs) International, CARE Bangladesh, and USAID, *SHOUHARDO 1st Phase Final Evaluation Report* (Tucson, Arizona: TANGO, 2009).

29 L. C. Smith et al., "Admissible Evidence in the Court of Development Evaluation? The Impact of CARE's SHOUHARDO Project on Child Stunting in Bangladesh," *World Development* no. 41 (2013): 196–216.

30 Ibid.

31 TANGO International et al., *SHOUHARDO 1st Phase Final Evaluation Report.*

32 Ibid.

33 Smith et al., "Admissible Evidence in the Court of Development Evaluation?"

34 TANGO International et al., *SHOUHARDO 1st Phase Final Evaluation Report.*

35 Ibid.

36 Smith et al., "Admissible Evidence in the Court of Development Evaluation?"

37 TANGO International et al., *SHOUHARDO 1st Phase Final Evaluation Report.*

38 Smith et al., "Admissible Evidence in the Court of Development Evaluation?"

39 TANGO International, CARE Bangladesh, and USAID, *CARE Bangladesh Mid-Term Review of SHOUHARDO II Multi-Year Assistance Program, Volume I – Main Report* (March 7, 2013), http://pdf.usaid.gov/pdf_docs/pdacx325.pdf.

40 L.C. Smith, *Quantitative Impact Evaluation of the SHOUHARDO II Project in Bangladesh,* commissioned by CARE Bangladesh (Tucson, AZ, USA: TANGO International, Inc., 2015).

41 TANGO International et al., *CARE Bangladesh Mid-Term Review of SHOUHARDO II Multi-year Assistance Program.*

42 S. R. Gillespie, *Scaling Up Community Driven Development: A Synthesis of Experience,* IFPRI Discussion Paper no. 181 (Washington, DC: IFPRI, 2004); H. Binswanger and S. Aiyar, "Scaling Up Community-Driven Development: Theoretical Underpinnings and Program Design Implications," Policy Research Working Paper no. 3039 (Washington, DC: World Bank, 2004).

43 J. Leavy et al., "What Matters Most? Evidence from 84 Participatory Studies with Those Living with Extreme

Poverty and Marginalization," *Participate* (Brighton, UK: IDS, 2013); G. Mansuri and V. Rao, "Localizing Development: Does Participation Work?" Policy Research Report (Washington, DC: World Bank, 2013); N. Nisbett et al., "Why Worry About the Politics of Childhood Undernutrition?" *World Development* 64 (2014): 420–433.

44 A. Joshi, "Do They Work? Assessing the Impact of Transparency and Accountability Initiatives in Service Delivery," *Development Policy Review* 31 (2013): 29–48.

45 Nisbett et al., "Why Worry About the Politics of Childhood Undernutrition?"

46 M. Bjorkman and J. Svensson, "Power to the People: Evidence from a Randomized Field Experiment on Community-Based Monitoring in Uganda," *Quarterly Journal of Economics* 124, no. 2 (2009): 735–769.

47 Stuart Gillespie et al., "Maternal and Child Nutrition 4: The Politics of Reducing Malnutrition: Building Commitment," *The Lancet* 382, no. 9891 (2013): 552–569, doi:10.1016/S0140-6736(13)60842-9.

Chapter 3

1 C. G. Victora, M. de Onis, P. C. Hallal, M. Blössner, and R. Shrimpton, "Worldwide Timing of Growth Faltering: Revisiting Implications for Interventions," *Pediatrics* 125, no. 3 (2010): e473–480; A. M. Prentice, K. A. Ward, G. R. Goldberg, L. M. Jarjou, S. E. Moore, A. J. Fulford, and A. Prentice, "Critical Windows for Nutritional Interventions against Stunting," *American Journal of Clinical Nutrition* 97, no. 5 (2013): 911–918.

2 C. G. Victora, L. Adair, C. Fall, P. C. Hallal, R. Martorell, L. Richter, and H. S. Sachdev, "Maternal and Child Undernutrition: Consequences for Adult Health and Human Capital," *The Lancet* 371, no. 9609 (2008): 340–357, doi:10.1016/S0140-6736(07)61692-4.

3 World Health Organization, *Global Strategy for Infant and Young Child Feeding* (Geneva: 2003).

4 C. G. Victora, R. Bahl, A. J. D. Barros, G. V. A. França, S. Horton, J. Krasevec, S. Murch, M. J. Sankar, N. Walker, and N. C. Rollins, "Breastfeeding in the 21st Century: Epidemiology, Mechanisms, and Lifelong Effect," *The Lancet* 387, 10017 (2016): 475–490, doi:10.1016/S0140-6736(15)01024-7.

5 Ibid.

6 Ibid.

7 N. C. Rollins, N. Bhandari, N. Hajeebhoy, S. Horton, C. K. Lutter, J. C. Martines, E. G. Piwoz, L. M. Richter, and C. G. Victora, "Why Invest, and What It Will Take to Improve Breastfeeding Practices?" *The Lancet* 387, 10017 (2016): 491–504, doi:10.1016/S0140-6736(15)01044-2.

8 Z. A. Bhutta, J. K. Das, A. Rizvi, M. F. Gaffey, N. Walker, S. Horton, P. Webb, A. Lartey, and R. E. Black, "Evidence-Based Interventions for Improvement of Maternal and Child Nutrition: What Can Be Done and at What Cost?" *The Lancet* 382, no. 9890 (2013): 452–477, doi:10.1016/S0140-6736(13)60996-4.

9 Victora et al., "Worldwide Timing of Growth Faltering."

10 World Health Organization (WHO), *Community-based Strategies for Breastfeeding Promotion and Support in Developing Countries* (Geneva: 2003).

11 M. Muller, *The Baby Killer: A War on Want Investigation into the Promotion and Sale of Powdered Baby Milks in the Third World* (London: War on Want, 1974).

12 WHO, *International Code of Marketing of Breast-milk Substitutes* (Geneva: 1981).

13 *Innocenti Declaration on the Protection, Promotion, and Support of Breastfeeding,* adopted by the WHO/UNICEF policy makers' meeting on Breastfeeding in the 1990s, Global Initiative at Spedale degli Innocenti, Florence, Italy, July 30–August 1, 1990.

14 UNICEF/WHO, *The Baby Friendly Hospital Initiative,* accessed February 10, 2016, http://www.unicef.org/programme/breastfeeding/baby.htm.

15 WHO, *Global Strategy for Infant and Young Child Feeding* (Geneva: 2003).

16 WHO, *International Code of Marketing of Breast-milk Substitutes;* Access to Nutrition Foundation, Access to Nutrition Index: Global Index 2016, accessed January 14, 2016, https://www.accesstonutrition.org/sites/2015.

17 E. G. Piwoz and S. L. Huffman, "The Impact of Marketing of Breast-Milk Substitutes on WHO-Recommended Breastfeeding Practices," *Food and Nutrition Bulletin* 36, no. 4 (2015): 373–386, doi:10.1177/0379572115602174; A. McFadden, F. Mason, J. Baker, F. Begin, F. Dykes, L. Grummer-Strawn, N. Kenney-Muir, H. Whitford, E. Zehner, and M. J. Renfrew, "Spotlight on Infant Formula: Coordinated Global Action Needed," *The Lancet* 387, no. 10017 (2016): 413–415, doi:10.1016/S0140-6736(16)00103-3.

18 WHO, *Country Implementation of the International Code of Marketing of Breast-milk Substitutes: Status Report 2011* (Geneva: 2011).

19 Rollins et al., "Why Invest, and What It Will Take to Improve Breastfeeding Practices?"

20 Ibid.

21 Pan American Health Organization and WHO, *Guiding Principles for Complementary Feeding of the Breastfed Child* (Washington, DC: PAHO, 2003).

22 WHO, *Guiding Principles for Feeding of Non-breastfed Children* (Geneva: 2005).

23 C. K. Lutter, L. Iannotti, H. Creed-Kanashiro, A. Guyon, B. Daelmans, R. Robert, and R. Haider, "Key Principles to Improve Programmes and Interventions in Complementary Feeding," *Maternal and Child Nutrition* 9 (2013): 101–115. doi:10.1111/mcn.12087.

24 UNICEF, *Improving Child Nutrition: The Achievable Imperative for Global Progress* (New York: 2013); Lutter et al., "Key Principles to Improve Programmes and Interventions in Complementary Feeding."

25 Victora et al., "Breastfeeding in the 21st Century."

26 Ibid.

27 International Food Policy Research Institute (IFPRI), *Global Nutrition Report 2014: Actions and Accountabilities to Accelerate the World's Progress on Nutrition* (Washington, DC: 2013).

28 WHO, WHA *Global Nutrition Targets 2025: Breastfeeding Policy Brief* (Geneva: n.d.).

29 IFPRI, *Global Nutrition Report 2014.*

30 S. Haroon, Sarah, J. K. Das, R. A. Salam, A. Imdad, and Z. A. Bhutta, "Breastfeeding Promotion Interventions and Breastfeeding Practices: A Systematic Review," *BMC Public Health* 13, no. 3 (2013): 1–18, doi:10.1186/1471-2458-13-S3-S20.

31 Rollins et al., "Why Invest, and What It Will Take to Improve Breastfeeding Practices?"

32 Ibid.

33 R. M. Ferreira, "A Review of Breastfeeding in Brazil and How the Country has Reached Ten Months' Breastfeeding Duration," *Cadernos de Saúde Pública* 19, supplement 1 (2003): S37–S45, http://dx.doi.org/10.1590/S0102-311X2003000700005; C. G. Victora, E. M. L. Aquino, M. do Carmo Leal, C. A. Monteiro, F. C. Barros, and C. L. Szwarcwald, "Maternal and Child Health in Brazil: Progress and Challenges," *The Lancet* 377, no. 9780 (2016): 1863–1876, doi:10.1016/S0140-6736(11)60138-4.

34 IFPRI, *Global Nutrition Report 2014.*

35 Victora et al., "Maternal and Child Health in Brazil: Progress and Challenges."

36 R. Pérez-Escamilla, L. Curry, D. Minhas, L. Taylor, and E. Bradley, "Scaling up of Breastfeeding Promotion Programs in Low-and Middle-Income Countries: The 'Breastfeeding Gear' Model," *Advances in Nutrition* 3, no. 6 (2012): 790–800.

37 Ibid.

38 Ibid; Ferreira, "A Review of Breastfeeding in Brazil and How the Country Has Reached Ten Months' Breastfeeding Duration."

39 C. K. Lutter and A. L. Morrow, "Protection, Promotion, and Support and Global Trends in Breastfeeding," *Advances in Nutrition* 4, no. 2 (2013): 213–219.

40 Ibid.

41 Bangladesh Demographic and Health Survey (DHS) 2004, accessed February 17, 2016, http://dhsprogram.com/pubs/pdf/fr165/fr-bd04[fr165].pdf; Bangladesh DHS 2007, accessed February 17, 2016, http://dhsprogram.com/pubs/pdf/FR207/FR207%5BApril-10-2009%5D.pdf.

42 UNICEF and Academy for Educational Development, *Infant and Young Child Feeding Programme Review: Consolidated Report of Six-Country Review of Breastfeeding Programmes* (New York: UNICEF, 2010), www.unicef.org/nutrition/files/IYCF_Booklet_April_2010_Web.pdf, accessed February 16, 2016.

43 Ibid.

44 Pérez-Escamilla et al., "Scaling up of Breastfeeding Promotion Programs in Low-and Middle-Income Countries."

45 WHO, *WHA Global Nutrition Targets 2025: Breastfeeding Policy Brief.*

46 Z. A. Bhutta, J. K. Das, A. Rizvi, M. F. Gaffey, N. Walker, S. Horton, P. Webb, A. Lartey, and R. E. Black, "Evidence-Based Interventions for Improvement of Maternal and Child Nutrition: What Can Be Done and at What Cost?" *The Lancet* 382, 9890 (2013): 452–477, doi:10.1016/S0140-6736(13)60996-4.

47 WHO, Complementary Feeding, accessed February 1, 2016, bit.ly/1IvoVCj.

48 Victora et al., "Worldwide Timing of Growth Faltering."

49 WHO, *Complementary Feeding: Report of Global Consultation, Geneva, 10-13 December 2001: Summary of Guiding Principles* (Geneva, 2002), accessed January 29, 2016, bit.ly/1DP5RJL.

50 K. G. Dewey, and S. Adu-Afarwuah, "Systematic Review of the Efficacy and Effectiveness of Complementary Feeding Interventions in Developing Countries," *Maternal and Child Nutrition* 4 (2008), doi:10.1111/j.1740-8709.2007.00124.x.

51 C. P. Stewart, L. Iannotti, K. G. Dewey, K. F. Michaelsen, A. W. Onyango, Contextualising Complementary Feeding in a Broader Framework for Stunting Prevention," *Maternal and Child Nutrition* Supplement 2 (2013): 27.

52 WHO, "Indicators for Assessing Infant and Young Child Feeding Practices. Part I: Definitions. Conclusions of a Consensus Meeting Held 6–8 November 2007 in Washington, DC, USA" (Geneva, 2008).

53 Ibid.

54 L. Haddad, N. Nisbett, I. Barnett, and E. Valli, *Maharashtra's Child Stunting Declines: What Is Driving Them? Findings of a Multidisciplinary Analysis* (Brighton: IDS and UNICEF, 2014).

55 Ibid.

56 Dewey and Adu-Afarwuah, "Systematic Review of the Efficacy and Effectiveness of Complementary Feeding Interventions in Developing Countries"; Pan American Health Organization and WHO, *Guiding Principles for Complementary Feeding of the Breastfed Child.*

57 D. Olney, K. Abdoulaye Pedehombga, M. T. Ruel, and A. Dillon, "A 2-Year Integrated Agriculture and Nutrition and Health Behavior Change Communication Program Targeted to Women in Burkina Faso Reduces Anemia, Wasting, and Diarrhea in Children 3–12.9 Months of Age at Baseline: A Cluster-Randomized Controlled Trial," *Journal of Nutrition* 145, no. 6 (2015): 1317–1324, doi:10.3945/jn.114.203539.

58 J. Baker, T. Sanghvi, N. Hajeebhoy, L. Martin, and K. Lapping, "Using an Evidence-Based Approach to Design Large-Scale Programs to Improve Infant and Young Child Feeding," *Food and Nutrition Bulletin* 34, Supplement 3 (2013): S146–S155.

59 Alive & Thrive, "Country Brief: Alive & Thrive's program approach and results in Ethiopia, July 2009 to May 2014," accessed January 20, 2016, http://aliveandthrive.org/resources/country-brief-alive-thrives-program-approach-and-results-in-ethiopia-july-2009-to-may-2014/.

60 Ibid.

Chapter 4

1 L. Allen, B. de Benoist, O. Dary, and R. Hurrell, *Guidelines on Food Fortification with Micronutrients* (Geneva: World Health Organization, 2006).

2 J. C. Sherwin, M. H. Reacher, W. H. Dean, and J. Ngondi, "Epidemiology of Vitamin A Deficiency and Xerophthalmia in At-risk Populations," *Transactions of the Royal Society of Tropical Medicine and Hygiene* 106, no. 4 (2012): 205–214.

3 M. B. Zimmermann, P. L. Jooste, and C. S. Pandav, "Iodine-deficiency Disorders," *Lancet* 372, no. 9645 (2008): 1251–1262.

4 R. E. Black, L. H. Allen, Z. A. Bhutta, L. E. Caulfield, M. de Onis, M. Ezzati, C. Mathers, and J. Rivera for the Maternal and Child Undernutrition Study Group, "Maternal and Child Undernutrition: Global and Regional Exposures and Health Consequences," *The Lancet* 371, no. 9608 (2008): 243–260.

5 H. Biesalski, "Quality Comes with a Price Tag: The Deadly Triangle of Hunger, Economics, and Child Development," in *Hidden Hunger,* English ed. translated by Patrick O'Mealy (Heidelberg, Germany: Springer Verlag, 2012).

6 J. Hoddinott, M. Rosegrant, and M. Torero, "Investments to Reduce Hunger and Undernutrition," paper prepared for the 2012 Global Copenhagen Consensus.

7 Allen et al., *Guidelines on Food Fortification with Micronutrients.*

8 Biesalski, "Quality Comes with a Price Tag."

9 A. Timmer, "Iodine Nutrition and Universal Salt Iodization: A Landscape Analysis in 2012," *IDD Newsletter* (International Council for Control of Iodine Deficiency Disorders) 40, no. 4 (2012): 5–9.

10 L. Laviolette and V. Mannar, "Scaling Up and Sustaining Nutrition Interventions: Lessons Learned from Success in the Asia-Pacific Region," White Paper (Seattle: National Bureau of Asian Research, 2008).

11 Z. P. Chen, "Sustained Elimination of IDD in China: An Update," *IDD Newsletter* (International Council for Control of Iodine Deficiency Disorders) 24, no. 3 (2006): 6–14.

12 Z. Chen, Z. Dong, and J. Lin, "Achieving and Sustaining USI: Effective Programme Development and Management: Lessons Learned from USI in China," *SCN News* 35 (2007): 33–37.

13 M. Qian, D. Wang, W. E. Watkins, V. Gebski, Y. Q. Yan, M. Li, and Z. P. Chen, "The Effects of Iodine on Intelligence in Children: A Meta-Analysis of Studies Conducted in China," *Asia Pacific Journal of Clinical Nutrition* 14, no. 1 (2005): 32–42.

14 R. Yip, Z. Chen, and J. Ling, "China Country Report" in *Towards the Global Elimination of Brain Damage due to Iodine Deficiency,* edited by B. S. Hetzel (New Delhi: Oxford University Press, 2005).

15 Chen, "Sustained Elimination of IDD in China: An Update."

16 Yip, Chen, and Ling, "China Country Report."

17 Ibid.

18 Chen, "Sustained Elimination of IDD in China: An Update."

19 K. Codling, Z. Chen, S. Hongmei et al., "China: Leading the Way in Sustained IDD Elimination," *IDD Newsletter* 42, no. 2 (2014): 2–5.

20 UNICEF, "Sustaining Universal Salt Iodization – China (2002)," www.unicef.org/evaluation/files/china2002saltiodization.doc, accessed October 23, 2015.

21 Z. Chen, "New Cretins Discovered in Southern Xinjiang, China," *IDD Newsletter* 23, no. 11 (2007): 18.

22 Y. Wu, X. Li, S. Chang, L. Liu, S. Zou, and D. B. Hipgrave, "Variable Iodine Intake Persists in the Context of Universal Salt Iodization in China," *Journal of Nutrition* 142, no. 9 (2012): 1728–1734.

23 Ibid.

24 Chen, "New Cretins Discovered in Southern Xinjiang, China."

25 Codling et al., "China: Leading the Way in Sustained IDD Elimination."

26 S. Li, Q. Zheng, J. Xu, J. Gorstein, and H. Wang, "Iodine Excess or Not: Analysis on the Necessity of Reducing the Iodine Content in Edible Salt Based on the National

Monitoring Results," *Asia Pacific Journal of Clinical Nutrition* 20, no. 4 (2011): 501–506.

27 Codling et al., "China: Leading the Way in Sustained IDD Elimination."

28 Timmer, "Iodine Nutrition and Universal Salt Iodization."

29 M. Andersson, V. Karumbunathan, and M. B. Zimmermann, "Global Iodine Status in 2011 and Trends over the Past Decade," *Journal of Nutrition* 142, no. 4 (2012): 744–750.

30 Timmer, "Iodine Nutrition and Universal Salt Iodization."

31 F. Ahmed and I. Darnton-Hill, "Vitamin A Deficiency," in *Public Health Nutrition,* edited by M. Gibney, B. M. Margetts, J. Kearney, and L. Arab (Oxford: Blackwell Science, 2010): 192–215.

32 N. Dalmiya, A. Palmer, I. Darnton-Hill, "Sustaining Vitamin A Supplementation Requires a New Vision." Lanc*et 368,* no. 9541 (2006): 1052–1054.

33 R. Klemm, P. Harvey, E. Wainwright, S. Faillace, and E. Wasantwisut, Scal*ing Up Micronutrient Programs: What Works and What Needs More Work?, A R*eport of the Innocenti Process (Washington, DC: Micronutrient Forum, 2009).

34 UNICEF Global Databases, Nutrition: Vitamin A Supplementation, http://data.unicef.org/nutrition/vitamin-a.html, accessed October 23, 2014.

35 UNICEF, *Tracking Progress on Child and Maternal Nutrition: A Survival and Development Priority* (New York: 2009).

36 UNICEF, *Tracking Progress on Child and Maternal Nutrition: A Survival and Development Priority;* J. H. Rah, R. Houston, B. D. Mohapatra, S. S. Kumar, F. Saiyed, S. Bhattacharjee, and V. M. Aguayo, "A Review of the Vitamin A Supplementation Program in India: Reasons for Success in the States of Bihar and Odisha," *Food and Nutrition Bulletin* 35, no. 2 (2014): 203–210.

37 M. Latham, "The Great Vitamin A Fiasco," Worl*d Nutrition 1,* no. 1 (2010): 12–45; J. B. Mason, T. Grenier, R. Shrimpton, D. Sanders, and J. Yukich, "Development. Malnutrition. Vitamin A. Let Food Be Our Medicine," *World Nutrition* 5, no. 11 (2014): 940–952.

38 Mason et al., "Development. Malnutrition. Vitamin A. Let Food Be Our Medicine."

39 S. Awasthi, R. Peto, S. Read, S. Clark, V. Pande, and D. Bundy, "Vitamin A Supplementation Every 6 Months with Retinol in 1 Million Pre-School Children in North India: DEVTA, A Cluster-Randomised Trial," *Lancet* 381, no. 9876 (2013): 1469–1477.

40 A. Imdad, K. Herzer, E. Mayo-Wilson, M. Y. Yakoob, Z. A. Bhutta, "Vitamin A Supplementation for Preventing Morbidity and Mortality in Children from 6 Months to 5 Years of Age," *Cochrane Database of Systematic Reviews* no. 12 (2010), doi:10.1002/14651858.CD008524.pub2.

41 C. S. Benn, P. Aaby, R. Arts, K. Jensen, M. Netea, and A. B. Fisker, "An Enigma: Why Vitamin A Supplementation Does Not Always Reduce Mortality Even Though Vitamin A Deficiency Is Associated with Increased Mortality," *International Journal of Epidemiology* 44, no. 3 (2015): 906–918.

42 N. W. Solomons, "Will Universal Periodic Vitamin A Supplementation Ever Reach Retirement Age?" *Food and Nutrition Bulletin* 35, no. 2 (2014): 200–202.

43 I. SaeterdalI, J. O. Mora, and L. M. De-Regil, "Fortification of Staple Foods with Vitamin A for Preventing Vitamin A Deficiency," *Cochrane Database of Systematic Reviews* no. 9 (2012), doi:10.1002/14651858.CD010068.

44 J. L. Fiedler and K. Lividini, "Managing the Vitamin A Program Portfolio: A Case Study of Zambia, 2013–2042," *Food and Nutrition Bulletin* 35, no. 1 (2014): 105–125.

45 B. de Benoist, E. McLean, I. Egli, and M. Cogswell, eds., *Worldwide Prevalence of Anaemia 1993–2005* (Geneva: World Health Organization, 2008).

46 R. J. Stoltzfus, R. Heidkamp, D. Kenkel, and J.-P. Habicht, "Iron Supplementation of Young Children: Learning from the New Evidence," *Food and Nutrition Bulletin* 28, no. 4 (supplement) (2007): S572–S584.

47 R. Galloway and J. McGuire, "Determinants of Compliance with Iron Supplementation: Supplies, Side Effects, or Psychology," *Social Science and Medicine* 39, no. 3 (1994): 381–390.

48 K. Bahl, E. Toro, C. Qureshi, and P. Shaw, *Nutrition for a Better Tomorrow: Scaling Up Delivery of Micronutrient Powders for Infants and Young Children* (Washington, DC: Results for Development Institute, 2013).

49 L. M. De-Regil, P. S. Suchdev, G. E. Vist, S. Walleser, and J. P. Peña-Rosas, "Home Fortification of Foods with Multiple Micronutrient Powders for Health and Nutrition in Children under Two Years of Age (Review)," *Evidence-Based Child Health* 8, no. 1 (2013): 112–201.

50 World Health Organization, *Guideline: Use of Multiple Micronutrient Powders for Home Fortification of Foods Consumed by Infants and Children 6–23 Months of Age* (Geneva, 2011).

51 World Vision, "Sprinkles: The Promise of Micronutrients to Change Children's Lives," *Impact* (Mississauga, Ontario, Canada, 2013).

52 K. G. Dewey, Z. Yang, and E. Boy, "Systematic Review and Meta-Analysis of Home Fortification of Complementary Foods," *Maternal and Child Nutrition* 5, no. 4 (2009): 283–321.

53 World Vision, "Sprinkles: The Promise of Micronutrients to Change Children's Lives."

54 Dewey, Yang, and Boy, "Systematic Review and Meta-Analysis of Home Fortification of Complementary Foods."

55 C. MacDonald and S. Altengeral, "National Scale-up of Micronutrient Powders in Mongolian Integrated Program: Innovations in Micronutrient Powder Programs: Opportunities to Reduce Child Anemia," presentation at IYCN Satellite Meeting, June 13, 2011, http://iycn.wpengine.netdna-cdn.com/files/FINALSprinklesGHCJun2011_v5061511.pdf.

56 World Vision, "Sprinkles: The Promise of Micronutrients to Change Children's Lives."

57 UNICEF, *Tracking Progress on Child and Maternal Nutrition.*

58 World Vision, "Sprinkles: The Promise of Micronutrients to Change Children's Lives."

59 MacDonald and Altengeral, "National Scale-up of Micronutrient Powders in Mongolian Integrated Program."

60 De-Regil et al., "Home Fortification of Foods with Multiple Micronutrient Powders."

61 S. Horton, M. Shekar, C. McDonald, A. Mahal, and J. K. Brooks, *Scaling Up Nutrition: What Will It Cost?* (Washington, DC: World Bank, 2010).

62 M. E. Jefferds, L. Irizarry, A. Timmer, and K. Tripp, "UNICEF–CDC Global Assessment of Home Fortification Interventions 2011: Current Status, New Directions, and Implications for Policy and Programmatic Guidance," *Food and Nutrition Bulletin* 34, no. 4 (2013): 434–443.

63 Bahl et al., *Nutrition for a Better Tomorrow.*

64 Jefferds et al., "UNICEF–CDC Global Assessment of Home Fortification Interventions 2011."

Chapter 5

1 WHO/UNICEF/WFP, *Global Nutrition Targets 2025: Wasting Policy Brief,* WHO Policy Brief 14.8 (Geneva: World Health Organization, 2014).

2 R. E. Black, L. H. Allen, Z. A. Bhutta, L. E. Caulfield, M. de Onis, M. Ezzati, C. Mathers, and J. Rivera for the Maternal and Child Undernutrition Study Group, "Maternal and Child Undernutrition: Global and Regional Exposures and Health Consequences," *The Lancet* 371, no. 9608 (2008): 243–260.

3 C. M. McDonald, I. Olofin, S. Flaxman, W. W. Fawzi, D. Spiegelman, L. E. Caulfield, et al., "The Effect of Multiple Anthropometric Deficits on Child Mortality: Meta-Analysis of Individual Data in 10 Prospective Studies from Developing Countries." *American Journal of Clinical Nutrition 97,* no. 4 (2013): 896–901.

4 R. E. Black, C. G. Victora, S. P. Walker, Z. A. Bhutta, P. Christian, M. de Onis, et al., "Maternal and Child Undernutrition and Overweight in Low-Income and Middle-Income Countries," *The Lancet* 382, no. 9890 (2013): 427–451.

5 R. Uauy, J.-F. Desjeux, T. Ahmed, M. Hossain, D. Brewster, D. Forbes, et al., "Global Efforts to Address Severe Acute Malnutrition," *Journal of Pediatric Gastroenterology and Nutrition* 55, no. 5 (2012): 476–481.

6 WHO/UNICEF/WFP, *Global Nutrition Targets 2025: Wasting Policy Brief.*

7 A. Briend, C. Prudhon, Z. W. Prinzo, B. Dealmans, and J. B. Mason, "Foreword: Putting Back the Management of Severe Malnutrition on the International Health Agenda," *WHO, UNICEF, and SCN Informal Consultation on Community-Based Management of Severe Malnutrition in Children,* SCN Nutrition Policy Paper No. 21 (Geneva: UN Standing Committee on Nutrition, 2006).

8 UNICEF, CMN (Coverage Monitoring Network), and ACF International, *The State of Global SAM Management Coverage 2012* (New York: UNICEF; London: ACF International, 2013.)

9 R. Uauy et al., "Global Efforts to Address Severe Acute Malnutrition"; S. Guerrero and E. Rogers, *Is Community-Based Treatment of Severe Acute Malnutrition (SAM) at Scale Capable of Meeting Global Needs?* Access for All, Volume 1 (London: Coverage Monitoring Network, 2013.)

10 Z. A. Bhutta, J. K. Das, A. Rizvi, M. F. Gaffey, N. Walker, S. Horton, P. Webb, et al., "Evidence-Based Interventions for Improvement of Maternal and Child Nutrition: What Can Be Done and at What Cost?" *The Lancet* 382, no. 9890 (2013): 452–477.

11 C. Schofield and A. Ashworth, "Why Have Mortality Rates for Severe Malnutrition Remained So High?" *Bulletin of the World Health Organization* 74, no. 2 (1996): 223–229.

12 E. Rogers, M. Myatt, S. Woodhead, S. Guerrero, and J. L. Alvarez, "Coverage of Community-Based Management of Severe Acute Malnutrition Programmes in Twenty-One Countries, 2012–2013," *PLoS One (Public Library of Science)* 10, no. 6 (2015).

13 Guerrero and Rogers, *Is Community-Based Treatment of Severe Acute Malnutrition (SAM) at Scale Capable of Meeting Global Needs?;* W. V. Damme and M. Boelaert, "Therapeutic Feeding Centres for Severe Malnutrition," *The Lancet* 59 (2002): 260–261.

14 S. Collins, N. Dent, P. Binns, P. Bahwere, K. Sadler, and A. Hallam, "Management of Severe Acute Malnutrition in Children," *The Lancet* 368 (2006): 1992–2000.

15 A. Briend and S. Collins, "Therapeutic Nutrition for Children with Severe Acute Malnutrition: Summary of African Experience," *Indian Pedriatrics* 47, no. 8 (2010): 655–659.

16 WHO/UNICEF, *WHO Child Growth Standards and the Identification of Severe Acute Malnutrition in Infants and Children: A Joint Statement by the World Health Organization and the United Nations Children's Fund,* WHO/UNICEF Joint Statement (Geneva: WHO/UNICEF, 2005).

17 WHO/UNICEF/WFP, *Global Nutrition Targets 2025: Wasting Policy Brief.*

18 WHO/UNICEF, *WHO Child Growth Standards and the Identification of Severe Acute Malnutrition in Infants and Children.*

19 H. Deconinck, A. Swindale, and C. Navarro-Colorado, *Review of Community-Based Management of Acute Malnutrition (CMAM) in the Post-emergency Context: Synthesis of Lessons on Integration of CMAM into National Health Systems* (Washington, DC: U.S. Agency for International Development, 2008); S. Collins and K. Sadler, "Outpatient Care for Severely Malnourished Children in Emergency Relief Programmes: A Retrospective Cohort Study," *The Lancet* 360 (2002): 1824–1830.

20 C. Dolan, T. Khara, A. M. Acosta, and J. Shoham, "Government Experiences of Scale-up of Community-based Management of Acute Malnutrition (CMAM): A Synthesis of Lessons" (Oxford, UK: Emergency Nutrition Network, 2012), http://files.ennonline.net/attachments/1374/cmam-conference-2012-synthesis.pdf, accessed December 15, 2015.

21 Ibid.

22 UNICEF, *Improving Child Nutrition: The Achievable Imperative for Global Progress* (New York, 2013). Note that CMAM was previously known as community-based therapeutic care, or CTC, and in some countries is currently called integrated management of acute malnutrition, or IMAM.

23 The Sphere Project, "Humanitarian Charter and Minimum Standards in Humanitarian Response," http://www.spherehandbook.org/en/how-to-use-this-chapter-3/, accessed January 8, 2016.

24 Collins et al., "Management of Severe Acute Malnutrition in Children."

25 UNICEF, *Improving Child Nutrition: The Achievable Imperative for Global Progress* (New York, 2013).

26 Dolan et al., "Government Experiences of Scale-up of Community-based Management of Acute Malnutrition (CMAM)."

27 ACF International, *SAM 2020: An Agenda for Scaling-up the Management of Severe Acute Malnutrition by 2020,* edited by S. Guerrero (London, 2015).

28 Guerrero and Rogers, *Is Community-Based Treatment of Severe Acute Malnutrition (SAM) at Scale Capable of Meeting Global Needs?*

29 UNICEF, *Improving Child Nutrition: The Achievable Imperative for Global Progress.*

30 WHO/UNICEF/WFP, *Global Nutrition Targets 2025: Wasting Policy Brief.*

31 V. M. Aguayo and K. Paintal, *Addressing Maternal and Child Undernutrition in Low-Income and Middle-Income Countries,* UNICEF South Asia Office Review of Interventions (Kathmandu: UNICEF, 2014).

32 International Food Policy Research Institute, *Global Nutrition Report 2014: Actions and Accountability to Accelerate the World's Progress on Nutrition* (Washington, DC, 2014).

33 Dolan et al., "Government Experiences of Scale-up of Community-based Management of Acute Malnutrition (CMAM)."

34 S. Kathumba, "Creating an Enabling Policy Environment for Effective CMAM Implementation in Malawi," Field Exchange 43, www.ennonline.net/fex/43/creating, accessed March 7, 2016.

35 Dolan et al., "Government Experiences of Scale-up of Community-based Management of Acute Malnutrition (CMAM)."

36 K. Maleta and B. Amadi, "Community-Based Management of Acute Malnutrition (CMAM) in Sub-Saharan Africa: Case Studies from Ghana, Malawi, and Zambia," *Food and Nutrition Bulletin* 35, no. 2 supplement (2014): S34–S38.

37 UNICEF, *Tracking Progress on Child and Maternal Nutrition: A Survival and Development Priority* (Geneva, 2009).

38 Concern Worldwide, *Concern Worldwide's Learning from 15 Years of Community Management of Acute Malnutrition Programming* (Dublin, 2015).

39 Maleta and Amadi, "Community-Based Management of Acute Malnutrition (CMAM) in Sub-Saharan Africa."

40 International Food Policy Research Institute, *Global Nutrition Report 2014, Malawi Nutrition Country Profile,* http://globalnutritionreport.org/files/2014/12/gnr14_cp_malawi.pdf, accessed December 2, 2015.

41 Briend and Collins, "Therapeutic Nutrition for Children with Severe Acute Malnutrition."

42 S. Chamois, "Decentralization and Scale up of Outpatient Management of SAM in Ethiopia (2008–2010)," Field Exchange 40, http://www.ennonline.net/fex/40/decentralisation, accessed March 7, 2016.

43 Dolan et al., "Government Experiences of Scale-up of Community-based Management of Acute Malnutrition (CMAM)."

44 WHO/UNICEF/WFP, *Global Nutrition Targets 2025: Wasting Policy Brief.*

45 UNICEF, *Evaluation of Community Management of Acute Malnutrition (CMAM): Ethiopia Country Case Study* (New York, 2012).

46 UNICEF, "Community-Based Nutrition Note: Ethiopia," www.unicef.org/ethiopia/2014-12-15-NUTRITION-based.pdf, accessed January 10, 2016.

47 International Food Policy Research Institute, *Global Nutrition Report 2014, Ethiopia Nutrition Country Profile,* http://globalnutritionreport.org/files/2014/11/gnr14_cp_ethiopia.pdf, accessed December 2, 2015.

48 United Nations Development Programme, *2014 Human Development Report,* http://www.undp.org/content/undp/en/home/librarypage/hdr/2014-human-development-report/, accessed December 2, 2015.

49 UNICEF, *Tracking Progress on Child and Maternal Nutrition.*

50 Deconinck et al., *Review of Community-Based Management of Acute Malnutrition (CMAM) in the Post-emergency Context.*

51 Ibid.

52 G. H. Maimouna, Y. Chegou, and E.-A. Ategbo, "Management of Acute Malnutrition in Niger: A Countrywide Programme," Field Exchange 43, http://www.ennonline.net/fex/43/management, accessed March 7, 2016.

53 T. K. Burki, "Malaria and Malnutrition: Niger's Twin Crises," *The Lancet* 382, no. 9892 (2013): 587–588.

54 Ibid.

55 Maimouna et al., "Management of Acute Malnutrition in Niger."

56 International Food Policy Research Institute, *Global Nutrition Report 2014, Niger Nutrition Country Profile,* http://globalnutritionreport.org/files/2014/11/gnr14_cp_niger.pdf, accessed December 2, 2015.

57 UNICEF, *Tracking Progress on Child and Maternal Nutrition.*

58 Maimouna et al., "Management of Acute Malnutrition in Niger."

59 Concern Worldwide, *Concern Worldwide's Learning from 15 Years of Community Management of Acute Malnutrition Programming.*

60 Dolan et al., "Government Experiences of Scale-up of Community-based Management of Acute Malnutrition (CMAM)."

61 Burki, "Malaria and Malnutrition: Niger's Twin Crises."

62 Dolan et al., "Government Experiences of Scale-up of Community-based Management of Acute Malnutrition (CMAM)."

63 Maleta and Amadi, "Community-Based Management of Acute Malnutrition (CMAM) in Sub-Saharan Africa."

64 Concern Worldwide, *Concern Worldwide's Learning from 15 Years of Community Management of Acute Malnutrition Programming.*

65 Maimouna et al., "Management of Acute Malnutrition in Niger."

66 Dolan et al., "Government Experiences of Scale-up of Community-based Management of Acute Malnutrition (CMAM)."

67 Ibid.

68 UNICEF, *Evaluation of Community Management of Acute Malnutrition (CMAM): Ethiopia Country Case Study.*

69 ACF International, *SAM 2020: An Agenda for Scaling-up the Management of Severe Acute Malnutrition by 2020.*

70 UNICEF, *Ready-to-Use Therapeutic Food for Children with Severe Acute Malnutrition,* Position Paper No. 1 (New York, 2013).

71 A. Ashworth, *Community-Based Rehabilitation of Severely Malnourished Children: A Review of Successful Programmes* (London: London School of Hygiene and Tropical Medicine, 2001).

72 UNICEF, *Ready-to-Use Therapeutic Food for Children with Severe Acute Malnutrition.*

73 S. Collins, K. Sadler, N. Dent, T. Khara, S. Guerrero, M. Myatt, et al., *Key Issues in the Success of Community-Based Management of Severe Malnutrition,* Technical Background Paper for WHO Consultation (Geneva: World Health Organization, 2005), http://www.who.int/nutrition/topics/backgroundpapers_Key_issues.pdf.

74 S. Arie, "Hungry for Profit", *BMJ,* no. 341 (2010): 5221.

75 Collins et al., *Key Issues in the Success of Community-Based Management of Severe Malnutrition.*

76 Dolan et al., "Government Experiences of Scale-up of Community-based Management of Acute Malnutrition (CMAM)."

77 UNICEF, *Ready-to-Use Therapeutic Food for Children with Severe Acute Malnutrition.*

78 Dolan et al., "Government Experiences of Scale-up of Community-based Management of Acute Malnutrition (CMAM)."

79 Collins et al., *Key Issues in the Success of Community-Based Management of Severe Malnutrition.*

80 A. Schoonees, M. Lombard, A. Musekiwa, E. Nel, and J. Volmink, "Ready-to-Use Therapeutic Food for Home-Based Treatment of Severe Acute Malnutrition in Children from Six Months to Five Years of Age," Cochrane Database of Systematic Reviews (Chichester, UK: John Wiley & Sons, 2013).

Chapter 6

1 D. J. Spielman and R. Pandya-Lorch, "Fifty Years of Progress," in *Millions Fed: Proven Successes in Agricultural Development,*

edited by D. J. Spielman and R. Pandya-Lorch (Washington, DC: International Food Policy Research Institute, 2009).

2 J. Hoddinott, M. Rosegrant, and M. Torero, "Investments to Reduce Hunger and Undernutrition," in *Copenhagen Consensus,* edited by B. Lomborg (Cambridge: Cambridge University Press, 2013).

3 World Bank, *Improving Nutrition through Multisectoral Approaches: Agriculture and Rural Development* (Washington, DC, 2013).

4 FAO, *The State of Food and Agriculture, 2010–2011: Women in Agriculture: Closing the Gender Gap for Development,* http://www.fao.org/docrep/013/i2050e/i2050e00.htm (accessed April 25, 2013); P. Pinstrup-Andersen, *The Food System and Its interaction with Human Health and Nutrition,* Brief 13 for 2020 Conference on Leveraging Agriculture for Improving Nutrition and Health (Washington, DC: International Food Policy Research Institute, 2011).

5 C. Doss, "The Effects of Intrahousehold Property Ownership on Expenditure Patterns in Ghana" *Journal of African Economies* 15 (2006): 149–180; E. Sraboni, H. J. Malapit, A. Quisumbing, and A. Ahmed, "Women's Empowerment in Agriculture: What Role for Food Security in Bangladesh?" *World Development* 61 (2014): 11–52; H. J. L. Malapit, S. Kadiyala, A. R. Quisumbing, K. Cunningham, and P. Tyagi, "Women's Empowerment Mitigates the Negative Effects of Low Production Diversity on Maternal and Child Nutrition in Nepal," *Journal of Development Studies* 51, no. 8 (2015).

6 F. Ahmed, "Vitamin A Deficiency in Bangladesh: A Review and Recommendations for Improvement," *Public Health Nutrition* 2, no. 1 (1999): 1–14.

7 V. N. Bushamuka, S. De Pee, A. Talukder, L. Kiess, D. Panagides, A. Taher, and M. Bloem, "Impact of a Homestead Gardening Program on Household Food Security and Empowerment of Women in Bangladesh," *Food and Nutrition Bulletin* 26 (2005): 17–25.

8 Ibid.

9 L. Iannotti, K. Cunningham, and M. T. Ruel, *Improving Diet Quality and Micronutrient Nutrition: Homestead Food Production in Bangladesh,* IFPRI Discussion Paper 00928 (Washington, DC: International Food Policy Research Institute, 2009).

10 M. T. Ruel, H. Alderman, the Maternal and Child Nutrition Study Group, "Nutrition-Sensitive Interventions and Programmes: How Can They Help to Accelerate Progress in Improving Maternal and Child Nutrition?" *The Lancet* 382, no. 9891 (2013): 536–551.

11 J. L. Leroy, M. T. Ruel, E. Verhofstadt, and D. Olney, "The Micronutrient Impact of Multisectoral Programs Focusing on Nutrition: Examples from Conditional Cash Transfer, Microcredit with Education, and Agricultural Programs," *Innocenti Review* 5: 1–91 (2008).

12 D. K. Olney, A. Talukder, L. L. Iannotti, M. T. Ruel, and V. Quinn, "Assessing Impact and Impact Pathways of a Homestead Food Production Program on Household and Child Nutrition in Cambodia," *Food and Nutrition Bulletin 30* (2009): 355–369; Iannotti, Cunningham, and Ruel, Impr*oving Diet Quality and Micronutrient Nutrition.*

13 Olney et al., "Assessing Impact and Impact Pathways of a Homestead Food Production Program."

14 E. Masset, L. Haddad, A. Cornelius, and J. Isaza-Castro, "Effectiveness of Agricultural Interventions That Aim to Improve Nutritional Status of Children: Systematic Review," *British Medical Journal* 244 (2012).

15 D. Olney, J. Behrman, E. Iruhiriye, M. van den Bold, and A. Pedehombga, "Helen Keller International's Enhanced Food Production Program in Burkina Faso: Results from a Process Evaluation," IFPRI Report (Washington, DC: International Food Policy Research Institute, 2013).

16 Olney et al., "Helen Keller International's Enhanced Food Production Program in Burkina Faso."

17 D. K. Olney, A. Pedehombga, M. T. Ruel, and A. Dillon, "A 2-Year Integrated Agriculture and Nutrition and Health Behavior Change Communication Program Targeted to Women in Burkina Faso Reduces Anemia, Wasting, and Diarrhea in Children 3–12.9 Months of Age at Baseline: A Cluster-Randomized Controlled Trial 1-3," *Journal of Nutrition* 145, no. 6 (2015): 1317–1324A.

18 D. K. Olney, L. Bliznashka, A. Pedehombga, A. Dillon, M. T. Ruel, and J. Heckert, "A Randomized Controlled Effectiveness Trial Showed that a 2-1 Y Integrated Agriculture and Nutrition Program in Burkina Faso Reduced the Prevalence of Underweight and Improved Dietary Intake and Empowerment among Participating Compared to Control Mothers" (International Food Policy Research Institute, Washington, DC, 2015, mimeo).

19 L. Bliznashka, D. K. Olney, M. T. Ruel, R. Rawat, E. Becquey, and O. Birba, "An Integrated Agriculture and Nutrition Program in Burkina Faso Has Positive Intra-Household Spillover Effects on Maternal and Child Nutritional Status, but No Sustained Long-Term Improvements in Household Welfare" (abstract submitted to Experimental Biology Conference, 2015, draft).

20 Olney et al., "A 2-Year Integrated Agriculture and Nutrition and Health Behavior Change Communication Program."

21 R. E. Black, C. G. Victora, S. P. Walker, Z. A. Bhutta, P. Christian, M. de Onis, M. Ezzati, S. Grantham-McGregor, and J. Katz, "Maternal and Child Undernutrition and Overweight in Low-Income and Middle-Income Countries," *The Lancet* 382 (2013): 427–451.

22 Swiss Contact, "Our Projects: Sustainable Cocoa Production Program," December 1, 2015, http://www.swisscontact.org/

en/indonesia/projects/projects/p/Project/show/sustainable-cocoa-production-program-scpp.html.

23 S. K. Vasal, "Quality Protein Maize Story," paper prepared for IFPRI conference "Improving Human Nutrition through the Role of International Agricultural Research," Los Baños, Philippines, October 5–7, 1999.

24 H. E. Bouis, *History of HarvestPlus* (International Food Policy Research Institute, Washington, DC, 2011, unpublished draft).

25 H. E. Bouis, C. Hotz, B. McClafferty, J. V. Meenakshi, and W. H. Pfeiffer, "Biofortification: A New Tool to Reduce Micronutrients," *Food and Nutrition Bulletin* 32 (2011): S31–S40.

26 J. Haas, J. Beard, L. E. Murray-Kolb, A. M. Del Mundo, A. Felix, and G. B. Gregoria, "Iron-Biofortified Rice Improves the Iron Stores of Nonanemic Filipino Women," *Journal of Nutrition 135* (2005): 2823–2830; L. M. Carvalho, M. M. Correa, and E. J. Pereira, "Iron and Zinc Retention in Common Beans (*Phaseolus vulgaris L.)* after Home Cooking," *Food and Nutrition Research* 56 (2012): 15618–15623; N. Petry, I. Egli, J. B. Gahutu, P. L. Tugirimana, E. Boy, and R. Hurrell, "Stable Iron Isotope Studies in Rwandese Women Indicate That the Common Bean Has Limited Potential as a Vehicle for Iron Biofortification," *Journal of Nutrition* 142 (2012): 492–497.

27 C. Hotz, C. Loechl, and A. Lubowa, "Introduction of β-Carotene-Rich Orange Sweet Potato in Rural Uganda Resulted in Increased Vitamin A Intakes among Children and Women and Improved Vitamin A Status among Children," *Journal of Nutrition* 142 (2012): 1871–1880; C. Hotz, C. Loechl, and A. De Brauw, "A Large-Scale Intervention to Introduce Orange Sweet Potato in Rural Mozambique Increases Vitamin A Intakes among Children and Women," *British Journal of Nutrition* 108 (2012): 163–176.

28 K. M. Jones and A. de Brauw, "Using Agriculture to Improve Child Health: Promoting Orange Sweet Potatoes Reduces Diarrhea," *World Development* 74 (2015): 15–24.

29 J. W. Low, M. Arimond, N. Osman, B. Cunguara, F. Zano, and D. Tschirley, "A Food-Based Approach Introducing Orange-Fleshed Sweet Potatoes Increased Vitamin A Intake and Serum Retinol Concentrations in Young Children in Rural Mozambique," *Journal of Nutrition* 137, no. 5 (2007): 1320–1327.

30 J. Fiedler and K. Lividini, *Zambia and Bangladesh Micronutrient Portfolio Analyses* (Washington, DC: HarvestPlus, 2014).

31 C. Hawkes and M. T. Ruel, *Value Chains for Nutrition,* Conference Paper 4 for 2020 Conference "Leveraging Agriculture for Improving Nutrition and Health" (Washington, DC: International Food Policy Research Institute, 2011).

32 A. Gelli, "Value Chains and Nutrition: A Framework to Support the Identification, Design, and Evaluation of Enterventions" (CGIAR Research Program on Agriculture for Nutrition and Health, International Food Policy Research Institute, Washington, DC), unpublished draft.

33 E. Kristjansson, V. Robinson, M. Petticrew, B. Macdonald, J. Krasevec, and L. Janzen, "School Feeding for Improving the Physical and Psychosocial Health of Disadvantaged Elementary School Children," *Cochrane Database Systematic Reviews* 1 (2007): CD004676.

34 E. A. Kristjansson, A. Gelli, V. Welch, T. Greenhalgh, S. Liberato, D. Francis, and F. Espejo, "Costs, and Cost-Outcome of School Feeding Programmes and Feeding Programmes for Young Children: Evidence and Recommendations," *International Journal of Educational Development* (in press).

35 D. Bundy, C. Burbano, M. Grosh, A. Gelli, M. Jukes, and L. Drake, *Rethinking School Feeding: Social Safety Nets, Child Development, and the Education Sector* (Washington, DC: World Bank, 2009).

36 J. Sumberg and R. Sabates-Wheeler, "Linking Agricultural Development to School Feeding in Sub-Saharan Africa: Theoretical Perspectives," *Food Policy 36* (2011): 341–349.

37 Bliznashka et al., *An Integrated Agriculture and Nutrition Program in Burkina Faso Has Positive Intra-Household Spillover Effects.*

38 Ruel, Alderman, and the Maternal and Child Nutrition Study Group, "Nutrition-Sensitive Interventions and Programmes."

39 World Bank, *2008 World Development Report: Agriculture for Development* (Washington, DC, 2007).

40 Ibid.

Chapter 7

1 J. Hoddinott, "Safety Nets and Social Protection: Opportunities for Mutual Learning between Asia and Latin America," paper presented at the conference "Fostering Growth and Reducing Poverty and Hunger in Asia and Latin America: Opportunities for Mutual Learning," Lima, March 22–25, 2010.

2 U. Gentilini and S. W. Omamo, *Unveiling Social Safety Nets* (Rome: World Food Programme, 2009).

3 International Labour Organization, *World Social Protection Report 2014/15* (Geneva: ILO, 2014).

4 H. Alderman and R. Yemtsov, "How Can Safety Nets Contribute to Economic Growth?" *World Bank Economic Review* 28, no. 1 (2013): 1–20.

5 SecureNutrition, case study briefs and presentations from the Global Forum on Nutrition-Sensitive Social Protection Programs, Moscow, September 2015, www.

securenutritionplatform.org/Pages/AboutSeminar.aspx?CID=37.

6 Food and Agriculture Organization of the United Nations, *Nutrition and Social Protection* (Rome, 2015).

7 J. Manley, S. Gitter, and V. Slavchevska, "How Effective Are Cash Transfer Programmes at Improving Nutritional Status?" *World Development* 48 (2013): 133–155.

8 E. Owusu-Addo and R. Cross, "The Impact of Conditional Cash Transfers on Child Health in Low- and Middle-Income Countries: A Systematic Review," *International Journal of Public Health* 59 (2014): 609–618.

9 R. de Groot, T. Palermo, S. Handa, L. P. Ragno, and A. Peterman, *Cash Transfers and Child Nutrition: What We Know and What We Need to Know,* Innocenti Working Paper 2015-07 (Florence: UNICEF Office of Research, 2015).

10 World Bank, *Improving Nutrition through Multisectoral Approaches,* Module D, "Improving Nutrition through Social Protection" (Washington, DC: World Bank, 2013), http://documents.worldbank.org/curated/en/2013/01/17211210/improving-nutrition-through-multisectoral-approaches.

11 J. R. Behrman and J. Hoddinott, "Programme Evaluation with Unobserved Heterogeneity and Selective Implementation: The Mexican PROGRESA Impact on Child Nutrition," *Oxford Bulletin of Economics and Statistics* 67, no. 4 (2005): 547–569; United Nations Development Programme, *Mexico: Scaling Up Progresa/Oportunidades— Conditional Cash Transfer Programme,* part of the series Poverty Reduction: Scaling Up Local Innovations for Transformational Change (New York: UNDP, 2001), http://www.undp.org/content/dam/undp/library/Poverty%20Reduction/Participatory%20Local%20Development/Mexico_Progresa_web.pdf.

12 World Bank, "Mexico's Oportunidades Program," Shanghai Poverty Conference case study summary, http://web.worldbank.org/archive/website00819C/WEB/PDF/CASE_-62.PDF.

13 Behrman and Hoddinott, "Programme Evaluation with Unobserved Heterogeneity and Selective Implementation"; United Nations Development Programme, *Mexico: Scaling Up Progresa/Oportunidades;* F. Lamanna, *Global Forum on Nutrition-Sensitive Social Protection Programs: Mexico—Social Protection System/Prospera Program: Case Study Brief,* 2015, https://www.securenutritionplatform.org/Documents/SecureNutrition_GlobalForum-case-study-briefs.zip.

14 Government of Mexico, *Oportunidades: A Program of Results* (Mexico City: Oportunidades Press and Media Office, 2008).

15 Behrman and Hoddinott, "Programme Evaluation with Unobserved Heterogeneity and Selective Implementation."

16 Ibid.

17 These gains correspond to 0.41 height-for-age Z-scores and 0.47 weight-for-height Z-scores; J. L. Leroy, A. García-Guerra, and L. M. Neufeld, "The Oportunidades Program Increases the Linear Growth of Children Enrolled at Young Ages in Urban Mexico," *Journal of Nutrition* 138 (2008): 793–779.

18 J. A. Rivera, D. Sotres-Alvarez, J.-P. Habicht, T. Shamah, and S. Villalpando, "Impact of the Mexican Programme for Education, Health, and Nutrition (PROGRESA) on Rates of Growth and Anemia in Infants and Young Children: A Randomized Effectiveness Study," *Journal of the American Medical Association* 291 (2004): 2563–2570.

19 G. Berhane, J. Hoddinott, N. Kumar, A. Taffesse, M. Diressie, Y. Yohannes, R. Sabates-Wheeler, M. Handino, J. Lind, M. Tefera, and F. Simma, *Evaluation of Ethiopia's Food Security Program: Documenting Progress in the Implementation of the Productive Safety Nets Programme and the Household Asset Building Programme* (Washington, DC: International Food Policy Research Institute, 2012).

20 D. O. Gilligan, J. Hoddinott, and A. S. Taffesse, An *Analysis of Ethiopia's Productive Safety Net Program and Its Linkages* (Washington, DC: International Food Policy Research Institute, 2008).

21 Ibid.

22 J. L. Leroy, M. Ruel, and E. Verhofstadt, "The Impact of Conditional Cash Transfer Programmes on Child Nutrition: A Review of Evidence Using a Programme Theory Framework," *Journal of Development Effectiveness* 1 (2009): 103–129.

23 L. C. H. Fernald, P. J. Gertler, and M. L. Neufeld, "Role of Cash in Conditional Cash Transfer Programmes for Child Health, Growth, and Development: An Analysis of Mexico's Oportunidades," *Lancet* 371 (2008): 827–837.

24 T. Barham, L. E. Brenzel, and J. A. Maluccio, *Beyond 80%: Are There New Ways of Increasing Vaccination Coverage? Evaluation of CCT Programs in Mexico and Nicaragua* (Washington, DC: World Bank, 2007).

25 T. Barham, *The Impact of the Mexican Conditional Cash Transfer on Immunization Rates* (Berkeley: Department of Agriculture and Resource Economics, University of California Berkeley, 2005).

26 P. Gertler, *The Impact of PROGRESA on Health* (Washington, DC: International Food Policy Research Institute, 2000).

27 M. C. Huerta, "Child Health in Rural Mexico: Has PROGRESA Reduced Children's Morbidity Risks?" *Social Policy and Administration* 40 (2006): 652–677.

28 Gertler, *The Impact of PROGRESA on Health.*

29 High Level Panel of Experts on Food Security and Nutrition, *Social Protection for Food Security* (Rome: Committee on World Food Security, 2012).

30 C. G. N. Mascie-Taylor, M. K. Marks, R. Goto, and R. Islam, "Impact of a Cash-for-Work Programme on Food Consumption and Nutrition among Women and Children

Facing Food Insecurity in Rural Bangladesh," *Bulletin of the World Health Organization* 88 (2010): 854–860.

31 A. Ahmed and J. Hoddinott, "Which Kinds of Social Safety Net Transfers Work Best for the Rural Ultra Poor?" (presentation at final seminar of the Transfer Modality Research Initiative, organized by IFPRI and WFP, Dhaka, Bangladesh, May 26, 2015).

32 J. L. Leroy, P. Gadsden, S. Rodríguez-Ramírez, and T. González de Cossío, "Cash and In-Kind Transfers in Poor Rural Communities in Mexico Increase Household Fruit, Vegetable, and Micronutrient Consumption but Also Lead to Excess Energy Consumption," *Journal of Nutrition* 140 (2010): 612–617.

33 United Nations General Assembly, "Transforming Our World: The 2030 Agenda for Sustainable Development," resolution adopted by the General Assembly on September 25, 2015, www.un.org/ga/search/view_doc.asp?symbol=A/RES/70/1&Lang=E.

Chapter 8

1 World Health Organization (WHO)/UNICEF, "JMP Progress on Sanitation and Drinking Water: 2015 Update and MDG Assessment," Accessed December 15, 2015, http://data.unicef.org/overview/water.html#sthash.PNcfJVEk.dpuf. Figures are for 2015 and 2014, respectively.

2 S. Cairncross, C. Hunt, S. Boisson, K. Bostoen, V. Curtis, I. C. H. Fung, and W. F. Schmidt, "Water, Sanitation and Hygiene for the Prevention of Diarrhoea," *International Journal of Epidemiology* 39, suppl 1 (2010): i193-i205.

3 A. E. Aiello, R. M. Coulborn, V. Perez, and E. L. Larson, "Effect of Hand Hygiene on Infectious Disease Risk in the Community Setting: A Meta-analysis," *American Journal of Public Health* 98, 8 (2008): 1372–1381.

4 W. A. Petri, M. Miller, H. J. Binder, M. M. Levine, R. Dillingham, and R. L. Guerrant, "Enteric Infections, Diarrhea, and Their Impact on Function and Development," *Journal of Clinical Investigation* 118, 4 (2008): 1277–1290; K. G. Dewey and D. R. Mayers, "Early Child Growth: How Do Nutrition and Infection Interact?" *Maternal and Child Nutrition* 7, suppl. 3 (2011): 129–142.

5 L. Liu, H. L. Johnson, S. Cousens, J. Perin, S. Scott, and J. E. Lawn, "Global, Regional, and National Causes of Child Mortality: An Updated Systematic Analysis for 2010 with Time Trends since 2000," The *Lancet 379*, 9832 (2012): 2151–2161.

6 T. F. Clasen, K. Bostoen, W. P. Schmidt, S. Boisson, I. C. Fung, and M. W. Jenkins, "Interventions to Improve Disposal of Human Excreta for Preventing Diarrhoea," *Cochrane Database of Systematic Reviews* 6 (2010); Waddington, H. B. Snilstveit, H. White, and L. Fewtrell, *Water, Sanitation and Hygiene Interventions to Combat Childhood Diarrhoea in Developing Countries,* International Initiative for Impact Evaluation Synthetic Review 1 (Washington, DC: 3ie, 2009); R. I. Ejemot, J. E. Ehiri, M. M. Meremikwu, and J. A. Critchley, "Handwashing for Preventing Diarrhoea," *Cochrane Database of Systematic Reviews* 1 (2008); Aiello, et al., "Effect of Hand Hygiene on Infectious Disease Risk in the Community Setting: A Meta-analysis."

7 A. Ahuja, M. Kremer, and A. Peterson Zwane, "Providing Safe Water: Evidence from Randomized Evaluation," *Annual Review of Resource Economics* 2 (2010): 237–256.

8 C. L. Fischer Walker, J. Perin, M. J. Aryee, C. Boschi-Pinto, and R. E. Black, "Diarrhea Incidence in Low- and Middle-Income Countries in 1990 and 2010: A Systematic Review," *BMC Public Health* 12 (2012): 220.

9 W. Checkley, G. Buckley, R. H. Gilman, A. M. O. Assis, R. L. Guerrant, and S. S. Morris, "Multi-Country Analysis of the Effects Of Diarrhoea on Childhood Stunting," *International Journal of Epidemiology* 37, 4 (2008): 816; R. L. Guerrant, R. B. Oriá, S. R. Moore, M. O. B. Oriá, and A. A. M. Lima, "Malnutrition as an Enteric Infectious Disease with Long-Term Effects on Child Development," *Nutrition Reviews* 66, 9 (2008): 487–505.

10 A. Pruss-Ustun, J. Bartram, T. Clasen, J. M. Colford, O. Cumming, and O. Curtis, "Burden of Disease from Inadequate Water, Sanitation and Hygiene in Low- and Middle-Income Settings: A Retrospective Analysis of Data from 145 Countries," *Tropical Medicine and International Health* 19, 8 (2014): 894–905.

11 WHO, "Global Health Observatory (GHO) data: soil-transmitted helminthiases – global prevalence estimates," accessed December 2, 2015, http://www.who.int/gho/neglected_diseases/soil_transmitted_helminthiases/en/.

12 P. O'Lorcain and C. V. Holland, "The Public Health Importance of Ascaris lumbricoides," *Parasitology* 121, Suppl. (2000): S51–S71.

13 S. Brooker, P. J. Hotez, and D. A. Bundy, "Hookworm-Related Anaemia among Pregnant Women: A Systematic Review," *PLoS Neglected Tropical Diseases* 2, 9 (2008): e291.

14 K. Ziegelbauer, B. Speich, D. Mäusezahl, R. Bos, K. Keiser, and J. Utzinger, "Effect of Sanitation on Soil-Transmitted Helminth Infection: Systematic Review and Meta-Analysis" *PLoS Medicine* 9, 1 (2012): e1001162.

15 P. S. Korpe and W. A. Petri, "Environmental Enteropathy: Critical Implications of a Poorly Understood Condition," *Trends in Molecular Medicine* 18, 6 (2012): 328–336.

16 P. G. Lunn, C. A. Northrop-Clewes, and R. M. Downes, "Intestinal Permeability, Mucosal Injury, and Growth Faltering in Gambian Infants," *The Lancet* 338 (1991): 907–910.

17 M. N. N. Mbuya and J. H. Humphrey, "Preventing Environmental Enteric Dysfunction through Improved Water, Sanitation, and Hygiene: An Opportunity for Stunting Reduction in Developing Countries," *Maternal and Child Nutrition* 12, Suppl. 1 (2016).

18 A. Lin., B. F. Arnold, S. Afreen, R. Goto, T. M. Huda, and R. Haque, "Household Environmental Conditions Are Associated with Enteropathy and Impaired Growth in Rural Bangladesh," *American Journal of Tropical Medicine and Hygiene* 89 (2013): 130–137.

19 D. Spears, "How Much International Variation in Child Height Can Open Defecation Explain?" World Bank Policy Research Working Paper 6351 (Washington, DC: World Bank, 2013).

20 D. Spears, A. Ghosh, and O. Cumming, "Open Defecation and Childhood Stunting in India: An Ecological Analysis of New Data from 112 Districts," *PLoS One* 8, 9 (2013): e73784.

21 A. D. Dangour, L. Watson, O. Cumming, S. Boisson, Y. Che, Y. Velleman, S. Cavill, E. Allen, and R. Uauy, "Interventions to Improve Water Quality and Supply, Sanitation and Hygiene Practices, and Their Effects on the Nutritional Status of Children," *Cochrane Database of Systematic Reviews* 8 (2013).

22 G. Fink, I. Gunther, and K. Hill, "The Effect of Water and Sanitation on Child Health: Evidence from the Demographic and Health Surveys 1986–2007," *International Journal of Epidemiology* 40, no. 5 (2011): 1196–1204.

23 WHO, *Improving Nutrition Outcomes with Better Water, Sanitation and Hygiene: Practical Solutions for Policies and Programmes* (Switzerland: 2015).

24 R. Sigler, L. Mahmoudi, and J. P. Graham, "Analysis of Behavioral Change Techniques in Community-led Sanitation Programs," *Health Promotion International* 30, 1 (2015): 16–28; K. Kar and R. Chambers, *Handbook on Community-Led Total Sanitation* (London: Plan UK, 2008).

25 P. Gertler, M. Shah, M. L. Alzua, L. Cameron, S. Martinez, and S. Patil, *How Does Health Promotion Work? Evidence from the Dirty Business of Eliminating Open Defecation,* NBER Working Paper 20997 (March 2015).

26 WASH Benefits, "WASH Benefits Research Objectives," accessed December 1, 2015, www.washbenefits.net/objectives.html.

27 MAL-ED, "Interactions of Malnutrition & Enteric Infections: Consequences for Child Health and Development," accessed December 1, 2015, http://mal-ed.fnih.org/.

28 The Sanitation Hygiene Infant Nutrition Efficacy (SHINE) Trial Team, "The Sanitation Hygiene Infant Nutrition Efficacy (SHINE) Trial: Rationale, Design, and Methods," *Clinical Infectious Diseases* 61, suppl. 7 (2015): S685–S702.

29 Sigler, Mahmoudi, and Graham, "Analysis of Behavioral Change Techniques in Community-led Sanitation Programs."

30 Ibid.

31 R. Chambers, "Going to Scale with Community-Led Total Sanitation: Reflections on Experience, Issues and Ways Forward," IDS Practice Papers (Brighton, UK: Institute of Development Studies, 2009): 1–52.

32 S. Sah and A. Negussie, "Community Led Total Sanitation (CLTS): Addressing the Challenges of Scale and Sustainability in Rural Africa," *Desalination* 000, 1–8 (2009); B. Bwire, "Breaking Shit Taboos: CLTS in Kenya," *Participatory Learning and Action* 61, 1 (2010): 91-96; P. A. Harvey, "Zero Subsidy Strategies for Accelerating Access to Rural Water and Sanitation Services," *Water Science Technology* 63: 1037–1043.

33 A. J. Pickering, H. Djebbari, C. Lopez, M. Coulibaly, and M. L. Alzua, "Effect of a Community-led Sanitation Intervention on Child Diarrhoea and Child Growth in Rural Mali: A Cluster-randomised Controlled Trial," *The Lancet Global Health* 3, 11 (2015): e701-e711.

34 UNICEF, "Evaluating the Impact of Community-Led Total Sanitation Programs in Mali- Baseline Analysis," preliminary draft report (2009); M. L. Alzua, A. J. Pickering, H. Djebbari, C. Lopez, J. C. Cardenas, M. A. Lopera, N. Osbert, and M. Coulibaly, "Key Findings of the Impact Evaluation of Rural Sanitation Programme in Mali" (academic poster).

35 UNICEF, *2014 Mali Annual Report* (New York: 2014).

36 Pickering, et al., "Effect of a Community-led Sanitation Intervention on Child Diarrhoea and Child Growth in Rural Mali: A Cluster-randomised Controlled Trial."

37 Ibid.

38 Ibid.

39 Ibid.

40 WHO and UNICEF, *Progress on Sanitation and Drinking-Water 2014* (Geneva: Joint Monitoring Programme for Water Supply and Sanitation, 2014).

41 I. Mahmud and N. Mbuya, *Water, Sanitation, Hygiene, and Nutrition in Bangladesh: Can Building Toilets Affect Children's Growth?* (Washington, DC: World Bank, 2016).

42 S. A. Ahmed, "Community Led Total Sanitation in Bangladesh: Chronicles of a People's Movement" (Write-shop paper, IDS, 2008).

43 Water and Sanitation Program, *Long Term Sustainability of Improved Sanitation in Rural Bangladesh,* Research Brief (Washington, DC: 2012).

44 WHO and UNICEF, *Progress on Sanitation and Drinking-Water 2014.*

45 P. Kov, S. Smets, D. Spears, and S. Vyas, *Growing Taller among Toilets: Evidence from Changes in Sanitation and Child Height*

in Cambodia, 2005–2010, Working Paper (New Delhi: Research Institute for Compassionate Economics, 2013); P. Hathi, S. Haque, L. Pant, D. Coffey, and D. Spears, *Place and Child Health: the Interaction of Population Density and Sanitation Behavior in Developing Countries,* Policy Research Working Paper 7124 (Washington, DC: World Bank, 2014); Lin et al., "Household Environmental Conditions are Associated with Enteropathy and Impaired Growth in Rural Bangladesh."

46 US Agency for International Development, *WASH and Nutrition: Water and Development Strategy,* Implementation Brief (Washington, DC, 2015).

47 L. C. Smith, F. Khan, T. R. Frankenberger, and A. K. M. Wadud, "Admissible Evidence in the Court of Development Evaluation? The Impact of CARE's SHOUHARDO Project on Child Stunting in Bangladesh," *World Development* 41 (2013): 196–216. This used a mixed-methods non- and quasi-experimental study design.

48 Ibid.

49 Ibid.

50 FHI 360, *Summary of Handwashing Initiative: Why Hand Washing is Critical to Child Health and Nutrition in Bangladesh—How to Make It a Reality,* Alive & Thrive Policy Brief (Washington, DC, 2012).

51 D. Spears and L. Haddad, "The Power of WASH," in *2014–2015 Global Food Policy Report* (Washington, DC: International Food Policy Research Institute, 2015).

52 Biran et al. found substantial increases in handwashing with soap using a scalable intervention. See A. Biran, W.-P. Schmidt, K. S. Varadharajan, D. Rajaraman, R. Kumar, K. Greenland, B. Gopalan, R. Aunger, and V. Curtis, "Effect of a Behaviour-change Intervention on Handwashing with Soap in India (SuperAmma): A Cluster-randomised Trial," *The Lancet Global Health* 2, 3 (2014): e145–e154.

53 L. Haddad, "WASH and Nutrition: Opportunities and Challenges from Farm to Faeces," Development Horizons Blog, November 12, 2015, http://www.developmenthorizons.com/2015/11/wash-and-nutrition-opportunities-and.html.

54 United Nations Sustainable Development Knowledge Platform, "Sustainable Development Goals," accessed January 12, 2016, https://sustainabledevelopment.un.org/sdgs.

Chapter 9

1 M. Ng, T. Fleming, M. Robinson, B. Thomson, N. Graetz, C. Margono, E. C. Mullany, et al., "Global, Regional, and National Prevalence of Overweight and Obesity in Children and Adults during 1980–2013: A Systematic Analysis for the Global Burden of Disease Study 2013," *The Lancet* 384 (2014): 766–781.

2 International Food Policy Research Institute, *Global Nutrition Report 2015: Actions and Accountability to Advance Nutrition and Sustainable Development* (Washington, DC: IFPRI, 2015); Ng et al., "Global, Regional, and National Prevalence of Overweight and Obesity."

3 A. M. Prentice, "The Emerging Epidemic of Obesity in Developing Countries," *International Journal of Epidemiology* 35 (2006): 93–99.

4 International Food Policy Research Institute, *Global Nutrition Report 2015.*

5 UNICEF, WHO, and World Bank, *Levels and Trends in Child Malnutrition: UNICEF–WHO–World Bank Joint Child Malnutrition Estimates* (New York: UNICEF; Geneva: WHO; Washington DC: World Bank, 2015).

6 S. S. Lim, T. Vos, A. D. Flaxman, G. Danaei, K. Shibuya, H. Adair-Rohani, M. A. AlMazroa, et al., "A Comparative Risk Assessment of Burden of Disease and Injury Attributable to 67 Risk Factors and Risk Factor Clusters in 21 Regions, 1990–2010: A Systematic Analysis for the Global Burden of Disease Study 2010," *The Lancet* 380 (2012): 2224–2260.

7 T. Lobstein, R. Jackson-Leach, M. L. Moodie, K. D. Hall, S. L. Gortmaker, B. A. Swinburn, W. P. T. James, Y. Wang, and K. McPherson, "Child and Adolescent Obesity: Part of a Bigger Picture," *The Lancet* 385, no. 9986 (2015): 2510–2520.

8 Ng et al. "Global, Regional, and National Prevalence of Overweight and Obesity."

9 J. Lachal, M. Orri, M. Speranza, B. Falissard, H. Lefevre, QUALIGRAMH, M. R. Moro, and A. Revah-Levy, "Qualitative Studies among Obese Children and Adolescents: A Systematic Review of the Literature," *Obesity Reviews* 14 (2013): 351–368.

10 B. M. Popkin, L. S. Adair, and S. W. Ng, "Global Nutrition Transition and the Pandemic of Obesity in Developing Countries," *Nutrition Reviews* 70 (2012): 3–21.

11 J. Goldstein, E. R. Jacoby, R. del Aguila, "Poverty Is a Predictor of Non-communicable Disease among Adults in Peruvian Cities," *Preventive Medicine* 41 (2005): 800–806; C. A. Monteiro, W. L. Conde, and B. M. Popkin, "Income-Specific Trends in Obesity in Brazil: 1975–2003," *American Journal of Public Health* 97 (2007): 1808–1812; R. Uauy, C. Albala, and J. Kain, "Obesity Trends in Latin America: Transiting from Under- to Overweight," *Journal of Nutrition* 131 (2001): 893S–899S.

12 C. A. Roberto, B. Swinburn, C. Hawkes, T. T.-K. Huang, S. A. Costa, M. Ashe, L. Zwicker, J. H. Cawley, and K. D. Brownell, "Patchy Progress on Obesity Prevention: Emerging Examples, Entrenched Barriers, and New Thinking," *The Lancet* 385, no. 9985 (2016): 2400–2409, doi:10.1016/S0140-6736(14)61744-X.

13 M. Cecchini, F. Sassi, J. A. Lauer, Y. Y. Lee, V. Guajardo-Barron, and D. Chisholm, "Tackling of Unhealthy Diets, Physical Inactivity, and Obesity: Health Effects and Cost-Effectiveness" *The Lancet* 376, no. 9754 (2016): 1775–1784.

14 Roberto et al., "Patchy Progress on Obesity Prevention."

15 World Health Organization, *Global Action Plan for the Prevention and Control of Noncommunicable Diseases 2013–2020* (Geneva: WHO, 2013); Corinna Hawkes, T. G. Smith, J. Jewell, J. Wardle, R. A. Hammond, S. Friel, A. M. Thow, and J. Kain, "Smart Food Policies for Obesity Prevention," *The Lancet* 385, no. 9985 (2016): 2410–2421, doi:10.1016/S0140-6736(14)61745-1.

16 World Health Organization, *Global Action Plan for the Prevention and Control of Noncommunicable Diseases.*

17 C. Lachat, S. Otchere, D. Roberfroid, A. Abdulai, F. M. Aguirre Seret, J. Milesevic, G. Xuereb, V. Candeias, and P. Kolsteren, "Diet and Physical Activity for the Prevention of Noncommunicable Diseases in Low- and Middle-Income Countries: A Systematic Policy Review," *PLoS Medicine* 10 (2013): e1001465.

18 World Health Organization, *Global Status Report on Noncommunicable Diseases 2014* (Geneva: WHO, 2014).

19 A. Asfaw, "Do Government Food Price Policies Affect the Prevalence of Obesity? Empirical Evidence from Egypt," *World Development* 35, no. 4 (2007): 687–701, doi:10.1016/j.worlddev.2006.05.005.

20 T. Lobstein and H. Brinsden, "Symposium Report: The Prevention of Obesity and NCDs: Challenges and Opportunities for Governments," *Obesity Reviews* 15, no. 8 (2014): 630–639.

21 C. Hawkes, J. Jewell, and K. Allen, "A Food Policy Package for Healthy Diets and the Prevention of Obesity and Diet-Related Non-communicable Diseases: The NOURISHING Framework," *Obesity Reviews* 14 (2013): 159–168.

22 Lobstein et al., "Child and Adolescent Obesity."

23 World Cancer Research Fund International, NOURISHING framework, "Offer Healthy Foods" (February 4, 2016), http://www.wcrf.org/int/policy/nourishing-framework/offer-healthy-foods.

24 C. Hawkes and T. Lobstein for the Polmark Consortium, "Regulating the Commercial Promotion of Food to Children: A Survey of Actions Worldwide," *International Journal of Pediatric Obesity 6,* no. 2 (2011): 83–94, doi:10.3109/17477166.2010.486836.

25 European Competitiveness and Sustainable Industrial Policy (ECSIP) Consortium; ECORYS, *Food Taxes and Their Impact on Competitiveness in the Agri-Food Sector: Final Report* (Rotterdam: July 12, 2014).

26 E. Sidaner, D. Balaban, and L. Burlandy, "The Brazilian School Feeding Programme: An Example of an Integrated Programme in Support of Food and Nutrition Security," *Public Health Nutrition* 16 (2013): 989–994.

27 Lobstein et al., "Child and Adolescent Obesity."

28 International Food Policy Research Institute, *Global Nutrition Report 2015.*

29 International Diabetes Federation, "Mexico," http://www.idf.org/membership/nac/mexico.

30 S. Barquera, L. Hernandez-Barrera, M. L. Tolentino, J. Espinosa, S. W. Ng, J. A. Rivera, and B. M. Popkin, "Energy Intake from Beverages Is Increasing among Mexican Adolescents and Adults," *Journal of Nutrition* 138, no. 12 (2008): 2454–2461; Euromonitor International, "Soft Drinks," http://www.euromonitor.com/soft-drinks.

31 World Health Organization, "Using Price Policies to Promote Healthier Diets" (Geneva: WHO, 2015).

32 M. Arantxa Colchero, B. M. Popkin, J. A. Rivera, and S. W. Ng, "Beverage Purchases from Stores in Mexico under the Excise Tax on Sugar Sweetened Beverages: Observational Study," *British Medical Journal* 352 (2016): h6704.

33 C. A. Monteiro, J.-C. Moubarac, G. Cannon, S. W. Ng, and B. Popkin, "Ultra-Processed Products Are Becoming Dominant in the Global Food System," *Obesity Reviews* 14 (2013): 21–28, doi:10.1111/obr.12107.

34 B. Popkin, C. Monteiro, and B. Swinburn, "Overview: Bellagio Conference on Program and Policy Options for Preventing Obesity in the Low- and Middle-Income Countries," *Obesity Reviews* 14 (2013): 1–8, doi:10.1111/obr.12108; Lobstein and Brinsden, "Symposium Report: The Prevention of Obesity and NCDs."

35 Roberto et al., "Patchy Progress on Obesity Prevention."

36 Colchero et al., "Beverage Purchases from Stores in Mexico."

37 S. Barquera, I. Campos-Nonato, L. Hernández-Barrera, M. Flores, R. Durazo-Arvizu, R. Kanter, and J. A. Rivera, "Obesity and Central Adiposity in Mexican Adults: Results from the Mexican National Health and Nutrition Survey 2006," *Salud Pública de México* 51 (2009, Supplement 4): S595–S603.

38 T. Rosenberg, "How One of the Most Obese Countries on Earth Took on the Soda Giants," *The Guardian* (November 3, 2015), http://www.theguardian.com/news/2015/nov/03/obese-soda-sugar-tax-mexico.

39 E. Donaldson, "Advocating for Sugar Sweetened Beverage Taxation: A Case Study of Mexico" (PhD dissertation, Johns Hopkins Bloomberg School of Public Health, Baltimore, 2015).

40 Rosenberg, "How One of the Most Obese Countries on Earth Took on the Soda Giants."

41 Donaldson, "Advocating for Sugar Sweetened Beverage Taxation."

42 Ibid.

43 O. T. Mytton, D. Clarke, and M. Rayner, "Taxing Unhealthy Food and Drinks to Improve Health," *British Medical Journal* 344 (2012). doi:10.1136/bmj.e2931.

44 Colchero et al., "Beverage Purchases from Stores in Mexico."

45 Rosenberg, "How One of the Most Obese Countries on Earth Took on the Soda Giants."

46 J. Angel Rivera, T. G. de Cossío, L. S. Pedraza, T. C. Aburto, T. G. Sánchez, and R. Martorell, "Childhood and Adolescent Overweight and Obesity in Latin America: A Systematic Review," *The Lancet Diabetes and Endocrinology* 2, no. 4 (2013): 321–332.

47 M. M. Finucane, G. A. Stevens, M. J. Cowan, G. Danaei, J. K. Lin, C. J. Paciorek, and G. M. Singh, "National, Regional, and Global Trends in Body-Mass Index Since 1980: Systematic Analysis of Health Examination Surveys and Epidemiological Studies with 960 Country-Years and 9.1 Million Participants," *The Lancet* 377 (2011): 557–567; Lim et al., "A Comparative Risk Assessment of Burden of Disease and Injury."

48 A. Ochoa-Avilés, S. Andrade, T. Huynh, R. Verstraeten, C. Lachat, R. Rojas, S. Donoso, B. Manuel-y-Keenoy, and P. Kolsteren, "Prevalence and Socioeconomic Differences of Risk Factors of Cardiovascular Disease in Ecuadorian Adolescents," *Pediatric Obesity* 7 (2012): 274–283; S. Andrade, A. Ochoa-Avilés, C. Lachat, P. Escobar, R. Verstraeten, J. Van Camp, S. Donoso, R. Rojas, G. Cardon, and P. Kolsteren, "Physical Fitness among Urban and Rural Ecuadorian Adolescents and Its Association with Blood Lipids: A Cross Sectional Study," *BMC Pediatrics* 14 (2014): 106.

49 A. M. Prentice, "The Emerging Epidemic of Obesity in Developing Countries," *International Journal of Epidemiology* 35 (2006): 93–99.

50 World Health Organization, "Diet, Nutrition, and the Prevention of Chronic Diseases: Report of a Joint WHO/FAO Expert Consultation," *WHO Technical Report Series* no. 916 (Geneva: WHO, 2002).

51 E. Waters, A. de Silva-Sanigorski, B. J. Hall, T. Brown, K. J. Campbell, Y. Gao, R. Armstrong, L. Prosser, and C. D. Summerbell, "Interventions for Preventing Obesity in Children," *Cochrane Database of Systematic Reviews* no. CD001871 (2011). doi:10.1002/14651858.CD001871.pub3.

52 R. Verstraeten, D. Roberfroid, C. Lachat, J. L. Leroy, M. Holdsworth, L. Maes, and P. W. Kolsteren, "Effectiveness of Preventive School-Based Obesity Interventions in Low- and Middle-Income Countries: A Systematic Review," *American Journal of Clinical Nutrition* 96, no. 2 (2012): 415–438.

53 S. Andrade, C. Lachat, A. Ochoa-Aviles, R. Verstraeten, L. Huybregts, D. Roberfroid, D. Andrade, J. Van Camp, R. Rojas, S. Donoso, G. Cardon, and P. Kolsteren, "A School-Based Intervention Improves Physical Fitness in Ecuadorian Adolescents: A Cluster-Randomized Controlled Trial," *International Journal of Behavioral Nutrition and Physical Activity* 11, no. 1 (2014): 153; S. Andrade, M. Verloigne, G. Cardon, P. Kolsteren, A. Ochoa-Avilés, R. Verstraeten, S. Donoso, and C. Lachat, "School-Based Intervention on Healthy Behaviour among Ecuadorian Adolescents: Effect of a Cluster-Randomized Controlled Trial on Screen-Time," *BMC Public Health* 15, no. 1 (2015): 942. doi:10.1186/s12889-015-2274-4; R. Verstraeten, "The Development of a School-Based Health Promotion Intervention in Ecuadorian Adolescents and Its Cluster Randomised-Controlled Evaluation Design" (doctoral thesis, Ghent University, Ghent, Belgium, 2014); A. M. Ochoa-Avilés, R. Verstraeten, L. Huybregts, S. Andrade, J. Van Camp, S. P. Donoso, P. L. Ramírez, C. Lachat, L. Maes, and P. Kolsteren, "A School-Based Health Promotion Intervention Improved Dietary Intake in Ecuadorian Adolescents: A Pair-Matched Cluster Randomized Controlled Trial," Universidad de Cuenca, Cuenca, Ecuador (unpublished manuscript).

54 Lobstein and Brinsden, "Symposium Report: The Prevention of Obesity and NCDs."

55 S. Chapman, "Advocacy for Public Health: A Primer," *Journal of Epidemiology & Community Health* 58 (2004): 361–365.

Chapter 10

1 The first three sections of this chapter are adapted from K. Tontisirin and S. Gillespie, "Linking Community-based Programs and Service Delivery for Improving Maternal and Child Nutrition," *Asian Development Review* 17, no. 1–2 (1999): 33–65.

2 UN Administrative Committee for Coordination/Sub-Committee on Nutrition (ACC/SCN), *Ending Malnutrition by 2020: An Agenda for Change in the Millennium,* Final Report of the ACC/SCN Commission on the Nutrition Challenges of the 21st Century (Geneva: 1999).

3 Ibid.

4 World Bank, World Development Indicators Database, accessed February 22, 2016, http://data.worldbank.org/indicator/SH.STA.MALN.ZS .

5 K. Tontisirin, V. Chavasit, T. Parinyasiri, et al., *Nutrition Impact of Agriculture and Food Systems: Thailand,* Country Policy Analysis (Geneva: UN System Standing Committee on Nutrition, 2013).

6 Thailand, Department of Health, *First National Nutrition Survey of Thailand* (Bangkok: Ministry of Public Health, 1960); Thailand, Bureau of Policy and Strategy, *Thailand Health Profile Report 2008–2010* (Bangkok: Ministry of Public Health, 2011).

7 Tontisirin et al., *Nutrition Impact of Agriculture and Food Systems: Thailand.*

8 Thailand, Department of Health, *First National Nutrition Survey of Thailand.*

9 R. Heaver and Y. Kachondam, *Thailand's National Nutrition Program: Lessons in Management and Capacity Development,* Health, Nutrition, and Population Discussion Paper (Washington, DC: World Bank, 2002).

10 Tontisirin et al., *Nutrition Impact of Agriculture and Food Systems: Thailand.*

11 Heaver and Kachondam, *Thailand's National Nutrition Program: Lessons in Management and Capacity Development.*

12 Ibid.

13 Ibid.

14 Ibid.

15 Tontisirin et al., *Nutrition Impact of Agriculture and Food Systems: Thailand.*

16 Heaver and Kachondam, *Thailand's National Nutrition Program: Lessons in Management and Capacity Development.*

17 C. J. Maguire, "Chiang Mai University Links with Rural Communities to Focus Research on Farming Problems and Foster Curriculum Change," in *Agricultural Innovation Systems: An Investment Sourcebook* (Washington, DC: World Bank, 2012).

18 Heaver and Kachondam, *Thailand's National Nutrition Program: Lessons in Management and Capacity Development.*

19 K. Tontisirin, "Alleviation of Malnutrition in Thailand," in *Partnerships for Social Development: A Casebook* (Future Generations in cooperation with John Hopkins University, 1995): 99–106; S. R. Gillespie, J. B. Mason, and R. Martorell, *How Nutrition Improves,* State-of-the-Art Series Nutrition Policy Discussion Paper 15 (Geneva: ACC/SCN, 1996).

20 J. von Braun, M. Ruel, and A. Gulati, *Accelerating Progress toward Reducing Child Malnutrition in India* (Washington, DC: International Food Policy Research Institute, 2008).

21 Heaver and Kachondam, *Thailand's National Nutrition Program: Lessons in Management and Capacity Development.*

22 Ibid.

23 Tontisirin et al., *Nutrition Impact of Agriculture and Food Systems: Thailand.*

24 International Food Policy Research Institute (IFPRI), *Global Nutrition Report 2015, Nutrition Country Profile: Thailand,* 2015, http://bit.ly/1ZJaVMe.

25 Heaver and Kachondam, *Thailand's National Nutrition Program: Lessons in Management and Capacity Development.*

26 L. Haddad, "Can Thailand Write Us a New Story for Nutrition Improvement in the 21st Century?" January 24, 2016, http://bit.ly/1LXPzZf.

27 Tontisirin et al., *Nutrition Impact of Agriculture and Food Systems: Thailand.*

28 Ibid.

29 Thai National Food Committee, *Strategic Framework for Food Management in Thailand* (Bangkok: Thailand Food Committee and National Bureau of Agricultural Commodity and Food Standards, 2012).

30 Tontisirin et al., *Nutrition Impact of Agriculture and Food Systems: Thailand.*

Chapter 11

1 C. A. Monteiro, M. H. Benicio, W. L. Conde, S. Konno, A. L. Lovadino, A. J. D. Barros, and C. G. Victora, "Narrowing Socioeconomic Inequality in Child Stunting: The Brazilian Experience, 1974–2007," *Bulletin of the World Health Organization* 88 (2009): 305–311.

2 Ibid.

3 S. I. Venanciol, S. R. Saldival, and C. A. Monteiro, "Secular Trends in Breastfeeding in Brazil," *Revista de Saúde Pública* 47, no. 6 (2013): 1–4.

4 C. G. Victora, E. M. L. Aquino, M. do Carmo Leal, C. A. Monteiro, F. C. Barros, and C. L. Szwarcwald, "Maternal and Child Health in Brazil: Progress and Challenges," *The Lancet* 377, no. 9780 (2011): 1863–1876.

5 Monteiro et al., "Narrowing Socioeconomic Inequality in Child Stunting: The Brazilian Experience, 1974–2007."

6 C. A. Monteiro, "The Spectacular Fall of Child Undernutrition in Brazil," *SCN News* 37 (2009).

7 R. E. Black, C. G. Victora, S. P. Walker, Z. A. Bhutta, P. Christian, et al., and the Maternal and Child Nutrition Study Group, "Maternal and Child Undernutrition and Overweight in Low-Income and Middle-Income Countries," *The Lancet* 382, no. 9890 (2013): 427–451.

8 C. A. Monteiro, M. H. Benicio, S. C. Konno, et al., "Causes for the Decline in Child Under-nutrition in Brazil, 1996–2007," *Revista de Saude Publica* 43, no. 1 (2009): 35–43.

9 C. G. Victora et al., "Maternal and Child Health in Brazil: Progress and Challenges."

10 S. A. Draibe, "A Política Social do Governo FHC e o Sistema de Proteção Social," *Tempo Social* 15, no. 2 (2003): 63–101.

11 OECD (Organization for Economic Co-operation and Development), *Strong Performers and Successful Reformers in Education: Lessons from PISA for the United States* (Paris: OECD, 2011), doi:10.1787/9789264096660-en.

12 S. Schwartzman, *Education-oriented Social Programs in Brazil: The Impact of Bolsa Escola* (Rio de Janeiro: Instituto de Estudos do Trabalho e Sociedade, 2005).

13 J. Paim, C. Travassos, C. Almeida, L. Bahia, and J. Macinko, "The Brazilian Health System: History, Advances, and Challenges," *The Lancet* 377, no. 9779 (2011): 1778–1797.

14 Monteiro et al., "Causes for the Decline in Child Under-nutrition in Brazil, 1996–2007."

15 M. Néri, *Miséria, Desigualdade e Políticas de Renda: O Real do Lula* (Rio de Janeiro: Fundação Getulio Vargas Social/ Instituto Brasileiro de Economia/Centro de Politicas Sociais, 2007), as cited in C. A. Monteiro et al., "Causes for the Decline in Child Under-nutrition in Brazil, 1996–2007."

16 A. Mejía Acosta, *Analysing Nutrition Governance: Brazil Country Report* (Brighton, UK: Institute of Development Studies, 2011).

17 B. R. Castiñeira, L. C. Nunes, and P. Rungo, "Impacto de los Programas de Transferencia Condicionada de Renta sobre el Estado de Salud: El Programa Bolsa Familia de Brasil," *Revista Española de Salud Pública* 83, no. 1 (2009): 85–97; R. Paes-Sousa, L. M. Pacheco Santos, and É. S. Miazaki, "Effects of a Conditional Cash Transfer Program on Child Nutrition in Brazil," *Bulletin of the World Health Organization* 89, no. 7 (2011): 496–503.

18 International Policy Centre for Inclusive Growth, *Structured Demand and Smallholder Farmers in Brazil: The Case of PAA and PNAE* (Brasilia: 2013).

19 S. Kleinert and R. Horton, "Brazil: Towards Sustainability and Equity in Health," *The Lancet* 377, no. 9779 (2011): 1721–1722.

20 J. Paim, C. Travassos, C. Almeida, L. Bahia, and J. Macinko, "The Brazilian Health System: History, Advances, and Challenges," *The Lancet* 377, no. 9779 (2011): 1778–1797.

21 R. Rocha and R. Soares, *Evaluating the Impact of Community-Based Health Interventions: Evidence from Brazil's Family Health Program,* Discussion Paper 4119 (Bonn: Institute for the Study of Labor, 2009); Brazil, Ministry of Health, *Saúde da Família no Brasil: Uma Análise de Indicadores Selecionados, 1998–2005/2006,* Série C Projetos, Programas e Relatórios (Brasilia, 2008).

22 R. Aquino and M. L. Barreto, "The Family Health Program in Brazil and the Adequacy of Its Coverage Indicator," *Cad Saude Publica* 24 (2008): 905–914; R. Aquino, N. F. de Oliveira, and M. L. Barreto, "Impact of Family Health Program on Infant Mortality in Brazilian Municipalities," *American Journal of Public Health* 99, no. 1 (2009): 87–93.

23 Paim et al., "The Brazilian Health System."

24 M. F. Rea, "A Review of Breastfeeding in Brazil and How the Country Has Reached Ten Months' Breastfeeding Duration, *Cadernos de Saude Publica* 19, suppl. 1 (2003): S37–S45.

25 WHO (World Health Organization), *Country Implementation of the International Code of Marketing of Breast-milk Substitutes: Status Report 2011* (Geneva, 2013).

26 C. G. Victora et al., "Maternal and Child Health in Brazil: Progress and Challenges"; International Food Policy Research Institute, *Global Nutrition Report 2014: Actions and Accountability to Accelerate the World's Progress on Nutrition* (Washington, DC, 2014); R. Pérez-Escamilla, L. Curry, D. Minhas, et al., "Scaling up of Breastfeeding Promotion Programs in Low-and Middle-Income Countries: The 'Breastfeeding Gear' Model," *Advances in Nutrition: An International Review Journal* 3, no. 6 (2012): 790–800.

27 UNICEF and WHO, *Countdown to 2015: Tracking Down Progress in Maternal, Neonatal and Child Survival—The 2008 Report* (New York, NY: UNICEF and WHO, 2008); WHO/UNICEF Joint Monitoring Programme for Water Supply and Sanitation," cited in International Food Policy Research Institute, *Global Nutrition Report 2014.*

28 C. G. Victora, "Diarrhea Mortality: What Can the World Learn from Brazil?" *Jornal de Pediatria* 85, no. 1 (2009): 3–5.

29 Monteiro et al., "Causes for the Decline in Child Under-nutrition in Brazil, 1996–2007."

30 UN Standing Committee on Nutrition, "Changing Food Systems for Better Nutrition," *SCN News* 40 (2013).

31 W. L. Conde and C. A. Monteiro, "Nutrition Transition and Double Burden of Undernutrition and Excess of Weight in Brazil," *American Journal of Clinical Nutrition* 100, no. 6 (2014): 1617S–1622S.

32 C. A. Monteiro, C. L. Wolney, and B. M. Popkin, "Is Obesity Replacing or Adding to Undernutrition? Evidence from Different Social Classes in Brazil," *Public Health Nutrition* 5, no. 1A (2002): 105–112.

33 C. G. Victora, M. L. Baretto, M. do Carmo Leal, et al., "Health Conditions and Health-policy Innovations in Brazil: The Way Forward," *The Lancet* 377, no. 9782 (2011): 2042–2053.

34 Brazil, Ministry of Health, *Dietary Guidelines for the Brazilian Population,* 2nd edition (Brasilia, 2014); C. A. Monteiro, G. Cannon, J. C. Moubarac, et al., "Dietary Guidelines to Nourish Humanity and the Planet in the Twenty-First Century: A Blueprint from Brazil," *Public Health Nutrition* 18, no. 13 (2015): 2311–2322.

35 FAO (Food and Agriculture Organization of the United Nations), IFAD (International Fund for Agricultural Development), and WFP (World Food Programme), *The State of Food Insecurity in the World 2014: Strengthening the Enabling Environment for Food Security and Nutrition* (Rome: FAO, 2014).

36 M. A. Ravallion, *A Comparative Perspective on Poverty Reduction in Brazil, China, and India,* World Bank Policy Research Working Paper 5080 (Washington, DC: World Bank, 2009).

37 H. Alderman and J. Hoddinott, "Growth-Promoting Social Safety Nets," in *The Poorest and Hungry: Assessments, Analyses, and Actions,* edited by J. von Braun, R. Vargas Hill, and R. Pandya-Lorch (Washington, DC: International Food Policy Research Institute, 2009); Ravallion, *A Comparative Perspective on Poverty Reduction in Brazil, China, and India.*

38 Mejía Acosta, *Analysing Nutrition Governance: Brazil Country Report.*

39 FAO, IFAD and WFP, *The State of Food Insecurity in the World 2014.*

40 Mejía Acosta, *Analysing Nutrition Governance: Brazil Country Report.*

41 FAO, IFAD and WFP, *The State of Food Insecurity in the World 2014.*

42 R. Uauy, "The Impact of the Brazil Experience in Latin America," *The Lancet* 377, no. 9782 (2011): 1984–1986.

Chapter 12

1 Annual GDP growth for 1996–2014 averaged 5.53 percent, with a low of 3.83 percent in 2002 and a high of 6.67 percent in 2006 (World Bank, World Development Indicators, data.worldbank.org, accessed March 12, 2016). Average per capita income in Bangladesh increased from US$599 during FY2007–2008 to US$848 during FY2011–2012 (Bangladesh Bureau of Statistics, *Preliminary Report on Household Income and Expenditure Survey—2010* [Dhaka, Bangladesh: 2011]). Bangladesh has a Human Development Index (HDI) value of 0.570, which places it within the medium human development group of countries (versus the low human development group). However, the country's HDI value is lower than the medium group's average of 0.630 and also below the average of 0.607 for countries in South Asia (UNDP, *Human Development Report 2015: Work for Human Development* [New York: 2015]).

2 D. D. Headey ("Developmental Drivers of Nutritional Change: A Cross-country Analysis," *World Development* 42 [2013]: 76–88) reports that underweight fell from 56.4 percent in 1997 to 46.1 percent in 2007, and stunting from 54.7 percent in 1997 to 36.0 percent in 2007.

3 D. D. Headey, J. Hoddinott, A. Disha, R. Tesfaye, and M. Dereje, "The Other Asian Enigma: Explaining the Rapid Reduction of Undernutrition in Bangladesh," *World Development* 66 (2015): 749–761.

4 For more information on these life histories, see P. Davis, "Patterns of Socio-economic Mobility in Rural Bangladesh: Lessons from Life History Interviews," in *Methodological Challenges and New Approaches to Research in International Development,* edited by L. Camfield (Basingstoke, UK: Palgrave Macmillan, 2014).

5 D. D. Headey et al.'s 2015 study used regression analysis to demonstrate that a little over one-half of the observed reduction in stunting in Bangladesh is linked to five interrelated trends, in the following order of importance: improvements in economic development in the form of wealth accumulation; improvements in maternal and paternal education; improved access to, and utilization of, prenatal and neonatal health services; improved sanitation; and demographic changes—such as reduced family size and increased birth intervals. Notably, the analysis was only able to explain just over half of the reductions in stunting (55.7 percent). This is likely due to variables not included in the model given the limitations on data available through successive rounds of the Demographic and Health Survey. The authors speculate on the role that increased food security and agricultural production may have played during this period.

6 L. Taylor, *The Nutrition Agenda in Bangladesh: 'Too Massive to Handle'? Analysing Nutrition Governance: Bangladesh Country Report* (Sussex, UK: Institute of Development Studies, 2012), www.ids.ac.uk/files/dmfile/DFID_ANG_Bangladesh_Report_Final.pdf.

7 S. M. Hossain, A. Duffield, and A. Taylor, "An Evaluation of the Impact of a US$60 Million Nutrition Programme in Bangladesh," *Health Policy and Planning* 20, no. 1 (2005): 35–40; D. Sack, S. K. Roy, T. Ahmed, and G. Fuchs, "Responses to: 'An Evaluation of the Impact of a US$60 Million Nutrition Programme in Bangladesh'," *Health Policy and Planning* 20, no. 1 (2005): 406–407; F. J. Levinson and J. Eliot Rohde, "Responses to: 'An Evaluation of the Impact of a US$60 Million Nutrition Programme in Bangladesh'," *Health Policy and Planning* 20, no. 1 (2005): 406–407; H. White, "Comment on Contributions regarding the Impact of the Bangladesh Integrated Nutrition Project," *Health Policy and Planning* 20, no. 6 (2005): 408–411; World Bank, *The Bangladesh Integrated Nutrition Project Effectiveness and Lessons,* Bangladesh Development Series Paper 8 (Dhaka, Bangladesh: 2005); B. Sen, P. Menon, A. U. Ahmed, and F. P. Chowdhury, *Food Utilization and Nutrition Security,* paper prepared for Bangladesh Food Security Investment Forum, May 26, 2010.

8 L. Taylor, *The Nutrition Agenda in Bangladesh: 'Too Massive to Handle'?*

9 Bangladesh National Nutrition Services, "Operational Plan (Final draft) in Health, Population and Nutrition Sector Development Program (HPNSDP) 2011–2016" (Dhaka, Bangladesh: 2011).

10 K. Saha, M. Billah, P. Menon, S. El Arifeen, and N. Mbuya, *Bangladesh National Nutrition Services: Assessment of Implementation Status,* World Bank Studies (Washington, DC: World Bank, 2015); World Bank, *Bangladesh Poverty Assessment: Assessing a Decade of Progress in Reducing Poverty 2000–2010,* Bangladesh Development Series Paper 31 (Washington, DC: 2013).

11 Bangladesh Bureau of Statistics, *Preliminary Report on Household Income and Expenditure Survey—2010* (Dhaka, Bangladesh: 2011); UBINIG (Policy Research for Development Alternative), Bangladesh, "Country Report: Situation of Nutrition and Food Sovereignty in Bangladesh," 2014, accessed April 12, 2016, http://aprnet.org/wp-content/uploads/2014/08/Nutrition-and-Food-Sov-in-Bangladesh.pdf.

12 F. I. Jahan, M. T. Islam, M. Rajib-ul-Hasan, A. R. Chowdhury, S. Seraj, M. S. Aziz, R. Jahan, M. A.

Khatun, R. Freedman, and M. Rahmatullah, "A Survey on Non-conventional Plant Parts Consumed during Monga: A Seasonal Famine Which Affects the Northern Districts of Bangladesh," *American-Eurasian Journal of Sustainable Agriculture* 4, no. 2 (2010): 230–236.

13 M. Hossain, F. Naher, and Q. Shahabuddin, "Food Security and Nutrition in Bangladesh: Progress and Determinants," *Electronic Journal of Agricultural and Developmental Economics* 2, 2 (2005): 103–132.

14 Hossain et al., "An Evaluation of the Impact of a US$60 Million Nutrition Programme in Bangladesh."

15 A. Rabbani, "Household Food Security in Bangladesh: Going beyond Poverty Measures," *Bangladesh Development Studies* 31, nos. 1 and 2 (2014): 103–125.

16 Davis "Patterns of Socio-economic Mobility in Rural Bangladesh: Lessons from Life History Interviews," 155.

17 D. Lewis, *Bangladesh: Politics, Economy and Civil Society* (Cambridge: Cambridge University Press, 2011).

18 A. U. Ahmed, J. F. Hoddinott, and S. Roy, *Which Kinds of Social Safety Net Transfers Work Best for the Ultra Poor in Bangladesh? Operation and Impacts of the Transfer Modality Research Initiative* (Dhaka, Bangladesh: International Food Policy Research Institute and World Food Programme, 2016).

19 M. Hossain, "Pumping up Production: Shallow Tubewells and Rice in Bangladesh," in *Millions Fed: Proven Successes in Agricultural Development,* edited by D. J. Spielman and R. Pandya-Lorch (Washington, DC: International Food Policy Research Institute, 2009).

20 F. Naher, A. Barkat-e-Khuda, S. S. Ahmed, and M. Hossain, "How Nutrition-friendly are Agriculture and Health Policies in Bangladesh?" *Food and Nutrition Bulletin* 35, no. 1 (2014): 133–146.

21 Ibid.; Hossain, "Pumping Up Production: Shallow Tubewells and Rice in Bangladesh"; Hossain et al., "Food Security and Nutrition in Bangladesh: Progress and Determinants."

22 D. D. Headey et al., "The Other Asian Enigma: Explaining the Rapid Reduction of Undernutrition in Bangladesh."

23 Bangladesh Bureau of Statistics, *Preliminary Report on Household Income and Expenditure Survey—2010.*

24 Ibid.; Hossain et al., "Food Security and Nutrition in Bangladesh: Progress and Determinants."

25 Naher et al., "How Nutrition-friendly Are Agriculture and Health Policies in Bangladesh?"

26 A. Ahmed, *Bangladesh Integrated Household Survey (BIHS), 2011–2012* (Washington, DC: International Food Policy Research Institute, 2013).

27 R. King, A. Kelbert, N. Chisholm, and N. Hossain, *Help Yourself! Food Rights and Responsibilities: Year 2 Findings from Life in a Time of Food Price Volatility,* Joint Agency Research Report (Brighton and Oxford, UK: IDS and Oxfam, 2014).

28 World Bank, *Maintaining Momentum to 2015? An Impact Evaluation of Interventions to Improve Maternal and Child Health and Nutrition Outcomes in Bangladesh* (Washington, DC: Operations Evaluation Department, World Bank, 2005).

29 A. M. R. Chowdhury, A. Bhuiya, M. E. Chowdhury, S. Rasheed, Z. Hussain, and Lincoln C. Chen, "The Bangladesh Paradox: Exceptional Health Achievement Despite Economic Poverty," *The Lancet* 382, no. 9906 (2013): 1734–1745.

30 NIPORT (National Institute of Population Research and Training), MA (Mitra and Associates), and ICF (ICF International), *Bangladesh Demographic and Health Survey 2011* (Dhaka, Bangladesh, and Calverton, Maryland, USA, 2013): 59.

31 D. D. Headey et al., "The Other Asian Enigma: Explaining the Rapid Reduction of Undernutrition in Bangladesh."

32 S. El Arifeen, A. Christou, L. Reichenbach, F. A. Osman, K. Azad, K. S. Islam, F. Ahmed, H. B. Perry, and D. H. Peters, "Community-based Approaches and Partnerships: Innovations in Health-service Delivery in Bangladesh," *The Lancet* 382, no. 9909 (2013): 2012–2026.

33 Ibid.; Chowdhury et al., "The Bangladesh Paradox: Exceptional Health Achievement despite Economic Poverty."

34 National Institute of Population Research and Training (NIPORT), Mitra and Associates, and ICF International, *Bangladesh Demographic and Health Survey 2014: Key Indicators* (Dhaka, Bangladesh, and Rockville, Maryland, USA, 2015).

35 Ibid.

36 D. D. Headey et al., "The Other Asian Enigma: Explaining the Rapid Reduction of Undernutrition in Bangladesh."

37 A. M. R. Chowdhury et al., "The Bangladesh Paradox: Exceptional Health Achievement despite Economic Poverty."

38 NIPORT, Mitra and Associates, and ICF International, *Bangladesh Demographic and Health Survey 2014: Key Indicators;* Helen Keller International (HKI) and James P Grant School of Public Health, *State of Food Security and Nutrition in Bangladesh: 2013* (Dhaka, Bangladesh, 2014).

39 The net enrollment rate of children in primary school increased from 72.4 percent in 1990 to 94.5 percent in 2010 (World Bank, World Development Indicators, Bangladesh Database, accessed April 12, 2016).

40 B. Baulch, "The Medium-term Impact of the Primary Education Stipend in Rural Bangladesh," *Journal of Development Effectiveness* 3, no. 2 (2011): 243–262.

41 J. Raynor and K. Wesson, "The Girl's Stipend Program in Bangladesh," *Journal of Education for International Development* 2, no. 2 (2006): 1–12; A. M. R. Chowdhury, S. R. Nath, and R. K. Choudhury, "Enrolment at Primary Level: Gender Difference Disappears in Bangladesh," *International Journal of Educational Development* 22 (2002): 191–203;

M. Huq and M. Rahman, "Gender Disparities in Secondary Education in Bangladesh," *International Education Studies* 1, no. 2 (2008): 115–128.

42 D. D. Headey et al., "The Other Asian Enigma: Explaining the Rapid Reduction of Undernutrition in Bangladesh."

43 UNICEF and World Health Organization (WHO), *Progress on Sanitation and Drinking Water: 2015 Update and MDG Assessment* (Geneva: WHO, 2015); R. L. Guerrant, J. B. Schorling, J. F. McAuliffe, and M. A. De Souza, "Diarrhea as a Cause and an Effect of Malnutrition: Diarrhea Prevents Catch-Up Growth and Malnutrition Increases Diarrhea Frequency and Duration," *American Journal of Tropical Medicine and Hygiene* 47, no. 1, part 2 (1992): 28–35.

44 S. S. Lim, T. Vos, A. D. Flaxman, G. Danaei, K. Shibuya, H. Adair-Rohani, M. A. AlMazroa, et al., "A Comparative Risk Assessment of Burden of Disease and Injury Attributable to 67 Risk Factors and Risk Factor Clusters in 21 Regions, 1990–2010: A Systematic Analysis for the Global Burden of Disease Study 2010," *The Lancet* 380, no. 9859 (2013): 2224–2260.

45 UNICEF and WHO, *Progress on Sanitation and Drinking Water: 2015 Update and MDG Assessment.*

46 D. D. Headey et al., "The Other Asian Enigma: Explaining the Rapid Reduction of Undernutrition in Bangladesh."

47 UNICEF and WHO, *Progress on Sanitation and Drinking Water: 2015 Update and MDG Assessment.*

48 Ibid., 20.

49 D. D. Headey et al., "The Other Asian Enigma: Explaining the Rapid Reduction of Undernutrition in Bangladesh."

50 E. Sraboni, H. J. Malapit, A. R. Quisumbing, and A. U. Ahmed, "Women's Empowerment in Agriculture: What Role for Food Security in Bangladesh?" *World Development* 61 (2014): 11–52.

51 N. Kabeer, "Conflicts over Credit: Re-evaluating the Empowerment Potential of Loans to Women in Rural Bangladesh," *World Development* 29, no. 1 (2001): 63–84.

52 In 2011, 41 percent of children under 5 were stunted, 16 percent wasted, and 36 percent underweight (NIPORT, MA, and ICF, *Bangladesh Demographic and Health Survey 2011*).

Chapter 13

1 K. Cunningham, A. Singh, D. D. Headey, P. Pandey Rana, and C. Karmacharya, *Stories of Change in Nutrition: Nepal* (Washington, DC: International Food Policy Research Institute, forthcoming); D. D. Headey and J. Hoddinott, "Understanding the Rapid Reduction of Undernutrition in Nepal, 2001–2011," *PLoS ONE* 10, no. 12 (2015): e0145738, doi:10.1371/journal.pone.0145738; Government of Nepal, Ministry of Health and Population, New Era, and ICF International, *Nepal Demographic and Health Survey* (Kathmandu, Nepal, and Calverton, MD, USA, 2011); World Bank, *Accelerating Progress in Reducing Maternal and Child Undernutrition in Nepal* (Kathmandu, Nepal, 2012); J. Crum, J. Mason, R. Pokharel, P. Hutchinson, S. Mebrahtu, P. Dahal, *Trends and Determinants of Maternal and Child Nutrition in Nepal: Further Analysis of the Nepal Health and Demographic Surveys, 1996–2011* (Kathmandu, Nepal: Government of Nepal, Ministry of Health and Population and UNICEF, 2013).

2 UNICEF, *Strategy for Improved Nutrition of Children and Women in Developing Countries,* Policy Review Paper E/ICEF/1990/1.6 (New York, 1990); Z. A. Bhutta, K. J. Das, A. Rizvi, M. F. Gaffey, N. Walker, S. Horton, P. Webb, A. Lartey, and R. E. Black, "Evidence-Based Interventions for Improvement of Maternal and Child Nutrition: What Can Be Done and at What Cost?" *Lancet* 382, no. 9890 (2013): 452–477, doi:10.1016/S0140-6736(13)60996-4.

3 Standing Committee on Nutrition, *Scaling Up Nutrition: Progress Report from Countries and Their Partners in the Movement to SUN* (Geneva: SUN Movement Secretariat, 2011); International Food Policy Research Institute (IFPRI), *Global Nutrition Report 2014: Actions and Accountability to Accelerate the World's Progress on Nutrition* (Washington, DC, 2014); IFPRI, *Global Nutrition Report 2015: Actions and Accountability to Advance Nutrition and Sustainable Development* (Washington, DC, 2015).

4 Stunting is an indicator of linear growth deficit calculated as children who have a height-for-age Z-score (HAZ) < -2.0 SD from the median of the reference population, based on the 2006 World Health Organization growth standards.

5 Maternal undernutrition is represented here as underweight, which is calculated as a body mass index (BMI) of less than 18.5. BMI is the ratio of weight (in kilograms) to height squared, for nonpregnant women.

6 Government of Nepal, Ministry of Health and Population et al., *Nepal Demographic and Health Survey.*

7 Headey and Hoddinott, "Understanding the Rapid Reduction of Undernutrition in Nepal, 2001–2011."

8 Cunningham et al., *Stories of Change in Nutrition: Nepal.*

9 V. Khanal, Y. Zhao, and K. Sauer, "Role of Antenatal Care and Iron Supplementation during Pregnancy in Preventing Low Birth Weight in Nepal: Comparison of National Surveys 2006 and 2011," *Archives of Public Health* 72, no. 1 (2014): 4, doi:10.1186/2049-3258-72-4; T. Powell-Jackson, and K. Hanson, "Financial Incentives for Maternal Health: Impact of a National Programme in Nepal," *Journal of Health Economics* 31, no. 1 (2012): 271–284, doi:10.1016/j.jhealeco.2011.10.010.

10 Nepal Health Economics Association, *Public Expenditure Review on Health Sector: 2003/2004 to 2005/2006* (Kathmandu, 2009); B. Ghimire and M. Gautam, "Social

Sector Budget Sees a Whooping 40pc Increase," *eKantipur*, July 15, 2013.

11 Nepal, Ministry of Health and Population, New Era, and USAID, *An Analytical Report on Female Community Health Volunteers of Selected Districts of Nepal* (Kathmandu, 2007).

12 Government of Nepal, Ministry of Health and Population et al., *Nepal Demographic and Health Survey*.

13 Powell-Jackson and Hanson, "Financial Incentives for Maternal Health."

14 Ibid.

15 Khanal, Zhao, and Sauer, "Role of Antenatal Care and Iron Supplementation during Pregnancy"; Headey and Hoddinott, "Understanding the Rapid Reduction of Undernutrition in Nepal, 2001–2011."

16 Nepal, National Hygiene and Sanitation Coordination Committee, "Nepal Country Paper," paper presented at the Sixth South Asian Conference on Sanitation, Dhaka, Bangladesh, January 11–13, 2016.

17 Ibid.

18 National Hygiene and Sanitation Coordination Committee (Nepal), Nepal Country Paper on the Sixth South Asian Conference on Sanitation, Dhaka, Bangladesh, 2016.

19 World Bank, *Accelerating Progress in Reducing Maternal and Child Undernutrition in Nepal*.

20 Government of Nepal, Central Bureau of Statistics, *Nepal Living Standard Survey 2010–2011: Statistical Report*, vols. 1 and 2 (Kathmandu, 2011); C. P. Acharya and R. Leon-Gonzalez, *The Impact of Remittance on Poverty and Inequality: A Micro-Simulation Study for Nepal*, GRIPS Discussion Paper 11-26 (Tokyo: National Graduate Institute for Policy Studies [GRIPS], 2012).

21 World Bank, *Accelerating Progress in Reducing Maternal and Child Undernutrition in Nepal*.

22 Government of Nepal, Ministry of Agricultural Development, *Agriculture Development Strategy 2015–2035* (Kathmandu, 2015).

23 World Bank, *Accelerating Progress in Reducing Maternal and Child Undernutrition in Nepal;* Headey and Hoddinott, "Understanding the Rapid Reduction of Undernutrition in Nepal, 2001–2011."

24 World Bank, *Nepal Public Expenditure Review*, Report No. 55388-NP (Kathmandu: World Bank Poverty Reduction and Economic Management Sector Unit, South Asia Region, 2010).

25 Nepal, Ministry of Education, *School Level Educational Statistics of Nepal*, Consolidated Report 2011 (2068) (Sanothimi, Bhaktapur, Nepal, 2012).

26 Government of Nepal, National Planning Commission, *Multi-Sectoral Nutrition Plan for Accelerating the Reduction of Maternal and Child Under-nutrition in Nepal* (Kathmandu, 2012).

27 Government of Nepal, Ministry of Health and Population et al., *Nepal Demographic and Health Survey*.

28 Ibid.

29 Ibid.

30 K. Cunningham, M. Ruel, E. Ferguson, and R. Uauy, "Women's Empowerment and Child Nutrition Status in South Asia: A Synthesis of the Literature," *Maternal and Child Nutrition* 11, no. 1 (2015): 1–19, doi:10.1111/mcn.12125; K. Cunningham, G. B. Ploubidis, P. Menon, M. Ruel, S. Kadiyala, R. Uauy, and E. Ferguson, "Women's Empowerment in Agriculture and Child Nutritional Status in Rural Nepal," *Public Health Nutrition* 18, no. 17 (2015): 3134–3145, doi:10.1017/S1368980015000683; H. Malapit, S. Kadiyala, A. Quisumbing, K. Cunningham, and P. Tyagi, "Women's Empowerment Mitigates the Negative Effects of Low Production Diversity on Maternal and Child Nutrition in Nepal," *Journal of Development Studies* 51, no. 8 (2014): 54–63.

Chapter 14

1 INEI (Instituto Nacional de Estadística de Informática, Perú), *Encuesta Demográfica y de Salud Familiar - ENDES*. Demographic and Health Surveys (Lima, 2014).

2 Ibid.

3 INEI, *Encuesta Demográfica y de Salud Familiar- ENDES 2014* (Lima, 2015): 311.

4 INEI, *Encuesta Demográfica y de Salud Familiar- ENDES* Continua 2004–2006 (Lima, 2007): 31.

5 A. Mejía Acosta, *Analysing Success in the Fight against Malnutrition in Peru*, IDS Working Paper 367 (Brighton, UK: Institute of Development Studies, 2011).

6 M. Tanaka and S. Vera, "Peru: La Dinamica 'Neodualista' de una Democracia sin Sistema de Partidos" in *Democracia en la Region Andina: Diversidad y Desafios*, edited by M. Cameron and J. P. Luna (Lima: Instituto de Estudios Peruanos, 2010).

7 Mejía Acosta, *Analysing Success in the Fight against Malnutrition in Peru*.

8 Scaling Up Nutrition Civil Society Network, "Peru: Working Together for Accountability for Nutrition" in *Think Piece on Accountability for Nutrition* (2015), http://bit.ly/1oPuNAt; Boston Consulting Group, "Ending Hunger Project: Peru Case Study," May 2015 (unpublished).

9 World Bank, "Realizing Rights through Social Guarantees: An Analysis of New Approaches to Social Policy in Latin America and South Africa," Report 40047 (Washington, DC: World Bank, 2008).

10 D. Stifel and H. Alderman, "The 'Glass of Milk' Subsidy Program and Malnutrition in Peru," *World Bank Economic Review* 20, 3 (2006): 421–448.

11 Mejía Acosta, *Analysing Success in the Fight against Malnutrition in Peru.* Before 2005, Peru's National Institute of Statistics and Informatics (Instituto Nacional de Estadística e Informática, INEI) was using the National Center for Health Statistics (NCHS)/WHO growth standards.

12 World Bank, World Development Indicators, GDP Growth Dataset, accessed April 4, 2016, http://data.worldbank.org/indicator/NY.GDP.MKTP.KD.ZG.

13 E. H. Vásquez, *Análisis de las Garantías Sociales en Educación, Salud, Alimentación y Pueblos Indígenas en el Perú* (Lima, Peru: Universidad del Pacífico, 2007).

14 IEH (Instituto de Estudios del Hambre/Institute of Hunger Studies), *A Comparative Study on Institutional Frameworks for Food Security and Nutrition at the National Level* (Madrid, 2012).

15 N. Jones, R. Vargas, and E. Villar, "Conditional Cash Transfers in Peru: Tackling the Multi-dimensionality of Poverty and Vulnerability" in *Social Protection Initiatives for Families, Women, and Children: An Analysis of Recent Experiences,* edited by A. Minujin (New York. New School and UNICEF, 2007).

16 E. Perova and R. Vakis, "5 Years in *Juntos:* New Evidence on the Program's Short and Long-Term Impacts," *Economia* 35, no. 69 (2012): 53–82.

17 C. T. Anderson, S. A. Reynolds, J. R. Behrman, B. T. Crookston, K. A. Dearden, J. Escobal, S. Mani, et al., "Participation in the Juntos Conditional Cash Transfer Program in Peru Is Associated with Changes in Child Anthropometric Status but Not Language Development or School Achievement," *Journal of Nutrition* 145, no. 10 (2015): 2396–2405.

18 Levinson and Balarajan, *Addressing Malnutrition Multisectorally.*

19 A. Mejía Acosta and L. Haddad, "The Politics of Success in the Fight against Malnutrition in Peru," *Food Policy* 44 (2014): 26–35.

20 Peru, Ministry of Social Development and Ministry of Labor and Employment Protection, "Articulation of Inter-sectoral Policies and Actions in Social Protection and Employment," presentation at seminar on Inter-sectoral Public Policies: Social Protection and Employment, Rio de Janeiro, Brazil, November 30–December 1, 2010.

21 F. J. Levinson and Y. Balarajan, *Addressing Malnutrition Multisectorally: What Have We Learned from Recent International Experience?* UNICEF Nutrition Working Paper (New York: UNICEF and MDG Achievement Fund, 2013).

22 INEI, *Encuesta Demográfica y de Salud Familiar- ENDES 2014.*

23 Levinson and Balarajan, *Addressing Malnutrition Multisectorally.*

24 J. Garrett, L. Bassett, and A. Marini, *Designing CCT Programs to Improve Nutrition Impact: Principles, Evidence, and Examples,* Working Paper 6 (Santiago, Chile: United Nations Food and Agriculture Organization [FAO] Hunger-Free Latin America and the Caribbean Initiative, 2009).

25 Perova and Vakis, "5 Years in *Juntos.*"

26 Ibid.

27 A. Sanchez and M. Jaramillo, "Impacto del Programa Juntos sobre Nutrición temprana," *Revista Estudios Economicos,* Report 23 (Lima, Peru: Banco Central de Reserva del Perú, 2012).

28 C. T. Anderson et al., "Participation in the Juntos Conditional Cash Transfer Program in Peru."

29 Mejía Acosta and Haddad, "The Politics of Success in the Fight against Malnutrition in Peru."

30 Banco Mundial, *Diagnostico del Impacto Social y Distributivo de la Descentralización de los Programas Sociales: Plan de Incentivos Municipales* (Lima: World Bank, 2013).

31 Levinson and Balarajan, *Addressing Malnutrition Multisectorally.*

32 L. Levard and V. Alby Flores, *Reconciling Agriculture and Nutrition: Case Study on Agricultural Policies and Nutrition in Peru* (Paris: Action contre la Faim, 2013).

33 Mejía Acosta, *"Analysing Success in the Fight against Malnutrition in Peru."*

34 Corporación Latinobarómetro, Latinobarómetro 2008 Banco de Datos, accessed on February 15, 2016. http://www.latinobarometro.org/latContents.jsp.

35 Mejía Acosta and Haddad, "The Politics of Success in the Fight against Malnutrition in Peru."

36 Ibid.

37 E. Perova and R. Vakis, *Welfare Impacts of the "Juntos" Program in Peru: Evidence from a Non-experimental Evaluation* (Washington, DC: World Bank, 2009).

38 C. Loret de Mola, R. Quispe, G. A. Valle, and J. A. Poterico, "Nutritional Transition in Children under Five Years and Women of Reproductive Age: A 15-Years Trend Analysis in Peru," *PLOS One* 9, no. 3 (2014): 1–10.

39 S. Gillespie, L. Haddad, V. Mannar, P. Menon, and N. Nisbett, "The Politics of Reducing Malnutrition: Building Commitment and Accelerating Progress" (web supplement), *The Lancet* 382, no. 9891 (2013): 552–569.

Chapter 15

1 World Bank, World Development Indicators 2014 (Washington, 2014).

2 P. Glewwe, S. Koch, and B. Nguyen, "Child Nutrition, Economic Growth, and the Provision of Health Services in Vietnam," in *Economic Growth, Poverty, and Household Welfare in Vietnam,* edited by P. Glewwe, N. Agrawal, and D. Dollar (Washington: World Bank, 2004). Note that this uses the World Bank's $1.25/day measurement (rather than the revised $2.00/day that was used in later years) for comparison with the poverty rates mentioned earlier in the chapter.

3 Ibid.

4 Ibid.

5 World Bank, *Vietnam Growing Healthy: A Review of Vietnam's Health Sector* 22210-VN (Hanoi, 2001).

6 Ibid., L. T. Hop, "Programs to Improve Production and Consumption of Animal Source Foods and Malnutrition in Vietnam," *Journal of Nutrition* 133 (2003): 4006S–4009S.

7 World Bank, Development Research Group, World Development Indicators 2015, accessed February 25, 2016, http://data.worldbank.org/datacatalog/world-development-indicators.

8 I. Bhushan, E. Bloom, N. H. Huu, and N. M. Thang, *Human Capital of the Poor in Vietnam* (Manila: Asian Development Bank, 2001); P. Glewwe et al., "Child Nutrition, Economic Growth, and the Provision of Health Services in Vietnam."

9 VDD (National Institute of Nutrition), Databank of Child Nutrition Situation in Viet Nam (2012), http://viendinhduong.vn/news/vi/106/61/a/so-lieu-thong-ke-ve-tinh-trang-dinh-duong-tre-em-quacac-nam.aspx.

10 World Bank, *Vietnam Health Sector Review* (Hanoi, 2001).

11 UNICEF, World Health Organization (WHO), and World Bank, 2013 Joint Child Malnutrition Estimates: Levels and Trends (New York, Geneva, and Washington, DC, 2015).

12 K. Lapping, P. Webb, E. Frongillo, and J. Coates, "Understanding the Sociopolitical and Epidemiological Dimensions of Malnutrition in Viet Nam," PhD thesis, Tufts University, 2012.

13 Ibid.

14 Ministry of Health and National Institute of Nutrition, *Plan of Action for Infant and Young Child Feeding 2006–2010* (Hanoi, 2006).

15 UNICEF, Global Databases 2015 based on Multiple Indicator Cluster Surveys (MICS), Demographic and Health Surveys (DHS), and other nationally representative surveys, accessed February 6, 2016, http://data.unicef.org/nutrition/iycf.html; N. Hajeebhoy, P. H. Nguyen, D. T. Tran, and M. de Onis, "Introducing Infant and Young Child Feeding Indicators into National Nutrition Surveillance Systems: Lessons from Vietnam," *Maternal and Child Nutrition* 9, Suppl. 2 (2013): 131–149.

16 A. Laillou, T. V. Pham, N. T. Tran, H. T. Le, F. Wieringa, F. Rohner, S. Fortin, et al., "Micronutrient Deficits Are Still Public Health Issues among Women and Young Children in Vietnam," *PLoS ONE* 7, no. 4 (2012): e34906, doi:10.1371/journal.pone.0034906.

17 International Food Policy Research Institute, *Global Nutrition Report 2015,* Nutrition Country Profile: Vietnam, http://ebrary.ifpri.org/utils/getfile/collection/p15738coll2/id/130055/filename/130266.pdf; World Health Organization, Nutrition: Global Targets Indicators 2014, http://www.who.int/nutrition/globaltargets_indicators/en/.

18 A. Laillou, et al., "Micronutrient Deficits Are Still Public Health Issues among Women and Young Children in Vietnam."

19 Ibid.

20 A. Laillou, J. Berger, B. M. Le, V. T. Pham, T. H. Le, C. K. Nguyen, D. Panagides, F. Rohner, F. Wieringa, and R. Moench-Pfanner, "Improvement of the Vietnamese Diet for Women of Reproductive Age by Micronutrient Fortification of Staple Foods and Condiments," *PLoS ONE* 7, no. 11 (2012): e50538, doi:10.1371/journal.pone.0050538

21 Scaling Up Nutrition, *2015 SUN Movement Annual Progress Report,* Vietnam Country Profile (Geneva).

22 L. T. Hop, "Programs to Improve Production and Consumption of Animal Source Foods and Malnutrition in Vietnam," *Journal of Nutrition* 133 (2003): 4006S–4009S; N. M. Thang, and B. M. Popkin, "Patterns of Food Consumption in Vietnam: Effects on Socioeconomic Groups during an Era of Economic Growth," *European Journal of Clinical Nutrition* 58 (2004): 145–153.

23 World Bank, *Vietnam Poverty Assessment: Well Begun, Not Yet Done: Vietnam's Remarkable Progress on Poverty Reduction and the Emerging Challenges* (Hanoi, 2012).

24 National Institute of Nutrition (VDD), National Nutrition Surveillance Dataset (2014), http://viendinhduong.vn/viewpdf.aspx?n=/TT%20tin%20Dd_2014/SDD_2014.pdf.

25 N. M. Thang and B. Popkin, "Child Malnutrition in Vietnam and Its Transition in an Era of Economic Growth," *Journal of Human Nutrition and Dietetics* 16, no. 4 (2003): 233–244.

26 K. Lapping, E. A. Frongillo, P. H. Nguyen, J. Coates, P. Webb, and P. Menon, "Organizational Factors, Planning Capacity, and Integration Challenges Constrain Provincial Planning Processes for Nutrition in Decentralizing Vietnam," *Food and Nutrition Bulletin* 35, no. 3 (2014): 382–391.

27 Ibid.

28 S. S. Lieberman, J. J. Capuno, and H. V. Minh, "Decentralizing Health: Lessons from Indonesia, the Philippines, and Vietnam," in *East Asia Decentralizes: Making*

Local Government Work (Washington: World Bank, 2005), 155–178.

29 K. Lapping, et al., "Organizational Factors, Planning Capacity, and Integration Challenges Constrain Provincial Planning Processes for Nutrition in Decentralizing Vietnam."

30 Ibid.

31 L. M. Do, T. K. Tran, B. Eriksson, M. Petzold, C. T. K. Nguyen, and H. Asche, "Preschool Overweight and Obesity in Urban and Rural Vietnam: Differences in Prevalence and Associated Factors," *Global Health Action* 8 (2015): 28615, doi:10.3402/gha.v8.28615.

32 P. V. Nguyen, T. K. Hong, T. Hoang, D. T. Nguyen, and A. R. Robert, "High Prevalence of Overweight among Adolescents in Ho Chi Minh City, Vietnam," *BMC Public Health,* 13 (2013): 141, www.biomedcentral.com/1471-2458/13/141.

Chapter 16

1 USAID (United States Agency for International Development), "Ethiopia: Nutrition Profile" (2014, updated February 8, 2016), https://www.usaid.gov/what-we-do/global-health/nutrition/countries/ethiopia-nutrition-profile.

2 International Food Policy Research Institute, *Global Nutrition Report Country Profile: Ethiopia,* Global Nutrition Report series (Washington, DC: IFPRI, 2014).

3 WHO, UNICEF, USAID, AED, UC DAVIS, and IFPRI, "Indicators for Assessing Infant and Young Child Feeding Practices. Part I: Definitions. Conclusions of a Consensus Meeting Held 6–8 November 2007 in Washington DC" (Geneva: World Health Organization, 2008).

4 IFPRI, *Global Nutrition Report Country Profile: Ethiopia.*

5 UNICEF (United Nations Children's Emergency Fund), "UNICEF Conceptual Framework," Nutrition in Emergencies, lesson 2.5, slide 4 (1990), http://www.unicef.org/nutrition/training/2.5/4.html; M. Ruel, H. Alderman, and Maternal and Child Nutrition Study Group, "Nutrition-Sensitive Interventions and Programmes: How Can They Help to Accelerate Progress in Improving Maternal and Child Nutrition?" *The Lancet* 382, no. 9891 (2013): 536–551.

6 N. Workie, W. Ramana, and N. V. Gandham, *The Health Extension Program in Ethiopia* (Washington, DC: World Bank, 2013).

7 UNICEF, Community Based Nutrition Briefing Note (December 2013), http://www.unicef.org/ethiopia/2014-12-15-NUTRITION-based.pdf.

8 R. Sauers, "New Fortified Wheat Flour Launched by Astco Food Complex" (March 17, 2015), https://www.usaid.gov/ethiopia/press-releases/new-fortified-wheat-flour-launched-astco-food-complex.

9 Global Alliance for Improved Nutrition (GAIN), "Ethiopia Universal Salt Iodization," http://www.gainhealth.org/knowledge-centre/project/ethiopia-universal-salt-iodization/.

10 Federal Democratic Republic of Ethiopia, *National Nutrition Program (2013–2015)* (Addis Ababa, Ethiopia: Government of Ethiopia, Ministry of Health, 2013).

11 IFPRI, *Global Nutrition Report Country Profile: Ethiopia.*

12 Water and Sanitation Program, "Learning by Doing: Working at Scale in Ethiopia," Water and Sanitation Program Learning Note (July 2011), www.wsp.org/sites/wsp.org/files/publications/WSP-Ethiopia-at-scale.pdf.

13 Federal Democratic Republic of Ethiopia, *National Nutrition Program.*

14 USAID, Nutrition Sensitive Agriculture Tool (Nutri-SAT) Ethiopian Pilot Study (2013), ethioagp.org/download/featured%20docs/Ethiopia%20Nutri-SAT%20pilot%20study%209_26_13.pdf.

15 USAID, "Ethiopia: Nutrition Profile" (2014).

16 Scaling Up Nutrition (SUN), Ethiopia, scalingupnutrition.org/wp-content/uploads/2015/10/SUN_Report2015_EN_Ethiopia.pdf; M. Beyero, J. Hodge, and A. Lewis, *Leveraging Agriculture for Nutrition in East Africa Country Report: Ethiopia* (Rome and Washington, DC: Food and Agriculture Organization of the United Nations and IFPRI, 2015).

17 D. Headey, *An Analysis of Trends and Determinants of Child Undernutrition in Ethiopia, 2000–2011,* Ethiopia Strategy Support Program (ESSP) II Working Paper 70 (Washington, DC, and Addis Ababa, Ethiopia: IFPRI and Ethiopian Development Research Institute [EDRI], 2014); D. Headey, "Nutrition in Ethiopia: An Emerging Success Story?" ESSP II Research Note 40 (Washington, DC: IFPRI, 2015).

18 D. Headey, *An Analysis of Trends and Determinants of Child Undernutrition in Ethiopia, 2000–2011.*

19 Food and Agriculture Organization of the United Nations, "Ethiopia: Economic Indicators," http://faostat.fao.org/CountryProfiles/Country_Profile/Direct.aspx?lang=en&area=238.

20 D. Headey, "Nutrition in Ethiopia: An Emerging Success Story?"

21 Ibid.

22 G. Berhane et al., *Evaluation of Ethiopia's Food Security Program: Documenting Progress in Implementation of the Productive Safety Nets Programme and the Household Asset Building Programme,* ESSP II–EDRI Report (Washington, DC: IFPRI, May 2013).

23 F. N. Bachewe, G. Berhane, B. Minten, and A. S. Taffesse, *Agricultural Growth in Ethiopia (2004–2014): Evidence and Drivers,* ESSP II Working Paper no. 81 (Washington, DC: IFPRI, 2015).

24 Ibid.

25 World Bank, "Ethiopia to Benefit from World Bank Support for Social Safety Net" (September 30, 2014), http://www.worldbank.org/en/news/press-release/2014/09/30/ethiopia-to-benefit-from-world-bank-support-for-social-safety-net.

26 A. Kuyvenhoven, J. Pender, and R. Ruben, "Development Strategies for Less-Favoured Areas," *Food Policy* 29, no. 4 (2004): 295–302.

27 L. A. German, J. Mowo, T. Amede, and K. Masuki, eds., *Integrated Natural Resource Management in the Highlands of Eastern Africa: From Concept to Practice* (London: Earthscan, 2012).

28 M. Beyero, J. Hodge, and A. Lewis, *Leveraging Agriculture for Nutrition in East Africa (LANEA): Country Report – Ethiopia* (FAO and IFPRI, 2015).

29 A. Warren, "Interview with Kebele Leader 1" (unpublished manuscript, Wolaita, SNNPR, Ethiopia: September 2015a).

30 Water and Sanitation Program, "From Burden to Communal Responsibility: A Sanitation Success Story from Southern Region in Ethiopia," WSP Field Note, Sanitation and Hygiene Series (January 2007).

31 Water and Sanitation Program, "Learning by Doing."

32 Water and Sanitation Program, "From Burden to Communal Responsibility."

33 D. Headey, *An Analysis of Trends and Determinants of Child Undernutrition in Ethiopia, 2000–2011;* D. Headey, "Nutrition in Ethiopia: An Emerging Success Story?"

34 Water and Sanitation Program, "Learning by Doing."

35 A. Warren, "Interview with Wolaita Zone Health Official" (unpublished manuscript, Wolaita, Sodo, Ethiopia: September 2015b).

36 Water and Sanitation Program, "From Burden to Communal Responsibility."

37 S. Baye H. Kloos, W. Mulat, A. Assayie, G. Gullis, A. Kumie, and B. Yirsaw, , "Assessment on the Approaches Used for Water and Sanitation Programs in Southern Ethiopia," *Water Resources Management* 26, no. 15 (2012): 4295–4309.

38 Ibid.

39 Water and Sanitation Program, "Learning by Doing."

40 Plan International, *Community-Led Total Sanitation in Ethiopia: Findings from a Situational Assessment* (Research Summary, February 2015).

41 O. Jones, *Monitoring Sanitation and Hygiene in Rural Ethiopia: A Diagnostic Analysis of Systems, Tools, and Capacity,* Water and Sanitation Program Technical Paper (June 2015).

42 Ethiopia Strategy Support Program (ESSP); IFPRI, "Helping to Make Programs Nutrition Sensitive," ESSP Outcome Note no. 9 (September 2015), http://essp.ifpri.info/files/2015/10/Outcome-Note_9_ESSP-and-the-PSNP.pdf.

43 G. Berhane, D. O. Gilligan, J. Hoddinott, N. Kumar, and A. S. Taffesse, "Can Social Protection Work in Africa? The Impact of Ethiopia's Productive Safety Net Programme," *Economic Development and Cultural Change* 63, no. 1 (2014): 1–26.

44 UNICEF, *UNICEF Annual Report: Ethiopia,* 2014.

45 Berhane et al., *Evaluation of Ethiopia's Food Security Program.*

46 A. Bossuyt, *Increasing Nutrition Outcomes of PSNP and HABP. Part 1, Main Report* (2014).

47 Federal Democratic Republic of Ethiopia, *Productive Safety Net Program Phase 4: Enhanced Social Assessment and Consultation Final Report* (Addis Ababa: Government of Ethiopia, Ministry of Agriculture, 2014).

48 World Bank, *Ethiopia: Productive Safety Nets Project Four* (Washington, DC, 2014), http://documents.worldbank.org/curated/en/2014/09/20198224/ethiopia-productive-safety-nets-project-4.

49 Ibid.

50 UNICEF, *UNICEF Annual Report: Ethiopia, 2014.*

51 S. Fan and C. Chan-Kang, "Returns to Investment in Less-Favored Areas in Developing Countries: A Synthesis of Evidence and Implications for Africa," *Food Policy* 29, no. 4 (2004): 431–444.

52 K. Hirvonen, "From Market to Mesob: Ensuring Access to Food Is Key to Improving Diets in Ethiopia" (March 8, 2016), http://www.ifpri.org/blog/market-mesob-ensuring-access-food-key-improving-diets-ethiopia.

Chapter 17

We thank the government of Odisha, India, especially the Department of Women and Child Development and the Department of Health, for their support of this study. We also thank several current and retired government officials and other stakeholders with knowledge about Odisha who provided information and perspectives. We are grateful to Development Corner (DCOR) Consulting, Odisha, for support of our qualitative research.

1 "Scheduled tribe" is an official designation of the Government of India applied to "tribal" populations; these populations are also referred to as *adivasis.*

2 NFHS 1992–1993, NFHS 1998–1999, NFHS 2005–2006, and RSOC 2013–2014. NFHS data are for children under 3 years of age. Data for 2013–2014 are for children under 5 years of age using the more recent RSOC, which was commissioned by the Ministry of Women and Child Development with technical and financial assistance from UNICEF India.

3 N. Raykar, M. Majumder, R. Laxminarayan, and P. Menon, *India Health Report: Nutrition 2015* (New Delhi: Public Health Foundation of India, 2015).

4 NFHS, *National Family Health Survey (NFHS-3): India,* vol. 1 (Mumbai: International Institute for Population Sciences, 2005).

5 Raykar et al., *India Health Report: Nutrition 2015.*

6 E. Cavatorta, B. Shankar, and A. F. Martinez, "Explaining Cross-State Disparities in Child Nutrition in Rural India," *World Development* 76 (2015): 216–237.

7 Two primary methods were used to examine changes in the past 25 years in nutrition outcomes among children in Odisha: (1) development of a timeline documenting changes in a variety of nutrition outcomes, determinants, and programs and policies, using multiple data sources; and (2) interviews with several stakeholders involved in shaping policies and programs over this 25-year period. The timeline of progress in nutrition outcomes and determinants, from 1991 to 2015, was developed using data from multiple rounds of the NFHS and other surveys. The policy and program timeline was based on a desk review of policy and program documents and stakeholder interviews, which were coded and analyzed to assess key drivers of change in programs and policies.

8 S. Gillespie, P. Menon, and A. L. Kennedy, "Scaling Up Impact on Nutrition: What Will It Take?" *Advances in Nutrition* 6 (2015): 440–451.

9 D. Thomas, B. L. Sarangi, A. Garg, A. Ahuja, P. Meherda, S. R. Karthikeyan, P. Joddar, R. Kar, J. Pattnaik, R. Druvasula, and A. D. Rath, "Closing the Health and Nutrition Gap in Odisha, India: A Case Study of How Transforming the Health System Is Achieving Greater Equity," *Social Science & Medicine* 145 (2015): 154–162.

10 Department of Health and Family Welfare, Government of Odisha, "Infant Mortality Rate Mission," http://203.193.146.66/hfw/IMR_Mission.asp?GL=8.

11 Department of Health and Family Welfare, Government of Odisha, *Navajyoti: A Strategy to Improve Maternal and Child Care with Focus on Prevention on Morbidity and Mortality Among New Borns* (Bhubaneswar, Odisha, India: Department of Health and Family Welfare, 2004).

12 Ibid.

13 Programme Evaluation Organisation Planning Commission, "Evaluation Study of National Rural Health Mission (NRHM) In 7 States" (New Delhi: Government of India, February 2011), http://planningcommission.nic.in/reports/peoreport/peoevalu/peo_2807.pdf.

14 Department of Health and Family Welfare, *NRHM Annual Report 2007–08* (Bhubaneswar, India: 2008).

15 Health and Family Welfare Department, Government of Odisha, "Annual Activity Report 2011–12," http://203.193.146.66/hfw/PDF/Annual_Report_2011_12_English.pdf.

16 Department of Health and Family Welfare, Government of Odisha, "Reproductive Child Health (RCH-II) Objectives," http://203.193.146.66/hfw/Reproductive_Child_Health.asp?GL=8.

17 Department of Women and Child Development, *Evidence Paper on Coverage of Nutrition Specific and Nutrition Sensitive Interventions for Under Two Children in the 15 HBDs, Compared to Those in Non-HBDs, and Among Vulnerable Population, and Its Correlation with Nutrition Outcomes* (Bhubaneswar, India: Department of Women and Child Development, 2015).

18 The Supreme Court directed the Government of India in December 2006 to sanction and operationalize a minimum of 1.4 million AWCs by December 2008 in a phased and even manner. This directive was then rolled out at the state level.

19 Odisha's Department of Women and Child Development launched Mission Shakti under ICDS in 2001, as a platform to form and promote self-help groups.

20 M. Sharma, B. L. Sarangi, J. Kanungo, S. Sahoo, L. Tripathy, A. Patnaik, J. Tewari, and A. D. Rath, "Accelerating Malnutrition Reduction in Orissa," *IDS Bulletin* 40 (2009): 78–85.

21 Gillespie et al., "Scaling Up Impact on Nutrition: What Will It Take?"

22 R. Avula, S. S. Kim, S. Chakrabarti, P. Tyagi, N. Kohli, and P. Menon, *Delivering for Nutrition in Odisha: Insights from a Study on the State of Essential Nutrition Interventions* (New Delhi: International Food Policy Research Institute, 2015).

23 R. N. Parhi and J. Saxton, *Pustikar Diwas: Convergent Action to Reduce Child Undernutrition in Odisha,* POSHAN Implementation Note 3 (New Delhi: International Food Policy Research Institute, 2014).

24 NITI Aayog, "Decentralization of ICDS Supplementary Nutrition Programme: Ensuring Timely and Quality Nutrition to All Beneficiaries in Odisha," in *Social Sector Service Delivery: Good Practices Resource Book* (New Delhi: NITI Aayog, 2015).

25 World Bank, *India Orissa in Transition: Challenges for 2006–2010* (New Delhi: World Bank, 2008).

Chapter 18

1 C. Johnson-Welch, K. MacQuarrie, and S. Bunch, "A Leadership Strategy for Reducing Hunger and Malnutrition in Africa: The Agriculture-Nutrition Advantage" (Washington, DC: International Research Centre for Women, 2005): 1–28; J. Bryce, D. Coitinho, I. Darnton-Hill, D. Pelletier, P. Pinstrup-Andersen, and Maternal and Child Undernutrition Study Group, "Maternal and Child Undernutrition: Effective Action at National Level," *The Lancet* 371, no. 9611 (2008): 510–526; S. Gillespie, L. Haddad, V. Mannar, P. Menon, N. Nisbett, and Maternal

and Child Nutrition Study Group, "The Politics of Reducing Malnutrition: Building Commitment and Accelerating Progress," *The Lancet* 382, no. 9891 (2013): 552–569.

2 A. Mejia Acosta and L. Haddad, "Sustaining Political Commitment in the Fight against Malnutrition in Peru," *Food Policy,* forthcoming; A. Mejia Acosta and J. Fanzo, *Fighting Maternal and Child Malnutrition: Analysing the Political and Institutional Determinants of Delivering a National Multisectoral Response in Six Countries: A Synthesis Paper* (Brighton, UK: Institute of Development Studies, 2012); R. Heaver, *Strengthening Country Commitment to Human Development: Lessons from Nutrition* (Washington, DC: World Bank, 2005); L. Haddad, N. Nisbett, and I. Barnett, *Maharashtra's Extraordinary Stunting Declines: What Is Driving Them? Findings of a Multidisciplinary Analysis* (Brighton, UK: Institute of Development Studies and UNICEF, 2014).

3 R. Hughes, R. Shrimpton, E. Recine, and B. Margetts, *A Competency Framework for Global Public Health Nutrition Workforce Development: A Background Paper* (World Public Health Nutrition Association, 2011).

4 J. Shiffman, "Issue Attention in Global Health: The Case of Newborn Survival," *The Lancet* 375, no. 9730 (2010): 2045–2049; J. Shiffman and S. Smith, "Generation of Political Priority for Global Health Initiatives: A Framework and Case Study of Maternal Mortality," *The Lancet* 370 (2007): 1370–1379.

5 J. Bor, "The Political Economy of AIDS Leadership in Developing Countries: An Exploratory Analysis," *Social Science and Medicine* 64, no. 8 (2007): 1585–1599, doi:S0277-9536(06)00634-4 [pii], 10.1016/j.socscimed.2006.12.005; C. Campbell, "Political Will, Traditional Leaders, and the Fight against HIV/AIDS: A South African Case Study," *AIDS Care* 22 (2010, Supplement 2): 1637–1643, doi: 10.1080/09540121.2010.516343 931121946 [pii].

6 N. Nisbett, E. Wach, L. Haddad, and S. El-Arifeen, "What Drives and Constrains Effective Leadership in Tackling Child Undernutrition? Findings from Bangladesh, Ethiopia, India, and Kenya," *Food Policy* 53 (2015): 33–45.

7 The authors conducted 89 semistructured interviews of leaders or potential leaders in four countries selected as a focus of the Transform Nutrition research program consortium. Consortium partners held stakeholder mapping sessions in each of the country capitals in 2011–2012 to build up a picture of organizational power and influence in each country. A list of influential figures within each organization was then created, with care to include champions with no institutional home. The list was then verified by attendees of the mapping workshops, and names were added as needed using a snowballing technique. Members of this list were then sampled purposively to ensure a sectoral and organizational balance, but the final list of interviewees was dependent on acceptance rates and availability within the research time frame. Interviews were recorded, transcribed, and thematically coded.

8 Please see Transform Nutrition's forthcoming "Stories of Change" full report for a longer discussion of the leadership environment in Zambia.

9 International Food Policy Research Institute (IFPRI), *Global Nutrition Report 2015: Actions and Accountability to Advance Nutrition and Sustainable Development* (Washington, DC, 2015), http://www.ifpri.org/publication/global-nutrition-report-2015; Central Statistical Office [Zambia], Ministry of Health [Zambia], and ICF International, *Zambia Demographic and Health Survey 2013–14* (Rockville, MD, USA, 2014).

10 S. Seco-Grutz, M. Sadlier, and D. Brunet, "Reflections on the Role of Donors in Scaling Up Nutrition in Zambia from 2010 to 2013: Successes, Challenges and Lessons Learnt," in J. Harris, S. Seco, C. Masi, and L. Haddad, eds., *Turning Rapid Growth into Meaningful Growth: Sustaining the Commitment to Nutrition in Zambia* (Brighton, UK: Institute of Development Studies, 2014).

11 IFPRI, *Global Nutrition Report 2015*.

12 S. Drimie, S. Kumar Chakrabarty, C. Dube, M. Smit-Mwanamwenge, R. Rawat, and J. Harris, "Intersectoral Coordination for Nutrition in Zambia," in J. Harris, S. Seco, C. Masi, and L. Haddad, eds., *Turning Rapid Growth into Meaningful Growth: Sustaining the Commitment to Nutrition in Zambia* (Brighton, UK: Institute of Development Studies, 2014).

13 Bryce et al., "Maternal and Child Undernutrition."

14 S. S. Morris, B. Cogill, and R. Uauy, "Effective International Action against Undernutrition: Why Has It Proven So Difficult and What Can Be Done to Accelerate Progress?" *The Lancet* 371, no. 9612 (2008): 608–621.

15 Heaver, *Strengthening Country Commitment to Human Development*.

16 E. B. Phiri for Eldis, "Making Policies Nutrition Sensitive in Zambia," May 28, 2015, http://www.eldis.org/go/blog/posts/making-policies-nutrition-sensitive-in-zambia#.VvYB0DEbv6g.

17 Nutrition Resource Platform, "IEC Campaign," http://164.100.72.205/care/cgi-bin/?q=IEC-Campaign, accessed April 4, 2016.

18 Global Alliance for Improved Nutrition (GAIN), *2011–2012 Annual Report* (Geneva, 2012), http://annualreport.gainhealth.org/annualreport.pdf.

19 D. L. Pelletier, E. A. Frongillo, S. Gervais, L. Hoey, P. Menon, T. Ngo, R. J. Stoltzfus, A. S. Ahmed, and T. Ahmed, "Nutrition Agenda Setting, Policy Formulation, and Implementation: Lessons from the Mainstreaming Nutrition Initiative," *Health Policy and Planning* 27, no. 1 (2012): 19–31.

20 Mejia Acosta and Fanzo, "Fighting Maternal and Child Malnutrition."

21 Mejia Acosta and Haddad, "Sustaining Political Commitment"; Mejia Acosta and Fanzo, "Fighting Maternal and Child Malnutrition."

22 H. Lyne de Ver, *Leadership, Politics and Development: A Literature Survey,* Background Paper no. 03 (Developmental Leadership Program, 2008).

23 M. Uhl-Bien, "Relational Leadership Theory: Exploring the Social Processes of Leadership and Organizing," *The Leadership Quarterly* 17 (2006): 654–676.

24 B. Brown, "Conscious Leadership for Sustainability: How Leaders with a Late-Stage Action Logic Design and Engage in Sustainability Initiatives" (PhD dissertation, Fielding Graduate University, Santa Barbara, CA, USA, 2011); T. Jordan, "Skillful Engagement with Wicked Issues: A Framework for Analyzing Meaning-Making Structures for Societal Change Agents," *Integral Review* 7, no. 2 (2011): 47–91, drawing on M. L. Commons et al., "The Existence of Developmental Stages as Shown by the Hierarchical Complexity of Tasks," *Developmental Review* 8, no. 3 (1998): 237–278; Robert Kegan, *The Evolving Self: Problem and Process in Human Development* (Cambridge, MA: Harvard University Press, 1982).

25 A. Pfaffenberger, "Optimal Adult Development: An Inquiry into the Dynamics of Growth," *Journal of Humanistic Psychology* 45, no. 3 (2005): 279–301; W. R. Torbert, "Cultivating Postformal Adult Development: Higher Stages and Contrasting Interverventions," in M. E. Miller and S. Cook-Greuter, eds., *Transcendence and Mature Thought in Adulthood: The Further Reaches of Adult Development* (New York: Rowman and Littlefield, 1994); J. Manners, K. Durkin, and A. Nesdale, "Promoting Advanced Ego Development among Adults," *Journal of Adult Development* 11, no. 1 (2014): 19–27.

26 E. Wielinga, W. Zaalmink, R. Bergevoet, F. Geerling-Eiff, H. Holster, L. Hoogerwerf, and M. Vrolijk, *Networking with Free Actors: Encouraging Sustainable Innovations in Animal Husbandry by Using the Free Actors in Networks Approach* (Wageningen, Netherlands: Wageningen University and Research Centre, 2008).

27 Gillespie et al., "The Politics of Reducing Malnutrition."

28 A. Leftwich and C. Wheeler, *Politics, Leadership and Coalitions in Development: Findings, Insights and Guidance from the DLP's First Research and Policy Workshop, Frankfurt, 10–11 March, 2011* (Developmental Leadership Program, June 2011).

29 D. J. te Lintelo, L. J. Haddad, J. Leavy, and R. Lakshman, "Measuring the Commitment to Reduce Hunger: A Hunger Reduction Commitment Index," *Food Policy* 44 (2014): 115–128.

30 Pelletier et al., "Nutrition Agenda Setting, Policy Formulation, and Implementation"; Shiffman, "Issue Attention in Global Health: The Case of Newborn Survival"; Shiffman and Smith, "Generation of Political Priority for Global Health Initiatives."

31 Gillespie et al., "The Politics of Reducing Malnutrition."

Appendix

1 J. Hagen-Zanker and R. Mallett, *How to Do a Rigorous, Evidence-Focused Literature Review in International Development: A Guidance Note,* Working Paper (London: Overseas Development Institute, 2013).

2 UN Standing Committee on Nutrition (UNSCN), The Nutrition Sensitivity of Agriculture and Food Policies: Individual Country Case Studies 2013, www.unscn.org/en/publications/country_case_studies/the_nutrition_sensitivity2.php; UNSCN, "Symposium on Realizing the Right to Adequate Food to Help Achieve the Millennium Development Goals: The SCN Four Country Case Studies," 2005, http://www.unscn.org/files/Publications/Country_Case_Studies/SYNTHESIS.pdf; ACC/SCN, (Administrative Committee on Coordination–Subcommittee on Nutrition), *Managing Successful Nutrition Programmes,* ACC/SCN State-of-the-Art Series, Nutrition Policy Discussion Paper No. 8 (Geneva: ACC/SCN, 1991).

3 UNICEF, *Tracking Progress on Child and Maternal Nutrition: A Survival and Development Priority* (Geneva, 2009); UNICEF, *Improving Child Nutrition: The Achievable Imperative for Global Progress* (New York, 2013).

4 Maternal and Child Undernutrition series in *The Lancet* 371, no. 9608 (2008), www.thelancet.com/series/maternal-and-child-undernutrition; Maternal and Child Nutrition series in *The Lancet* 382, no. 9890 (2013), www.thelancet.com/series/maternal-and-child-nutrition.

5 International Food Policy Research Institute (IFPRI), *Global Nutrition Report 2014: Actions and Accountability to Accelerate the World's Progress on Nutrition* (Washington, DC, 2014); IFPRI, *Global Nutrition Report 2015: Actions and Accountability to Advance Nutrition and Sustainable Development* (Washington, DC, 2015).

Glossary

acute malnutrition (wasting): normally the result of acute (short-term) insufficient food intake and frequent illness. Wasting is assessed by anthropometric measurements (weight-for-height) mainly in children younger than 5 years of age, but also in adults (body mass index).

anthropometry: the use of body measurements, such as height, weight, and mid-upper arm circumference, along with age and sex, to determine nutritional status.

Baby Friendly Hospital Initiative: a global program that recognizes and awards birthing facilities that offer an optimal level of care for infant feeding and bonding between mothers and their babies.

behavior change communication: an intervention or set of activities involving communication strategies and channels to promote positive behaviors among individuals, communities, or societies.

body mass index: a measure calculated by dividing weight (in kilograms) by height (in meters) squared, and used to classify individuals on a scale from underweight to obese.

breast-milk substitutes: foods that are marketed or presented as partial or total replacement for breast-milk.

chronic malnutrition (stunting): normally an indicator of chronic (long-term) insufficient energy or micronutrient intake, which results in irreversible growth retardation and cognitive and mental impairment in children in the first years of life. Children younger than 5 years of age are classified as stunted if they have a height-for-age Z-score that is more than 2 standard deviations below the median of an international reference population of the same age and sex.

complementary feeding: the introduction of safe, age-appropriate soft and solid food to a baby starting at 6 months of age, for the period of transition from breastfeeding to the gradual introduction of new foods until a baby is eating the same foods as the rest of the family. The period of complementary feeding, usually between 6 and 23 months of age, is the most nutritionally vulnerable period for a child and coincides in many developing countries with a rapid acceleration in the incidence of stunting (particularly among children 6–12 months of age).

dietary diversity: the number of food groups consumed by a household or individual over a specific time period. The most commonly used indicator of dietary diversity is the proportion of children 6–23 months of age who receive foods from four or more food groups daily.

exclusive breastfeeding: the practice of giving an infant only breastmilk and no other food or water for the first 6 months of life.

fortification: adding vitamins or minerals (micronutrients) to foods, usually staples, to improve their nutritional content or to restore nutrients lost during food processing.

growth monitoring and promotion: the monitoring of monthly weight gain or decline of children and their families and the prescription of an intervention, such as counseling on feeding practices, to promote growth or ameliorate growth problems.

International Code of Marketing of Breast-milk Substitutes: a global health policy framework adopted by the World Health Assembly of the World Health Organization to promote breastfeeding and restrict the marketing of breast-milk substitutes such as infant formula.

iron-deficiency anemia: the most common type of anemia, a condition in which the blood does not have an adequate number of healthy red blood cells. When the body is deficient in iron, it cannot produce enough hemoglobin, a substance that enables red blood cells to carry oxygen to the body's tissues.

low birth weight: a birth weight below 2,500 grams.

malnutrition: an abnormal physiological condition caused by inadequate, unbalanced, or even excessive consumption of macronutrients (carbohydrates, protein, and fats) or micronutrients (vitamins and minerals) and/or poor utilization of consumed food due to illness.

macronutrients: nutrients that contribute most of the energy to a diet, including carbohydrates, fats, and protein.

micronutrients: essential nutrients that are consumed in smaller amounts. These include various vitamins along with minerals such as calcium, iron, potassium, selenium, sodium, zinc, and folic acid.

micronutrient malnutrition: lack of vitamins and minerals necessary for health. From a public health perspective, the most significant micronutrient deficiencies in developing countries are deficiencies of iron, vitamin A, zinc, and iodine.

micronutrient powders or Sprinkles: single doses of vitamins and minerals in powder form that can be sprinkled onto any ready-to-eat semi-solid food. These are often used to increase an individual's consumption of micronutrients without changing his or her dietary habits.

minimum meal frequency: indicator used to assess the proportion of breastfed and non-breastfed children 6–23 months of age who receive solid, semi-solid, or soft foods (also including milk feeds for non-breastfed children) the minimum number of times or more per day—that is, two times for 6–8 months, three times for 9–23 months, and four times for 6–23 months (if not breastfeeding).

minimum acceptable diet (composite indicator): proportion of children 6–23 months of age who had both minimum meal frequency and dietary diversity (in both breastfed and non-breastfed children).

moderate acute malnutrition: the condition of a wasted child who has a weight-for-height between -2 and -3 standard deviations from the median of a reference population.

noncommunicable diseases: diseases that are not infectious nor transmittable; also known as chronic diseases of long duration. The most common types of noncommunicable diseases globally are cardiovascular diseases (for example, heart attacks and stroke), cancers, chronic respiratory diseases (such as chronic obstructed pulmonary disease and asthma), and diabetes.

obesity: a condition of excess body fat. A person is generally considered obese when his or her body mass index is more than 30, though some countries use lower cutoff points.

overweight: generally defined as having a body mass index of 25–30.

ready-to-use (therapeutic) foods: processed "medicinal foods" with appropriate nutrient content for rapidly improving children's nutritional and health status.

severe acute malnutrition: the condition of a wasted child who has a weight-for-height below the cutoff point of -3 standard deviations from the median of a reference population of the same age and sex.

undernourishment: having food intake that is insufficient to meet dietary energy requirements for an active and healthy life (the Food and Agriculture Organization of the United Nations defines this as an average food intake less than 1,800 kilocalories a day). Insufficient food intake is one cause of undernutrition. Hunger is usually defined as the discomfort associated with a lack of food.

stunting: low height-for-age in children. This indicator is most often expressed as a Z-score or as a percentage of individuals stunted. Individuals with Z-scores below -2 standard deviations from the median of a reference population are classified as stunted and below -3 standard deviations as severely stunted.

total fertility rate: the number of children that would be born to a woman if she were to live to the end of her childbearing years and have children according to current age-specific fertility rates.

underweight: low weight-for-age in children. A composite measure of stunting and wasting, this indicator is most often expressed as a Z-score or as a percentage of individuals underweight. Individuals with Z-scores below -2 standard deviations from the median of a reference population are classified as underweight and below -3 standard deviations as severely underweight.

wasting: low weight-for-height in children. This indicator is most often expressed as a Z-score or as a percentage of individuals wasted. Individuals with Z-scores below -2 standard deviations from the median of a reference population are classified as wasted and below -3 standard deviations as severely wasted.

Z-score: a statistical measure of a child's nutritional status. A Z-score essentially measures the standard deviation, or the distribution of data. A weight-for-age Z-score (WAZ), for example, is the number of standard deviations of the actual weight of a child from the median weight of children of his or her age in a particular sample. A WAZ score of 0 would mean that the child's weight is the same as the median weight of all children of his or her age in the sample. When applied to international reference populations, Z-scores can be used to determine degrees of underweight, stunting, and wasting.

Contributors

Nazneen Akhtar is an independent researcher, based in Bangladesh.

Rasmi Avula is a research fellow in the Poverty, Health, and Nutrition Division at the International Food Policy Research Institute, based in India.

Elisabeth Becker is a doctoral candidate in sociology at Yale University, based in the USA.

Namukolo Covic is a research coordinator in the Poverty, Health, and Nutrition Division at the International Food Policy Research Institute, based in Ethiopia.

Kenda Cunningham is an independent consultant, based in the UK.

Peter Davis is an independent social research consultant, based in the UK.

Scott Drimie is adjunct associate professor in the Nutrition Division at the University of Stellenbosch, based in South Africa.

Shams El Arifeen is director of the Centre for Child and Adolescent Health at the International Centre for Diarrhoeal Disease Research, Bangladesh (icddr,b), based in Bangladesh.

Karine Gatellier is a nutrition convenor at the Institute of Development Studies, based in the UK.

Stuart Gillespie is a senior research fellow in the Poverty, Health, and Nutrition Division at the International Food Policy Research Institute, and CEO of Transform Nutrition, based in the UK.

Jay Goulden is a consultant on program strategy and innovation, based in the UK.

Lawrence Haddad is a senior research fellow in the Poverty, Health, and Nutrition Division at the International Food Policy Research Institute, based in the UK.

Jody Harris is a senior research analyst in the Poverty, Health, and Nutrition Division at the International Food Policy Research Institute, based in the UK.

Derek Headey is a senior research fellow in the Poverty, Health, and Nutrition Division at the International Food Policy Research Institute, based in the USA.

Judith Hodge is an independent consultant on global food and nutrition security for the International Food Policy Research Institute, based in the UK.

Chandni Karmacharya is a research officer at the Nutrition Innovation Lab at the Johns Hopkins Bloomberg School of Public Health, based in Nepal.

Meagan Keefe is the associate director of the Program of African Studies at Northwestern University, based in the USA.

Neha Kohli is a senior research analyst in the Poverty, Health, and Nutrition Division at the International Food Policy Research Institute, based in India.

Purnima Menon is a senior research fellow in the Poverty, Health, and Nutrition Division at the International Food Policy Research Institute, based in India.

Nicholas Nisbett is a cluster leader and research fellow at the Institute of Development Studies, based in the UK.

Angélica Ochoa-Avilés is professor and researcher at the University of Cuenca, based in Ecuador.

Pooja Pandey Rana is deputy chief of party for Suaahara at Helen Keller International, based in Nepal.

Rajul Pandya-Lorch is chief of staff in the Director General's Office and head of the 2020 Vision Initiative at the International Food Policy Research Institute, based in the USA.

Samantha Reddin is communications manager for Transform Nutrition at the Institute of Development Studies, based in the UK.

Akriti Singh is a doctoral student at the Friedman School of Nutrition Science and Policy at Tufts University, based in the USA.

Kraisid Tontisirin is an emeritus professor of pediatrics at Ramathibodi Hospital and a senior adviser at the Institute of Nutrition, Mahidol University, based in Thailand.

Mara van den Bold is a senior research analyst in the Poverty, Health, and Nutrition Division at the International Food Policy Research Institute, based in the USA.

Roos Verstraeten is a researcher at the Institute of Tropical Medicine, based in Belgium.

Elise Wach is research and evaluation adviser at the Institute of Development Studies, based in the UK.

Andrea Warren is a doctoral candidate in public health at the University of South Carolina, based in the USA.

Jessica White is nutrition evaluation program manager at the Institute of Development Studies, based in the UK.

Sivan Yosef is a senior program manager in the Director General's Office at the International Food Policy Research Institute, based in the USA.

Laura Zseleczky is a research analyst in the Director General's Office at the International Food Policy Research Institute, based in the USA.

Advisory Committee

Alan Berg is a former senior nutrition adviser at the World Bank, based in the USA.

Charlotte Dufour is nutrition, food security, and livelihoods officer at the Food and Agriculture Organization of the United Nations (FAO), based in Italy.

Bonnie McClafferty is the director of the Agriculture for Nutrition Global Program at the Global Alliance for Improved Nutrition (GAIN), based in the USA.

Purnima Menon is a senior research fellow in the Poverty, Health, and Nutrition Division of the International Food Policy Research Institute (IFPRI), based in India.

Robert Mwadime is the chief of party of the US Agency for International Development's Community Connector project managed by FHI360, based in Uganda.

Marie Ruel is director of the Poverty, Health, and Nutrition Division at the International Food Policy Research Institute (IFPRI), based in the USA.

Werner Schultink is the chief of nutrition and associate director of the Programme Division of UNICEF, based in the USA.

Meera Shekar is a senior nutrition specialist at the World Bank, based in the USA.

Patrick Webb is the Alexander MacFarlane Professor of Nutrition at Tuft University's Friedman School of Nutrition Science and Policy, based in the USA.